SELLING S

G000092472

The Health Service Executive has now become a Sickness Industry, the largest and most incompetent run enterprise in the country.

Daily we hear of, or see, the medical profession 'SELLING SICKNESS'

Both sick and healthy people are being sent down a cul-de-sac when the use of chemical manufactured drugs and medicines are prescribed or taken into the human body, the most intricate system in the world.

Many are undernourished and sick, because of eating factory made, additive filled food, much of which is foodless.

RONNIE PLANT

Published by St John Publishing
Wellingtonbridge, Co. Wexford, Ireland.
Email: plantrf@eircom.net

Printed in Republic of Ireland by Hogan Print
Enniscorthy, Co. Wexford.
Email: design@hoganprint.com

ISBN 978-0-9551051-8-0

SELLING SICKNESS!

*There has never been a period in the history
of mankind when the value of pure,
additive-free foods and drinks
was more essential than now.*

*The majority give little, if any thought,
to what is put into the phenomenal and
remarkable system, which is the human body.*

CONTENTS

SELLING SICKNESS!

It is a well known fact that this title or heading
is real in the Sickness Industry, which has
only recently grown out of our once
managable Health Service.

Within these pages there is ample evidence
provided to accredit this as we go down the
wrong road of treating illness of mind and body.
Perhaps one should add soul!

Ronnie Plant

Selling Sickness!

Many who had reason to visit a doctor, consultant or hospital, have experienced the art of sickness being sold to them. Frequently they are plausibly informed that a prescription is being given for an invented or thought up ailment, such as cholesterol. The majority do not realise this, placing full trust in the medic.

This book, *Selling Sickness!*, contains an amount of evidence of this. Much more is on record regarding what must be regarded as very serious and unscrupulous conduct, being carried on by professionals, who in the past were looked upon as being trustworthy and honest. Here are blatant examples of the gross overuse of the doctor's prescription pad. Healthy people, who are on no medication or chemical drugs, are being turned into infirm patients unethically.

Set out here is a clear example of the '**selling of sickness**' to a healthy person who is on no chemical drugs or medication. Visiting a consultant, by appointment, regarding an eye problem, brought on probably because of increasing years, the lady referred to was not too happy with the manner of his prognosis. Mentioned was what appeared to be an element of indifference, with nothing other than a further or future appointment being made, despite records of previous eye examination and tests at hand. Here again is evidence of the money garnering, health referral conveyor system, referred to more than once in this book.

Without either asking or being asked, with no hint or advance notice, the woman was told, *"I'm putting you on cholesterol tablets and will be writing to your doctor. After being on these tablets for two months you will need to arrange a liver scan".* There was no warning of the serious side effects or harm these drugs can cause, other than the liver directive. The advance notice regarding the need for a scan is because the statin drugs prescribed can seriously affect the liver as well as other parts of the body system. Cholesterol levels were not checked, with no other reference made to the issuing of the prescription. It is appalling and scandalous that **SICKNESS SELLING** is carried out extensively. Their is no apparent check or control on the blatant over prescribing or of how the doctors, such as the person referred to, can issue prescriptions with little thought and no valid reason. Few, if any, visit a doctor and come away without a prescription.

The instance referred to is only one of many given by people who visit me as a practicing Naturopath, where natural way of living and health giving advice is promoted. Like the bankers of not so long ago, the G.Ps. have free rein, with no restraint, restriction or control over much of their revenue obtaining methods. The profession has certainly organised the highly lucrative business of **SELLING SICKNESS**, as they do now.

CURE AND REMEDY FOR THE 'SICK'
SICKNESS INDUSTRY WE HAVE

It is obvious that the Health Service Executive (H.S.E.), now turned into the Sickness Industry, has expanded in recent years to such an extent that it has run amok in it's leadership, management and control.

Examples of the carry-on over the years substantiate this claim or statement.

• In the years 2005 to 2008 the budgetary figures rose from €11 billion to over €14 billion, over a 30% increase. In 1997 the allotted amount was barely €3.7 billion.

• From 2005 to 2009 the H.S.E./Sickness Industry staff rose from 101,975 to over 111,000.

• The wage bill in that period escalated from a little over €4 billion to over €5.3 billion .

• Hospital consultant numbers increased from 1960 to 2225.

• **Vaccines:** Excluding the extreme costs of the Swine flu vaccine, much left unused and which had to be destroyed, the H.S.E. last year spent €36 million on this highly questionable treatment, by use of vaccines.

• The figure given for those receiving methadone treatment in 2007 is 6,008. In 2010 the target had increased to 8,800. This is a preventative treatment and here is a prime example of failure, a further specimen of how selling of sickness is promoted.

• In 2007 there were supposedly over 529,000 long term illness claims. We are given an approximate figure of over 1,000,000 for 2010, almost a doubling up. The thought of this fact alone must challenge the thinking or mentality of those at the top who profess to run the enterprise which is The Sickness Industry.

• The number of prescriptions issued in 2009 was over 16 million, yes, 16,195,000. The projected figure for 2010 was almost 18.5 million, yes, 18,500,000. The doctor's prescription pad is without doubt an extremely costly and cash till culture, with authority to issue these costly recommendations left entirely to the medics. Like the bankers who were given a free hand to run the banking business, the obvious unchecked and uncurbed methods of the medical profession are somewhat similar. It appears that they are answerable to nobody.

♦ The drug bill for the year 2000 was €579 million. In 2009 this figure had increased to a mind boggling €2.1 billion.

♦ In November 2011 we hear the now familiar statement of overspend on annual budget. This time it is only €400 million!

In this book, **'Selling Sickness!',** much information is given, an amount of it highly critical, of how the Health Service Executive has in little over a decade become a monstrous, uncontrolled Sickness Industry, which must not be allowed to trade as it does.

The remedy or remedies to dismantle or bury this establishment, which is so lucrative for all too many, are set out, some of it repetitively and in varying ways, throughout the pages of this book. If you wish to learn more about this later turn to, *The Sickness Industry which is The Health Service Executive* caption.

With only a percentage of a percentage of the H.S.E. budget of billions of euro, much of it squandered, being spent on **Prevention** and **Health Education**, would it ever occur to the legislators that this is number one for the health of all. Education about our eating, drinking, sleeping and exercise habits, with emphasis on change of lifestyle, is the method all, including those who govern, should pursue. If these rulers, whom I refer to, have not read *'The Expert World Cancer Research Report'*, as set out under caption in these pages, I respectfully suggest that they do so. Unless they are fools the realisation must be that the carousel must be stopped. That is, of course, if they have any common sense, which in present day leadership appears to be extremely scarce. It would certainly be much cleverer to pull the plug on the money draining Sickness Industry and advise all about my two slogans.

Given here, verbatim, is part of the proposed remedy or remedies; *'The answer, the principal remedy for many suffering from ill health is so simple that it is ludicrous that the professionals who treat the sick have not and do not wish to recognise the logic behind my slogans, which I highlight daily. Of course there would be no money in it for the medical profession or the chemical drug manufacturing conglomerates. The prescription pads would be almost unwanted. The back to basic mottos or advice are* **'We Are As We Eat, Drink, Sleep And Exercise',** *also* **'A Change Of Lifestyle Works Wonders'.** *The lifestyle change to include pure natural, non-processed, additive free foods and .drinks, little or no alcohol, no caffeine, sugar or sugary products, no fast or microwave 'foods', with everything taken into the body to be nutritious and sustaining, is a major part, often a complete answer to many health problems. Already I can hear rumblings or questions being asked, especially about the food costs. I suggest that the caption* **'Eat Well on a Limited Budget'** *be read. To continue with the solution to be rid of the much sickness we have, also the Sickness Industry, please read on.*

Learning to read the ingredients labels on the food, often foodless, we are offered, should be a compulsory requirement. Exercise also proper sleep and sleep pattern is vital for wellbeing. The main requisite is discipline. If all who can do so put into practice the advice, information or suggestions offered in this book, at the same time following my slogans, the thriving, money guzzling Sickness Industry would be killed off, with hospitals and surgeries working minimum hours, a number of them having to be closed, being unwanted. I know, I have seen what I write about work for thousands, including myself, now in my eighties. A change of lifestyle is all that is needed by the majority'. **I have not got the money or clout to promote what is set out. Our Government, instead of pouring money into what is like a bottomless pit, the Health Service Executive/Sickness Industry, should act ——NOW. BILLIONS OF EURO CAN BE SAVED.**

ACKNOWLEDGEMENTS AND THANKS

Some years ago, after much research and learning, I put together the book Health is Wealth, an A to Z Encyclopaedia of Over the Counter Natural Remedies and Good Food. Little did I realise that it would be such a huge success or that its publication would result in the making of so many friends. The many records of subsequent better health of all who put into practice what I advocate, was certainly unforeseen before writing or publishing the encyclopaedia. **In paraphrasing the words of the Androzzo's hit song of 1945 I feel grateful that 'I have helped somebody as I passed along, as I showed somebody they were travelling wrong'.**

Invitations were received to give talks in both Ireland and the U.K., also being interviewed and speaking on many radio stations. The culmination of or reaction to all this has been a continuing amount of telephone calls, letters, cards, mass bouquets also visits to express thanks, or from the many who seek advice and help which might lead to better health of mind or body. I feel that it should be added here that no reward is sought, only asking for the person's prayers. If they insist, they are asked to give to my favourite charity, St. Vincent de Paul. From many of these good people I have learned much.

Hundreds have told of their terrible or dreadful experiences as a result of being prescribed chemical based drugs and medicines. Vaccinations in many cases turned into appalling episodes. Why do I dwell on this when declaring my thanks? It is set out here simply to offer my sincere thanks and appreciation to all whom I am indebted to for so much information given, which has been added to what has been recorded and collated over the years, some of which is set out in this volume *'Selling Sickness!'* to expose or reveal *Why the Sickness Industry thrives.*

It would be impossible to set down the names of all who shared with me their time when passing on counsel, knowledge, or expressing their views about how they, their families, relatives, or in some instances friends whom they had passed on natural health information to, had attained better health, being more energetic by using natural foods, supplements and remedies. I repeat my 'Thank You' again and again.

I must add that since putting together and launching **Health is Wealth**, my first foray into writing a book, much has been learned about compiling, writing, publishing, distributing and selling. To all I say, "There is the material for a book of some kind in every person. If I can do it then anybody can".

To all the kind people in the various radio stations I send a special word of thanks for their help. I am especially grateful to Marie Cleary, Carmel Downes, Eimear Hogan, Fiona Kearney, Anna Kehoe, Margaret Lowndes, Andrea Martin, and Clair Whitty for all their observations, corrections and advice. To my doctor friends whom I have argued and debated with about the scandal which is the Sickness Industry, so often referred to in this book, and the wrong road they take in treating and prescribing, I proffer a special word of thanks. Their names are omitted for reasons left unexplained and which they and the reader will accept on reading the volume. To Charlie Keegan, Bernard Browne and Tomás Hayes I am indebted for their encouragement and for giving me so much of their valuable time.

I cannot thank sufficiently my patient, loved and loving wife Freda. Here again this good lady's help and understanding has been wonderful, especially the much time and sometimes composure given to speaking with the many who telephone our home, not to mention the tea and scones provided for the many visitors.

Ronnie Plant

NATURAL AND HERBAL REMEDIES

AND THE ON-GOING PROTEST TO STOP THEM BEING BANNED

IF THE EUROPEAN UNION (E.U.), THE AMERICAN GOVERNMENT, ALSO THE MILLIONS IN BOTH JURISDICTIONS WITH VESTED INTERESTS IN LEGALISED CHEMICAL DRUGS, HAVE THEIR WAY AND SAY, WE WILL BE WITHOUT NATURAL AND HERBAL REMEDIES IN THE FUTURE. THIS WILL INCLUDE VITAMINS, MINERALS, FOOD SUPPLEMENTS ALSO MUCH MORE WHICH IS NATURAL AND INVALUABLE TO HELP KEEP US IN BETTER HEALTH.

REGULARLY WE SEE ARTICLES PUBLISHED IN SUPPOSEDLY RESPECTABLE MEDICAL JOURNALS, ALL OF THEM PEER REVIEWED, THAT PURPORT TO SHOW US HOW TRULY USELESS – EVEN DANGEROUS – DIETARY SUPPLEMENTATIONS, WITH NATURAL AIDS TO HEALTH, SUCH AS VITAMINS AND FOOD SUPPLEMENTS CAN BE. MUCH OF WHAT IS WRITTEN IN THE ARTICLES IS DECEITFULLY COMPOSED AS THE ANTI-VITAMIN AND SUPPLEMENT DRIVE GETS MORE RIDICULOUS.

A NEW *'BRITISH MEDICAL JOURNAL'* PRESS RELEASE, EMBLAZONED ACROSS ITS PAGES, TELLS US; *COMPLEMENTARY MEDICINES CAN BE DANGEROUS FOR CHILDREN.* WHEN LOOKED AT, THE REPORTED PROOF IS UTTERLY RIDICULOUS. THIS IS TYPICAL SCAREMONGERING BY THE MEDICAL PROFESSION AND THE MIGHTY ORTHODOX CHEMICAL DRUG PROVIDERS, ALL PART OF THE SICKNESS INDUSTRY. THEY REALISE THE DANGERS OF A GROWING PERCENTAGE OF THEIR EASY MONEY OBTAINING TECHNIQUES BEING ERODED.

ACTUALLY, ALL OF THE VITAMIN BASHING HAS SERVED A USEFUL PURPOSE, BY REVEALING WHAT MAY BE CHEMICAL DRUG PHARMA'S NEW GAME PLAN: TO MUSCLE IN ON THE LUCRATIVE DIETARY/FOOD SUPPLEMENT MARKET. COUPLED WITH THE LIKELY RIDICULOUSLY AND UNSCIENTIFICALLY LOW MAXIMUM PERMITTED LEVELS OF VITAMINS AND MINERALS IN SUPPLEMENTS, AS PROMISED BY THE E.U., THE IDEA APPEARS TO BE TO SCARE PEOPLE AWAY FROM SUPPLEMENTS AND TO MAKE HIGH DOSE SUPPLEMENTS UNAVAILABLE OVER THE COUNTER. MOST PEOPLE WILL THEN HAVE LITTLE OPTION OTHER THAN TO USE CONVENTIONAL CHEMICAL DRUGS WHEN THEY BECOME ILL, AND SOME OF THESE, AGAINST THEIR BETTER JUDGEMENT, WILL BE LED TO BELIEVE THIS IS THE SAFEST COURSE OF ACTION.

AT THE SAME TIME, PEOPLE WHO REALLY WANT TO USE HIGHER DOSE THERAPEUTICALLY-ACTIVE NATURAL PRODUCTS, WILL ONLY BE ABLE TO DO SO IF THEY ARE PRESCRIBED BY A MEDICAL DOCTOR. THIS IS GOOD FOR THE PHARMA. INDUSTRY, GOOD FOR ORTHODOX MEDICINE, ALSO THE DOCTORS

WHO PRESCRIBE IT, BUT BAD FOR THE GENERAL PUBLIC, ESPECIALLY FOR THOSE WHO USE ONLY NATURAL REMEDIES WHICH ARE TRIED AND TRUSTED. FIRST, ONE NEEDS TO BE SICK TO GET THEM, WHICH IS A KICK IN THE TEETH FOR PREVENTATIVE HEALTH CARE. SECOND, MOST MEDICAL DOCTORS KNOW LITTLE, IF ANYTHING, ABOUT MICRONUTRIENTS OR NUTRITION AS THEY RECEIVE NO TRAINING ON THIS AT MEDICAL SCHOOL OR COLLEGE. THE REALITY IS THAT THE MILLIONS OF PEOPLE WHO HAVE BENEFITED FROM FOOD/DIETARY SUPPLEMENTATION KNOW BETTER. THEY'VE EXPERIENCED THE RESULTS THEMSELVES AND CANNOT BE DISSUADED BY PRO-PHARMA, ANTI-VITAMIN PROPAGANDA.

LUCKILY WE HAVE A VERY KNOWLEDGABLE AND GOOD TEAM FIGHTING THE ISSUES, WITH SUCCESS SO FAR. THE ALLIANCE FOR NATURAL HEALTH NEED HELP, PATRONAGE AND THE AID OF ALL WHO ARE INTERESTED IN, USE, OR PROMOTE THE USE OF ANYTHING NATURAL IN THE SEARCH FOR BETTER AND GOOD HEALTH. REGULARLY THEY ISSUE NEWS LETTERS ALSO AN AMOUNT OF OTHER VALUABLE HEALTH INFORMATION. ALL OF THIS CAN LEAD TO COMMON SENSE PREVAILING, IN DEMANDING WHAT ARE THE RIGHTS OF ALL INDEPENDENT AND FAIR MINDED NATURAL HEALTH SUPPORTERS. ANY PERSON DESIRING TO DONATE TO THE FUND SET UP TO FIGHT FOR THE LEGAL RIGHT OF FREEDOM TO RETAIN NATURAL VITAMINS, MINERALS AND HERBAL REMEDIES, MAY DO SO BY SENDING CHEQUE OR P.O. TO: A.M.H.-INTL., ATRIUM, CURTIS ROAD, DORKING, RH4 1XA UK.

THE ALLIANCE FOR NATURAL HEALTH WEBSITE IS: WWW.ANHCAMPAIGN.ORG AND THE E-MAIL ADDRESS IS: INFO@ANHCAMPAIGN.ORG

INTRODUCTION.

Within the pages of this guide *Selling Sickness!* are set out facts about the using and over use of food additives. Similarly expounded is the over use of the doctors cash till, which is the prescription pad, the margarine 'scandal' of hydrogenated oil and fat use and the cholesterol bamboozle or con. Combined with this is the invention of, also the selling of, sickness as carried on by the chemical drugs-manufacturing conglomerates and all too many within the Sickness Industry we have now. Questions are set out, with many of them answered, as to why we have the colossal increase in sickness and ill-health. Written about are claims and facts about pills and medicines which are being forced on us by the might of the chemical drug-manufacturing industry, many with side effects, fatalities, withdrawal symptoms and much else which we hear about regularly, with some of it repressed when it suits the bureaucrats. Embodied are facts about our Sickness Industry, which is the Health Service Executive of Ireland and the National Health Service of the U.K. It is very obvious that our Health Service Executives, who employ consultants, doctors and other health specialists, using tax payers money, can only do so on the terms laid down by the professionals referred to. It appears to many ordinary people in life that these people wish to do little or nothing and be paid handsomely. It begs the question, **"Do they want to work anymore?"**

Few in every day life, other than medical consultants within the Health Service Executive/Sickness Industry or some of the fat cats who are leaders in business or industry, can expect remuneration of well over €5000 per week. Again the person in the street, the taxpayer, is helpless in a hopeless situation. I repeat, *"The sense of outrage of the taxpayer is not there anymore".* In these pages the really serious situation of our food supplies is emphasised, with huge price rises and shortages forecast. We learn of grain prices rising as the totally immoral idea of using food-growing land to produce bio fuel materials, such as rape and other seeds, is impressed on us.

Governments in both the U.K. and Ireland have never had to plan for food supplies to feed the nation. There has always been a surplus, but in recent years with much restraint on the farmer, as to what is produced, things are changing rapidly. Those who promote and tout the European Union Directive which brought in the ludicrous directive of leaving excellent growing land as 'set-aside' can be looked on as being insane. They should be named and shamed. The health and needs of those who put them in power, the general public, the voter, are way down the list. Many who govern are far removed from the realities of life, or so it appears. To use a cliché, **'Common sense is all too often not common'**.

Before the multinational supermarkets of this world began to dictate what we must eat and drink, the farmer automatically produced the necessities to cater for our needs. Now the food selling leaders, and other hypermarkets, have screwed our farmers, including milk and horticultural producers, into the ground. They bring food across the world, some thousands of miles, much of it produced by cheap labour. They can dictate to us as they wish. Like the almighty drug-manufacturing companies, the food retailers will be on a cash cow result, another gravy train. An example of this is the retail increase in prices of milk and dairy products. Not so long ago there was a milk price war amongst the food selling conglomerates, resulting in many disheartened milk producers leaving the dairy enterprise. The supermarket hierarchy are highly experienced in methods of arranging this type of scenario, with a bonanza in sight, just as the drug companies connived the 'Flu Pandemic' that never was. The results are the netting of billions. See *Flu - The Supreme Deception* caption.

Read in this book about how some of our health charities, such as the Diabetes Federation of Ireland, Diabetes U.K., Asthma U.K. and Ireland, Spina Bifida and others, all started by small groups of individuals in a private capacity, have now grown into businesses which are part of the Sickness Industry. All this and much else throughout these pages as the gullible public stand idly by and do nothing. I repeat, **"They have lost the will to fight many issues"**.

Only today I read that some 'experts' have stated that the health of the country was excellent. First of all there are no experts, only those who set themselves up to be so, and secondly it is clear that these statements are idiotic. This is what one has come to expect from the so-called experts. **If these maestro's findings are correct then why are our hospitals full, with waiting lists for operations and treatment? Why are so many people waiting months for appointments to be even made? Why are the doctor's surgeries full, with waiting lists here too? The gullible public listen to these *'experts'* and stay silent.** Nowhere do we hear of the easy and simple way to avoid ill health. The answer to this is set out repeatedly within these pages. **Sad to relate the word prevention, or the use of preventative medicine, is unheard of by those who govern our country, or who run the Health Service Executive, now the Sickness Industry**.

The Sickness Industry, which is mentioned frequently in this book, is now our biggest money-spinner by far. Over the past 25 years it has mushroomed, as the pharmaceutical industry produces endless amounts of chemical drugs, none of which cure, with different branded names being prescribed, all appearing on the shelves and being promoted daily. The Sickness Industry as we know it now is made up of the Health Service Executive of Ireland, the National Health Service Executive of the U.K., Private Hospitals, the mighty Pharmaceutical Drug Combines, Chemists and Pharmacy stores and shops, Hospitals, Nursing Homes, Doctors, Consultants, Nurses and all others who work within the industry. Even small shops, filling stations and market stalls are in on the act as they sell thousands of off the shelf legalised drugs, where a prescription is not required. Up to the 1980's we had nothing like this. There was no queuing, or need to make appointments. Our surgeries and hospitals were not used, as is the case now. Today, we are a sick nation as we are daily sold illness by the huge Sickness Industry we now have. Many who attend the doctor, surgery or hospital often go there being healthy, only to be put on drugs permanently, all of which makes them ill for the rest of their lives. **All too many are foolish enough to accept the medication offered without question. Again I'm being repetitive when I say we are a sick and under nourished nation as the Sickness Industry thrives.**

FACTS OR SCARE-MONGERING

In my writings, also in the talks I give in Ireland and the U.K., there is no scare mongering, just facts being given. Manufacturers of food and drinks, drug companies, the medical profession and others are written about for what they are or produce.

The only companies or people who come back to lambaste or try to tear a strip off me are those with vested interests in what I have written about or decry. Some of them are nasty, threatening all sorts of things. Legal proceedings and solicitors letters are mentioned. Over the past 40 years I have told them all, **"Meet me in any court of law and I'll be delighted"**. I will bring with me 200 or indeed more of my witnesses if required. Nobody has bothered to take up the challenge. Only two or three have come back to berate me a second time. They were given an earful of true facts, being sent on their way, hopefully realising that what I write about or say is true.

At no time do I advise anybody to come off prescribed drugs. It is up to the person concerned to use their common sense, as I have done over the years. Talk with the GP or health advisor, then, make your own decision. Your health is your own responsibility. It should be that of nobody else.

CHASTISEMENT

Here is further serious food for thought in the world we live in today. Taken from Proverbs, chapter 29, verse 15. *"The rod of correction imparts wisdom, but a child left to himself disgraces his mother"*. Many do not realise or stop to think that every child has a brain, a spine and a backside. In the past a slap on the backside conveyed a message via the spine to the brain that this was chastisement. Now it is common practice for children to be shouted at almost endlessly, as the parent or guardian becomes stressed, while all of the time the person being shouted at or castigated carries on as if deaf to the scolding voice. What children need is much love, also encouragement.

THE WAY TO A WOMAN'S HEART
'THE WAY TO A WOMAN'S HEART IS THROUGH THE DOOR OF A GOOD RESTAURANT'.

This is very true and it leads me to record one of my most often complaints of eating when away from home. We are constantly told that we should eat plenty of fruit. Note the menus in almost all hotels, restaurants or eating-places. Seldom if ever will one find the two words Fruit Salad. We will be offered gooey, sugary desserts. Hotel staff have often told me that there is little demand for Fruit Salad. So much for healthy eating, which includes eating a varied selection of fresh fruit. People should become aware of its excellence.

PRAYER BEFORE MEALS

A simple way of showing gratitude to GOD before meals is to form the habit of saying this lovely Gaelic thanksgiving.
Beannaigh an bia,
Beannaigh an deoch,
agus Beannaigh sinne a Thiarna.
When translated this means,
'Bless the food, Bless the drink and Bless us all O Lord.'

SCIENCE AND SICKNESS

I do not fear contradiction when I state that there is as much scientific proof on natural medicine and remedies, as sold by the health food store, as there is on prescribed and over the counter conventional chemical medicines, as all too excessively turned out by the drug-manufacturing companies. We do not hear this for the simple and also natural reason, no pun here, that there is no immediate money in what is more genuine – the purely natural, for either the pharmaceutical chemical drugs-manufacturing industry or the medical profession.

All the scientific, pharmaceutical and medical results of tests are bought and paid for. Nothing natural will be considered. The results of testing the natural cannot buy into patenting medicines. This is where the end product is for the drug-manufacturing companies. **MONEY!** The natural, whether food or medicine, is ignored by the Sickness Industry.

There is not one chemical drug that cannot be matched in the health food store or by a qualified and good Herbalist, Homeopathic doctor or other alternative health practitioner. There will be no side or after effects and certainly no dangers when used as prescribed, let's say when used properly. The difference is, the chemical drugs in almost all instances are useless, with the natural remedy being successful in over ninety percent of all instances of taking.

THE DO-GOODERS

Those interested in better health are pestered, besieged daily, being told to eat this, avoid that, do this, do that, as the do-gooders and advisers, all too many of them with monetary or vested interests, try to get the message across. We hear all this nonsense about fats. Nobody knows which fats are good or otherwise, as different views are aired regularly. My simple advice is to be sensible. If food is processed, with colours, additives or preservatives, leave it on the shelf and especially if with ingredients listed which have unpronounceable names.

Processed and packaged meats are to be avoided. Fresh meat from the butcher, as displayed in open form, is good. Where we need variation to obtain a balanced diet, natural foods are the answer. Be sensible.

A STORY

An excellent cook and food provider for a large family, who provided only natural and additive free food and drink, tells a story. Things have got to a peculiar stage now where I will probably be told I am not politically correct to call this friend a housewife! Should it be home manager?

This good lady explains how for several years she had been asking her elderly mother-in-law to join in the weekly shopping visit to the local supermarket. The answer was always an emphatic, *"No I do not like them places".* On being asked one day as usual, surprisingly the senior citizen said, *"I will come".* Away they went on the trip. Helping the mother from the car, the daughter-in-law took her into the store, showing her and explaining where to meet in about 45 minutes. During the session and while proceeding down one of the aisles of 'foods' and much else stacked on the shelves, the daughter and mother-in-law met. The younger of the two asked *"Well, what do you think Mother?"*.   The retort was *"I never saw so much stuff we do not want. Having looked at the ingredients labels, I am convinced much of it should be destroyed. I have never been ill in my life, now in my 90's, never using any of that kind of stuff"*. Certainly much food for thought was given here.

MIND YOURSELF

Our health is our own responsibility – our very own. I make no apologies for repeating this. It is as the eleventh commandant 'Man mind thyself, woman do thou likewise'.

EAT AND DRINK WELL

All should bear in mind that we can have very much better health by using natural foods, drinks and remedies. Combining these with exercise and proper sleep pattern can eliminate the use of medication. I have seen the benefits of natural food, also alternative and complementary medicine, with the health of the most sceptical, the doubters, improved. Many thousands whom I have helped and advised accordingly are now firm believers and ardent supporters of the natural way of living, including the use of natural remedies. **Better health comes from good food.** It is a simple exercise to purchase food that is natural and health giving, as opposed to that which contains factory made ingredients. Leave the junk food on the shelf. We are reliably informed that this can be over 75% of what is on the supermarket shelves. Do you read the ingredients labels? Do you understand what is nutritious, natural, unadulterated, healthy, not processed? It takes only a very short time to learn.

IS TV YOUR GOD?

I am told that the TV is my Shepherd
I shall not want.
It makes me lie down on the sofa
It leads me away from the Faith
It destroys my soul
It leads me in the path of sex and
violence for the sponsor's sake
Yea, though I walk in the shadow of
Christian responsibilities there will be no
interruption, for the TV is with me
Its cable and remote control, they comfort me.
It prepares a commercial for me. In the
presence of my worldliness, it anoints my
head with humanism and consumerism
My covering runneth over
Surely laziness and ignorance shall follow me
all the days of my life
and I shall dwell in the house watching TV for ever.

Acknowledgements to 'The Curate's Diary' and Rev Fr Thady Doyle

BOOKS

The celebrated educationalist, **Charles William Eliot,** so rightly said; *"Books are the quietest and most constant of friends, they are the most accessible and wisest councillors, and the most patient of teachers".* Any person young or old who does not read books frequently is missing much. Reading the doom and gloom in newspapers can make one disheartened.

Our libraries are under utilised, their shelves are packed tightly with much good reading matter. They are a great source of much that is good. Any place where there are children and no books is not a home. Reading is one of the most enjoyable leisures in life. I remember as a small boy reading **'Ireland's Own'.** From this wonderful publication I learned much, especially Irish history. Many can say likewise. It led me to seeking out books and much literature of varying kinds. It also made me seek out libraries, book shops, including second-hand ones, which are excellent places to browse and pick up book bargains. In the course of all this I met many nice people. Reading is something where parents must set example to the youth, just as my parents did. Even to have only 20 or 30 books in the home, is a huge incentive for all to browse and learn. These to include dictionary, thesaurus, encyclopaedia, also something about art, literature, sport, classical mythology, cookery books, Oxford concise medical dictionary, or whatever else comes to mind or is affordable. The biggest selling book in the world, The Bible, is a must. Books are a big part of the University of Life.

AN APPLE

An apple each day keeps the doctor away.
It is as true a maxim as any ever expressed.

THE KNOW-ALLS

Of all those whom I speak with, who have health problems, there are some who are time wasters. They annoy me. They are on medication, perhaps taking up to eight or ten different prescribed drugs, none of which will cure them. They visit me because they are feeling unwell. From the commencement of interview, I realise that here are the type of people who will not accept advice. They listen as it falls on deaf ears. With fixed ideas and a love for the chemical company's drugs, which they are on, they are not for changing. It often ends up with this kind of patient advising me, giving the impression they know it all! Many do not wish to learn about natural remedies and subsequent better health. Here is one of the many reasons why we have a sick nation. Listening to good advice gives further food for thought. *'There are none so blind as those who will not see, there are none so deaf as those who will not hear'*

(St John Chrysostom, 345 – 407)

PRAYER OF SAINT THOMAS AQUINAS

Here is a prayer, which I use before commencing to write, prepare for a talk or lecture. It is something that can be used before study or especially when preparing for or sitting exams. Parents and young people whom I have given it to have later thanked me.

LORD GOD, You, who make eloquent the tongues of infants
please refine my speech
and pour forth upon my lips the goodness of your blessing
Please GOD grant me keenness of mind
capacity to remember
skill in learning
subtlety to interpret
and eloquence in speech
May you guide the beginning of my work
direct its progress, and bring it to completion
You who are true GOD and true Man
who lives and reigns, world without end
Amen.

WATCH IT

Most people are not aware that if leaving a battery operated watch unused or stored, it can be switched off simply by pulling out what was once called the winder stem, now used to adjust the hands. To restart just push in the stem and adjust the hands. This may not be food for though but it saves money. Leaving it out disconnects the power. I pass this information on because when my watch stopped today I had another on standby but the battery in that was dead too. One learns everyday, as I did.

A HEALTHY TALK

The following is an extract from a talk which I gave at a corporate health function. It was made into a brochure by a friend who is very computer literate. Thousands of these brochures have been handed out at natural health functions and talks. It may be repeated in some of what is written in this book, *Selling Sickness!,* but I feel it will further get the message across, that to live naturally is best. This talk gave much food for thought, proving that we must give very much more thought to the foods, often foodless, we are offered and indeed eat.

The talk given was as follows:

"If we wish to enjoy better health then number one is to adopt my motto, **WE ARE AS WE EAT, DRINK, SLEEP AND EXERCISE**, *learn to be disciplined, positively practicing these four things.*

Do you read the ingredient labels of the food being purchased? Take time to do so. Discover that much of what we are offered as food and drink is 'foodless', non-sustaining, having been put together in factories. Eat natural, non-processed, additive, colour and preservative free food. There is much which is natural in the supermarkets. There is a big selection of everything natural in both the health food shops and the fruit and vegetable stores. Use plenty from the latter, including the humble spud.

Breakfast is vital, laying the foundation in the morning for the first day of the rest of your life. Porridge cannot be bettered as a breakfast food. It is one of two natural, off the shelf, packaged breakfast cereals, with nothing added, nothing taken away. The other is shredded wheat, slightly processed I admit. I counted 84 branded breakfast cereals, before giving up. **With the exception of the oatmeal and shredded wheat, all had additives of some type**. *Sugar and salt were in most. They are a danger to good health. A good suggestion is to add fruit, bran, and seeds, such as sunflower, sesame, linseed or pumpkin, to the porridge. Sweeten, if desired by adding sultanas, raisins or currants, which have been soaked overnight, or use a spoonful of pure honey, but not supermarket purchased honey.*

Use meat, eggs or fish every third day as the base for main meal. Eat Salads regularly, especially side salads. Steam the vegetables. Grill or stew the meat. Grill, poach or steam the fish. Do not use tin foil, or cling film, ever. The frying pan is out, as is frying. All too many make good food bad in the kitchen. Wholemeal bread, plenty of raw onions, soft cheese, such as Brie or Danish Blue, all being natural, makes a wonderful sandwich – a meal in itself. Use Honey Roast ham from the butcher instead of cheese, if you wish to. Support your local butcher before it is too late.

Avoid anything with sugar or sweeteners. If you must sweeten, use pure honey, except if diabetic. The use of sugars or artificial sweeteners are amongst the chief causes of ill-health. **They should have health warnings on the packaging. Today, we use 80 times more sugar than was used over a century ago. This is why diabetes for instance, is endemic.**

Cooking oils or anything containing cooking oils are also to be avoided. The oil is usually hydrogenated. At last we have it out in the open, that hydrogenated oil may be the cause of clogging up veins and arteries, causing serious circulation problems, being detrimental to ones health. Margarine has been made with hydrogenated oil since early in the last century, until recently. All my life I have advised people to use butter sparingly. It is pure and natural. Instead of eating bread and butter, all too many eat butter and bread. Simply smear the butter on.

Drink pure water, up to seven or eight glasses daily. I use a reasonably priced inline filter system, which removes, amongst other impurities, the chemicals chlorine and 94% of the fluoride, which should not be in our water. It is easily fitted, being relatively cheap, giving excellent pure water and can be obtained from Simply Water, Environment House, Brighton Green, Dublin 6. Telephone 01.492.0414.

Forget about fizzy and so-called energy drinks. Many are sugarised, or worse still include the much rejected aspartame or other additives, some of which can be 'harmful' to health, especially in the long term. Some fizzy drinks constituents may be one of the causes of diabetes, obesity and ill-health. Read the ingredient labels and more importantly, leave these drug-like liquids on the shelf. Using cokes, lucozade, energise, red bull or such tasty bud-appealing liquids to quench thirst or to re-energise is a fallacy. The energy boost is very, very short lived. Within a very short time the longing is there for more of the same, all this being arguably harmful to the consumer's health. It has been discovered that Bisphenol A and perhaps other chemicals used in the make-up of plastic bottles, to contain these liquids, is leaching into the drinks. We have been informed this can be detrimental also perhaps being one of the causes of obesity.

Pure water is a thirst quencher and as already stated, it is one of nature's greatest medicines, acting as a lubricant.

Most people do not realise the importance of regular and proper sleep patterns, with sufficient sleep. It is vital for all aspects of better health.

When exercise is mentioned, many cringe, almost wince, or to put it bluntly do not wish to know. This is foolish thinking. Walking costs nothing. I know, I walk up to four miles daily and this is not just a saunter. Even 30 minutes daily is a big aid to feeling well.

A liquidiser is a must in every home. We mix a small amount of broccoli and carrot with an amount of varied fruit, natural additive free yoghurt, with added Stute or Biona Brand Organic 100% pure red grape juice and a little water. Vary this daily to find out what you enjoy best.

A good Multivitamin, such as Quest Brand Improved Once-a-Day, is a great aid for vitality. All over the age of 35 should take Calcium Bone Formula to help prevent Osteoporosis. Calcium on its own is useless, probably harmful. The health food store can provide a calcium bone formula. This includes magnesium, which is necessary to make the calcium easily ingested. Within this formula also is boron and zinc, all vitally *necessary for good bone health. See **Calcium** Caption*

*Our bodies, sad to relate, are treated with contempt, disregard, or to put it nicely, disrespect. The whole human system is the most intricate in the world, being supernatural, a wonder, but taken for granted until it is too late. I reiterate, **"We spend the first half of our lives harming the body and the second half trying to undo the damage."***

***Hippocrates**, the Father of Modern Medicine, laid down the dictum **"THAT FOOD BE YOUR MEDICINE AND MEDICINE BE YOUR FOOD"**. Can you imagine the doctor issuing a prescription informing you of this? They are only interested in drugs, with many over-prescribing them. Here is one of the chief reasons why we are a sick nation.*

All should remember that our health is our own responsibility and that of nobody else. We hear of the Government, the Minister for Health, the Health Service Executive and others being blamed. We have only ourselves to blame. If all disciplined themselves to follow the nine words of my motto, they would be amazed at the results, like the many who have taken my advice over the years. Daily, I receive thanks through letters, telephone calls, thank you cards, emails and have had many Mass Bouquets. People tell me of how they have been able to leave aside the pharma-drugs, chemical medicines and other now unneeded chemical remedies. Those who have followed my advice, making valiant efforts to change the lifestyle, have told me of the amazing difference to their lives.

*Nothing will convince me otherwise, having proved it myself, also through the many I have helped to better health, time and time again, over the past 47 years, but that **"WE ARE AS WE EAT, SLEEP, DRINK AND EXERCISE".***

CALCIUM
IGNORE THE SCARE-MONGERING OF THE MEDICAL PROFESSION.

We have had 'experts' raise a scare about the use of calcium. They are part of the medical profession. They have now told us who practice the natural line of thought what we always knew, that calcium, unless properly formulated, can be injurious to health. The Health Food Store has always promoted and sold calcium for prevention of, and as an aid for porous bones, better known as osteoporosis

The chemists and drug companies, combined, had to bring calcium into their range of chemical, so-called remedies. Only in the past ten to fifteen years or perhaps more recently, has this happened. It is blatantly obvious that they know little about the so-natural calcium, or its use. They produce calcium, some on its own, or with chemical additives in the

22

formula. It is their contention that including vitamin D3 with the calcium helps it work. This is partly wrong. Visit any Health Food Store and read the ingredients labels on Calcium Bone Formula, Ultimate Bone Support or others offered to help cope with or prevent Osteoporosis. Note that the ingredients are as has been advised for years, many years. In order to work properly the bone formula must have almost half as much magnesium, with vitamin K, boron, zinc, manganese, copper also five hundred international units or more of vitamin D3.

Walk into the chemist shop and ask for calcium. Note the difference, as the formula reads of chemicals and synthetic ingredients as turned out by the synthetic drugs manufacturers. They are far removed from the entirely safe formulation from the Health Food Store, with the latter's products having no side effects.

I have purposely gone into chemist's shops, going out of my way to seek advice about calcium. That given was at all times wrong. Leaflets giving warnings of side-effects and care needed are included with the packaging of the chemical made-up calcium. You will find none of this with properly formulated bone aids, including those containing calcium, in the Health Food Store. There one will find natural remedies, including the excellent bone formulas mentioned, all tried and trusted, for many years. Trained personnel will give excellent advice.

Like so much drugs produced by the chemical manufacturers, their calcium mix on offer needs a gigantic re-formulation in order to make it totally safe. I repeat, **"Visit the Health Food Store to be sure of safe and excellent calcium containing products."** One would imagine that the 'experts' would have looked into all this, before issuing their unacceptable statement regarding the alleged 'harm' of calcium. Of course one would not expect them to visit the Health Food Store. This would be beneath their dignity. They have all to learn about the natural and the wonderful remedies produced and sold there.

Osteoporosis is known as being a silent crippler. It can be helped and prevented by taking a proper formulated calcium bone formula, like those mentioned, which, I repeat, are available from the health food store.

RESVERATROL

This is a wonderful anti-aging agent. It is found in certain red wines, pure organic red grape juice, grapes, blueberries, raspberries, pure untreated cranberries, also pure cranberry juice. Taking Resveratrol daily, also following my slogan "We are as We Eat, Drink, Sleep and Exercise", is an excellent combination to avoid aging. It helps one feel good and with much better energy levels. I repeat, **"We will grow old, but we don't have to feel older"**.

HEALTH INVESTMENT

My interest is to be healthy. I will probably die from a common cold! Amongst my other interests is to be able to help others to be healthy. Health is true wealth, invest in it.

THE FOOD LABELLING STUPIDITY OF OUR LEGISLATORS

Do you understand the law, direction or sense of how food is labelled now? It has become so complex, over elaborated, with some of it misleading, that it is absurd, with much of it meaningless to the layperson. Most housewives, especially older people, do not understand in the slightest way what is set out on the labelling. They have not got the time to sit down and study all of the blurb, much of it nonsense.

One cannot expect mothers with children to devote precious time to trying to understand the labelling farce we have. The nutritional value in all too much is nil. Most women interviewed have not got the understanding or in many cases the inclination, to recognise what is good and what can be dangerous to health. The whole set up on labelling is simply not in lay-mans language.

Many breakfast cereals, fizzy drinks, juice drinks and products which claim to be good sources of vitamins, often with dubious health claims, are examples of 'foods' which can be of no value nutritionally. Commercial processors include sugar, aspartame and many other undesirable additives. When the ingredients label sets out a list of the added vitamins or minerals, all of which have had to be added to the pretentious, foodless food, to try making it of some use to the body, which it is not, it is best left on the shelf.

Sadly all too many mothers give in to the whims or tastes of children. Youngsters, in their innocence, accept the hype or propaganda of the advertising professionals, or the jargon which is aimed at them, then demanding the food, often to be compared to garbage, which they have seen promoted on T.V. and elsewhere

Health claims are made in many advertisements, which are at variance with either common sense or what is on the label.

Unfortunately the majority of parents are too busy or have no interest in these all too often highly promoted variations, regarding so-called foods and drinks. The young people fall for this kind of hype which is beamed at them, much of it spurious. In my talks I have questioned thousands on this subject. No more than two or three per cent understand the rigmarole, figures or writing set out. This includes the ingredients, energy, protein, fat, carbohydrates, fibre, sodium or salt. Sodium and salt are the same thing to all except the very odd person, yet often given separate headings.

Fats are one thing which people try to understand but without much success. **Few can differentiate between trans-fats, low fat, saturated fats and the others fats we read and hear about, including the essential fatty acids. We learned recently that the addition of trans-fats to processed fast foods may be unlawful and probably has been for some considerable time.** 'Food' producers do not have to declare the trans-fats presence in the so-called foods produced. On re-reading this, again it is highly obvious that all who eat processed and fast foods are being made fools of by the producers, the processors.

Until the 1950's there was little if any control over the use of food additives. There was no need for regulation. There were little factory made ingredients. Our food was mostly natural, unprocessed. About 1960 the European Economic Commission, the forerunner of the European Union (EU), started issuing Directives on additives. **The food processing industry was taking off.** In 1984 the Food Labelling Regulations were an eye opener. The amounts of ingredients were as nothing compared to now, but for the first time the purchaser could read, whatever about understanding, what was in the food on the shelves of the food store.

Pages could be written about present day labelling or the way it is being done. Most of it has got out of hand, with little understanding of the wording or collation. Having so many bodies that add their piece frequently, it is difficult to understand whom, if any single group, organisation or body is totally responsible. The media tells us that a survey showed that the Food Safety Authority of Ireland (F.S.A.I.) considers existing food labelling to be informative, stating that 27% of consumers said they read the labels when shopping for food. I thought to myself this is idiocy, or my questioning of people and their answers are highly questionable.

I set out for three days, visiting over 15 supermarkets to question shoppers and asking, *"Do you read the ingredient labels or seek other information from them?"* My findings were even worse than found at my talks. Just four per cent read them. Many look at them, try to read them, but don't understand. There is a very big difference between just looking at the labels and reading them to gather information. **So much for the F.S.A.I. survey. I feel they like to appear as being busy and this survey speaks much about their short-comings.** They too don't wish to rock the boat or make further work for themselves. Their 27% referred to, was nonsense.

The independent food expert, Professor Michael Crawford of London Metropolitan University maintains that the Food Safety

Authority's (F.S.A's.) food safety agenda is transparent, *"It is nothing but a smoke screen for industry"*. My belief is similar and I have written and said this many times in the past.

Many told me of how they look at the sell by or use by dates but seldom look at anything else on the labels simply because they just don't understand the jargon. Maybe to the third level or higher educated people, who devise what is on the labels, it might be clear, but certainly not to the ordinary persons in the streets or the food stores. My wife, family or myself don't read them anymore because when shopping we have learned to use our common sense, purchasing only nutritious, additive free and pure, natural food and drinks.

A few days after the F.S.A. survey mentioned was printed by the media, we hear of the British Environment secretary calling for a more sensible approach to food safety, as part of a drive to cut waste and reduce imports. He said that people should take more notice of 'best before' labels, advising them to decide for themselves whether the food is still good to eat or not.

Since coming to the years of discretion, or when I realised how vital one's health is to enjoy living properly, it has been the policy to *'Buy Irish'* if at all possible. Take the misleading shams of labelling as it is now and try to buy Irish. The relevant authorities, such as Bord Bia, do something, but it is certainly not good enough. There should be a law to protect their Bord Bia Q A logo. It appears that anyone can use **'Irish Quality Assured'** on many food products where it should not be allowed. Read the labels on certain smoked products, such as bacon rashers, to discover that the ingredients are exactly the same only to find that a Bord Bia logo is on one and not on another. One presumes that the other is of foreign origin. My advice is **"Be Irish, Buy Irish"**, even if you have to shop around. Now we find further scares about smoke or 'smoked' meats, crisps and other 'smoked' products.

Typical of the nonsense of food labelling is that of salmon. How can one tell the difference between Irish Smoked Salmon and Smoked Irish Salmon? **Slight change of wording, is like a sleight change of hand.** It appears it is the first requisite to make life more difficult for the purchaser. In many incidences like this, the labelling is farcical. Here, if the word Irish is placed first, it is imported salmon. The other way it is Irish salmon. Even rereading this myself I am not convinced, but it is crookedly true or a lie, according to how it is interpreted. As mentioned elsewhere in this book the salmon is factory farmed, fed colour and food with additives, some artificial, being given chemicals which make the salmon flesh unnatural. Even the artificial smoking of food, including fish, is now being treated as a serious matter, with questions to be answered about whether or not it is carcinogenous.   See **Salmon** also **Smoked Foods and the 'Dangers'** captions.

We hear of the organisation Food and Drinks Ireland (F. D. I.), backed by the huge food ingredients manufacturers Kerry and Glanbia, lobbying against the introduction of a mandatory national labelling scheme, which is to include a traffic light system in the U.K. As is usual the big moneyed industrialists have won out, so it is back to the drawing board. The procrastination virus has again set in. I sometimes suffer from this myself but not regarding pure food.

Previous to this we heard of the U.K. food firms taking on the official watchdog, which in this instance is supposed to be The Food Standards Agency.   The food barons there too don't wish to have the labelling proposals foisted on them. We now learn that the food industry there has also won the day. How many more years will it be before the general public will be able to read and understand food labelling, as the food industry again and again makes the Government bow to and agree to their vagaries, sometimes conceited. The power of lobbying is colossal.

Like much in politics and big business the huge lobbies must be appeased, changes will not be made, with the proposed new laws being withdrawn.   At the end, the all too innocent public, especially the housewife and those who eat the often 'foodless' food offered, will be none the wiser, just as the majority are left unaware now.

Now in my 80's, I often remark to myself and to other old friends, who are codgers like me, *"How did we manage?"* All agreed that we lived reasonably healthy lives because we ate sensibly. We ate and drank natural unprocessed, additive, colour and preservative free foods and drinks. Synthetic or chemically produced vitamins and minerals, as added now, in an endeavour to make food of the stuff produced, were unheard of, as was anything processed. The addition of these chemical vitamins is a modern idea, now used to try putting some goodness into the manufactured and processed 'rubbish' type foods we are offered.   I repeat **"All too much of what is sold as food is foodless"**.

I don't know if I am right in referring to myself and old friends as codgers. The definition of this word is **'Eccentric elderly men'**. My friends may take exception! I trust they will forgive me, but then I may be right in my description of some of them.

As if one needs confirmation that what I say here about food labels is correct, here is the latest. The E.U. Health Commissioner tells us that food companies must provide key nutritional information, such as fat content on labelling of packaging. This makes things even more complicated because of the many varying types of fat available.

A new E.U. law designed to tackle the obesity problem is also being drafted. The new regulation is aimed at simplifying the countless and varying laws throughout Europe. **The Irish Obesity Task Force's 93 recommendations, as compiled by some 27 members of an Oireachtas Committee in 2005, have not been acted upon**. We now hear of new E.U. laws working on the same subject. Will the E.U. laws supersede the Irish ones, not yet acted upon, or will the joint recommendations be acted on? The taxpayer again pays for this carry on. See *Obesity* caption

The E.U. also informs us that shoppers are confused because of bombarding them with *"too much"* and sometimes *"all too often"*, misleading information. What a pity I did not have this information some time ago. I would not have had to dig up my file notes regarding the farce which is *'Food labelling'*. We now await the outcome with interest.

One highly relevant question to be answered before spending millions on formulating another set of food labelling rules or proposed laws is, *IF THE FOOD AND DRINKS MANUFACTURING AND DISTRIBUTING CONGLOMERATES WOULD NOT ACCEPT WHAT WAS PROPOSED LAST TIME, WHAT IS THE POINT OF CONTINUING FURTHER?*   Giving in to the all-powerful food and drinks industrialists, including their many lobbyists, points to weak governing, another case of the tail wagging the dog. Big business wins time after time. The general public, whom this matter concerns in a huge way, are left to look on at another unacceptable episode which has gone on for years, with no satisfactory rules regarding food labelling in sight. All too much of the factory made, processed, so called food and drinks are 'rubbish' and to add insult to 'injury', the giant producers, let's call them moguls, have rubbished their customers, the general public, by not allowing proper and informative labelling.

To add to my vexation about all of this crazy, mindless, and terribly confusing make up of the food labelling system, I now get further heat under the collar. It transpires that beers, spirits and wine products will not have to conform to or obey the supposedly strict compulsory labelling requirements. We are told openly that this comes about because of a lobbying campaign by the drinks firms.

No doubt their lobby groups, such as The Food and Drink Industry Ireland and the Drinks Manufacturers of Ireland (D.M.I.) also their counterparts in the U.K., all of which are funded by the drinks industry, are smirking. It is entirely wrong that they can get away with not having to list the ingredients in alcohol beverages on the cans or bottles. It is more than wrong, it is disgraceful. One cannot help being with thoughts about brown envelopes, one of Irelands ways of lobbying! Don't tell me that it is a thing of the past! Often it does not have to be done in a brown envelope. Just subscribe to a relevant political party and be home and dry. It cannot be overlooked that this information about another E.U. law being drafted comes from Brussels. It begs the question, **"Who governs us? Is it our democratically elected Government or the nameless, faceless Brussels Eurocrats?"** All who voted 'YES' to Europe have helped to bring much which is idiocy on us. Of course many were duped into voting thus, having originally voted 'NO'.

As with much else serious regarding the health and well being of our nation, the food labelling laws are certainly not being made simple for the ordinary person, as the politicians grovel and kowtow to the food and drinks industry barons.

FIRST PRAYER OF THE DAY
DOES IT EVERY OCCUR TO ASK GOD FOR HELP?
HERE IS A PRAYER TO START EACH DAY WITH

LORD GOD, I welcome this new day
It is your gift to me –the first day of the rest of my life
I thank you for the gift of being alive this morning
I thank you for the sleep that has refreshed me
I thank you for the chance to begin life all over again
LORD, this day is full of promise and opportunity
Help me to waste none of it
LORD GOD, this day is full of mystery and of the unknown
Help me to face it without anxiety
During this day, may I become a more thoughtful person
a more prayerful person
a more generous and kindly person
and a more healthy person
LORD, bless this day for all of us Amen

THE WEATHER

An old proverb, often attributed to Mark Twain, that everybody talks about the weather, but nobody does anything about it, could be linked to our Health Services. We hear much on airwaves and through the media, with fault finding and complaining about the Sickness Industry the taxpayer is burdened with. The weather is the main topic of conversation in the Western world. Because of its unpredictability, it is all too often a deterrent to walking and taking exercise, Whatever the weather, if properly clad, walking is one of the most enjoyable forms of exercise. We should remember *'THERE IS NO SUCH THING AS BAD WEATHER, JUST DIFFERENT KINDS OF GOOD WEATHER'*. Every day is a good day, every hour is a bonus. Live life, all of it, to the full, whatever the weather.

'HEALTH IS WEALTH',
AN A TO Z ENCYCLOPAEDIA OF OVER THE COUNTER NATURAL REMEDIES AND GOOD FOOD

Some years ago, after nearly 40 years of research, and five and a half years of putting it together, I wrote the Encyclopaedia *'Health is Wealth. An A to Z of Over the Counter Natural Remedies and Good Food'*. It is a tremendous success in so many ways, being up there amongst the best sellers. Since then the many stories told to me about ill-health, side effects, the harm caused by and the uselessness of prescribed chemical drugs, much overly so, are sad.

Thinking of the blatant overuse of antibiotics, also the too easily obtained chemical so-called drug remedies off the shelf, makes my blood pressure rise considerably.

Within days of *'Health is Wealth'* being launched, there were invitations to give talks, some call them lectures. I lecture nobody but I do advise and speak with groups, varying from 10 people at an Active Retirement Group meeting, to 290 at a corporate health function. Many friends were made, much knowledge was gained by myself, and I hope many have been helped physically and mentally by the talks and advice given. The vast majority of those whom I spoke with knew little about natural foods, or over the counter natural remedies, as sold by the health food store and now by some chemists. Synthetic vitamins, minerals, pills and medicines as churned out by the drug-manufacturing companies and sold by the chemists, the filling station or the supermarket meant just the same to them as the natural remedies. The billions spent by the pharmaceutical drug industry promoting their chemicals, almost all of them being of little or no use, all too many of them harmful, is scandalous, one could add immoral. The food industry is similar in some ways. See the **Bibliography** section on how to obtain **Health is Wealth.**

PRAISE

*Chas. W. Schwab, the chief aide and confidante of the Scots/American industrialist and philanthropist Andrew Carnegie, said, **"I have yet to see the person who could not do good work if praised and given merit for achievement".** Ella Wheeler Wilcox, well known American poetess, is on record as saying, **"A pat on the back is only a few vertebrae removed from** *a kick in the seat of the pants, but is miles ahead in results".* *If with people working under you try rewarding them for good service, even if only by praising them. It boosts morale.*

THE SUGAR BEET SAGA

Irish sugar beet growing farmers received little notice when told that production of sugar beet would cease in Ireland. The whole restructuring plan to cut the level of production across the E.U. was presented and carried out extremely fast, especially in Ireland. Farming, which is a business, whether in a large or small way, was certainly not treated as such, with most farmers having to make hasty decisions as to their future, as part of their livelihood was whisked from them.

A figure of five million tonnes was that given by the E.U. as being needed to cut from production. The figure to date shows it has only been reduced by a fraction of that amount. The Irish farmers were left to their own devices and one can safely say made to look foolish, again being the losers. The Irish Farmers Association also the Beet Growers Association made their voices heard in a limp and certainly un-business like manner. Here again our sense of outrage was missing.

Now, years later, the E.U. bureaucrats who were largely responsible for the closure of the farm reliant sugar beet industry acknowledge that they were totally wrong. A profitable business, giving much employment, directly and indirectly, was shut down, closed impulsively. Farmers and those who depended on the growing of beet for a livelihood could do no more than stand and stare. Disgraceful is too nice a word to describe the exit by Greencore, the owners, who took the major part of the compensation on offer.

One thing can be said about the Irish, it is that they are great losers, probably the best in the world. Sure we have plenty of practice. Here is another case of being ruled by the E. U., the non-democratic, faceless bureaucrats, who run our country in so many ways. In this instance they were responsible for giving entirely wrong information also supporting figures which turned out to be misleading, all of which led to the closure of the one remaining sugar beet factory. The best that can be said about this saga is that sugar is an evil commodity as are most artificial sweeteners, which should be avoided, if one wishes to be reasonably healthy.

LAUGHTER

Joseph Addison (1672 – 1719) never forgot the amazing power of laughter and remarked, *"Man is distinguished from all other creatures by the faculty of laughter, laughter is contagious. Why not start an epidemic today!"*

Laughter is one of our greatest remedies, just as whistling was. Laughing is a feel good factor. Whistling used to be too but now one seldom hears a person whistle. I well remember when the latest hit tunes would be whistled as we walked. Recently I tried to whistle some of the present day so called hits but found it impossible. There is just no melody, no rhythm. The beat and tempo is gone from the oomph-omph 'music', now loud in every sense. At least we can laugh and it is one of the greatest medicines.

There is a time to laugh and when the time comes, do not miss it. We must learn to express ourselves and enjoy life. Laughter is a victory over a world of ills that plague humanity, and when we can laugh at ourselves, that is some victory.

Laughter is a good remedy for relieving the strains of life, loosening tightened nerves, and increasing the strength for the performance of duties. It is certainly more enjoyable than the pharmaceutical kind of chemical medicine all too readily available. There are times when it can be much more beneficial too and there are certainly no side effects!

Laughter is a potent stress buster, bringing relaxation and helping to lower blood pressure. Try memorising jokes and sharing them. Jimmy Cricket, the comedian, is an example of all that is good about laughing as he says, *"Come'ere there's more"* and tells us *"I am so healthy I would make you sick".*

A recent article in that wonderful magazine **'Ireland's Own'** sets out the benefits of laughter. The author tells us that children laugh up to 400 times a day. Adults only manage a meagre four or five times. There is much food for thought here. We are told of how laughter helps the heart and assists one to lose weight, eases pains, reduces the risk of heart attack, stimulates blood flow, boosts the immune system, with many other health giving facts included. **'Ireland's Own'** gives us many laughs. It is one of Ireland's treasures. All those who read it agree that *'The Week Wouldn't Be The Same Without It!'*

Some years ago, I went into a store on the Old Kent Road, in South London. It had a lovely little restaurant or tearooms attached. When I first found it, I was on my way home from work at about 6.30am on a beautiful summer morning. I called in for breakfast because they did very nice natural foods. The place was fairly crowded but what struck me was that all were so glum and serious looking. I called out, good and loud, **"Good**

morning all, what a day to be alive". Within a few seconds all were chattering, laughing, the atmosphere completely different. Many times after this I visited that café, always to be greeted by the welcome *"Here is the man who knows how to get the best out of life".*

TISSUE SALTS
Marvellous, wonderful, simple, so natural remedies, all taken from the earth.

In my associate book, the encyclopaedia **'Health Is Wealth'**, there are three pages devoted to Tissue Salts. I wish not to be repetitive and to copy as little as possible from **'Health Is Wealth'**, but must explain that the many telephone calls and letters received, extolling the goodness of Tissue Salts, should be mentioned here. These came from people who learned of their excellence through the writings in **'Health Is Wealth'**. They told of how these Tissue Salts cured cracked and chapped lips, dandruff, mouth ulcers, acne, cramps, chilblains, earache, flatulence, hives and hundreds of minor or niggling ailments. There are 12 of these salts from the earth, all purely natural, not being drugs in any sense of the word. Visit your health food store and be surprised at what can be likened to the opening of a 'Pandora's Box' when Tissue Salt information is given. You may also write to New Era Laboratories Ltd., Hedon Road, Hull, England. HU9 5NJ, who will send further information. Please give reference as to how you heard about these simple homeopathic remedies, all of which work and *cure*.

WE CAN ALL HELP TO BE HEALTHIER

There is not a doubt that our Doctors, Consultants, Nurses and all who deal with the health of our nation need very much education about **Disease Prevention**. This to include natural healing and simple methods, such as ingraining into the minds of the public the understanding behind my slogans, *'We are as we eat, drink, sleep and exercise,'* or *'Change the lifestyle'.*

I can almost see the GPs shake their heads, with some of them throwing a fit. I ask all of them what can be more natural than proper nutrition? **Hippocrates**, whom doctors when training take an oath to, said *"Let food be thy medicine and medicine be thy food."* It is certainly not in the advice or jargon of the medical voices today. Drugs and more drugs are their only answer. As set our in this book more than once, *'Change of*

33

lifestyle' is not in their vocabulary. With nearly 50 years of helping people who have been ill, I have restored many to good and better health, often by only a change of modern living. Many only need to learn about the simple things of life, also to be disciplined to avoid alcohol, smoking and the foodless food and drinks offered.

Nobody will change my outlook. I repeat, that if all were to put into practice my slogan's *'WE ARE AS WE EAT, DRINK, SLEEP AND EXERCISE'* also using the three words *'CHANGE YOUR LIFESTYLE,* the health of all would improve immensely. Our hospitals would be quarter full or three quarters empty according to one's line of thought. Our doctors and the medicos generally, would be on short time. The pharmaceutical industry would see many conglomerates liquidated. It is a sad state of affairs, but a fact, that over 40% of present day exports from Ireland come from the medical device and chemical drug-manufacturing companies, so our economy would therefore be decimated. Our Government will not rock the boat. Our health is not their concern except to ensure that the Sickness Industry thrives, as it continues to grow, mostly by making healthy people ill or by inventing new illnesses, as is being done. All must ask, *'Which is more important, money or health?'* My answer to that is, *"It is crystal clear that the state of health of the economy comes before the health of the inhabitants of the nation"*.

As far as I am concerned health is wealth. It is without doubt our most valuable asset. **"Would you trust anybody with a priceless blessing such as your health?"** The majority are doing this as they accept without question the prescriptions being doled out, or the over the counter chemical drugs all so easily obtained, as if they are of little consequence, also the need for other things such as surgery, which is very often not required. An example of this is that a friend of mine, who was told that he had cancer of the prostate, decided to forego the operation suggested. He treated himself the natural way, taking Saw Palmetto, Zinc/Copper, Pulsatilla, Lycopene and Pumpkin seeds. Now, almost six years later he has little discomfort. This is only one of many similar type cases which can be related. Certainly we can all help ourselves to be healthier. **One can start by giving thought to how the body is treated, or more often mistreated.**

Nothing in the world makes people so afraid as the influence of the independent mind" **Albert Einstein 1879 –1955**

SUICIDE – WHAT IS THE CURE?

In my book **'Health is Wealth'** was a caption on Suicide. When I commenced writing it I was almost reluctant to do so. I felt that here was a subject where I could hurt a family, or others, who had the traumatic experience of losing a loved one. There was the desire to be nice, not to offend anyone. That feeling has not changed over the years. What has changed is my mind-set, as I feel a wave of anger at the approach made to the problem of Suicide by so many of those in authority.

Much is said and written, with little being done, much leading to my anger. **Almost daily we see headings such as "HSE cannot predict if Suicide reduction target will be met", "Money sought for Suicide prevention" "Time to combat teenage Suicide", "Antidepressant and chemist shop drugs involved in one third of fatal overdoses", "Eighty per cent of Suicide victims took antidepressant drugs", "Alcohol is a major factor in young Suicides,"** with many other headings which can be quoted. All are seriously worrying.

We now have a **'World Suicide Prevention Day'**, with campaigners holding a candlelight vigil as they seek more action. Seminars, meetings, talks and other get-togethers on the subject are being held.

"We can talk until the cows come home" to use an Irish adage, but all agree that those with suicidal thoughts or tendencies will not hear, they will be on a different wavelength. They need help in mind and body.

Recently I was invited to speak at a seminar titled '**Suicide-What Is The Cure?** I came away feeling annoyed, exasperated, one could say helpless. Why? Because I got the biggest ovation on the night with most of those attending coming to speak with me afterwards, saying "**How much they were in agreement".** My exasperated feeling of helplessness came from the fact that there were 26 listeners and I wished to get my message to the whole world. Another source of annoyance was that a speaker on the night was scathing of the Government because they did not provide or fork out €1,000,000 promised to Suicide prevention programmes from the '**Dormant Accounts Fund.'** The Government very often gets the blame, but not for the right reasons. What is the point of providing money if there is no valid arrangement as to how it would be spent? **I would berate the Government for not educating the people, and I mean everybody, about their eating, drinking, sleeping and exercise habits. Here is the cardinal reason why suicide is so prevalent.**

Change of lifestyle is all that is needed for many to attain very much better health of body and mind. Having made my introductory remarks, including in them some of what you have read, I continued, *"This* is my message to all, young and old. I will not be convinced otherwise. Daily as I speak with the many who seek my advice I note their lifestyle. I am told of some of the problems, but not in any order, which can be lack of energy, depression, anxiety, headaches or migraine, being overweight, high blood pressure and many and varied other health troubles. Wrongly worrying to some of them is the fact that the doctor has told them their cholesterol levels are high.

Question these nice people, many troubled and fretful, but not outwardly, to discover that what they are eating and putting into their bodies is slowly killing them. This includes additive-filled 'foods' also chemical medicines. So it is with many today. Visit the supermarket and view the additive laden 'foods' on the shelves, see the nosh, the fare turned out and offered as food, much of it foodless.

Try to read the ingredients labels where all too often one requires a magnifying glass. Ask the store assistant, manager or proprietor to explain what the additives are. They have not got a clue, no more than the gullible customer who unwittingly purchases the stuff, all too often trash.

We have thousands of factory made additives of which many are artificial, including preservatives, stabilisers, humectants, acidity regulators, flavour enhancers, colours, bulking aids, fillers, artificial sweeteners, emulsifiers, gelling agents and much more, mostly added to attract the taste buds and cheapen the so called food.

Taking many of these things as food is mostly why people are ill. Taking these things leads to ill health. If one is not healthy in body, one is not healthy in mind. A sick mind can all too often lead to suicide.

Walk into the deli, chippie, filling station, the newsagents, and other shops and stores. See the rows upon rows of fizzy and sugarised drinks. Read the ingredients labels of the so-called energy drinks and be amazed. Note the mars and nutri-grain bars, snickers also the other many and varied sugar or additive-filled snacks being purchased by so many, especially young people. Only last week when in a Tesco supermarket, I measured the length and height of the fizzy drink and bottled water section in the store. It was 22 metres long, yes nearly 70 feet, and seven feet high, over two metres. It contained thousands of plastic bottles of additive-filled and sugary drinks. This was one of their smaller stores.

I have gone out of my way to queue at 'deli' counters just to see what is being purchased. The smell of frying oil and curry is often enough to make one ill. Note the white 'cotton wool type rolls' and what is put into them. One sees being purchased what may be the breakfast and lunch combined, with a roll containing a piece of overcooked *chicken or perhaps with the end of a sausage or two protruding. The meal would frequently be washed down by a bottle of sugary liquid such as lucozade or coke, this being held in the other hand by the purchaser. A mars bar, snickers snack or perhaps nutri-grain or similar is for afters. Imagine what all these things may do to the system. There is certainly no nutrition in them. Visit cafes, delis, restaurants or even some hotels and see what is being offered as 'food'. I make a point of collecting menus from some of these eating-houses. I have over 150 of them on file. What is offered by many is non-sustaining with little if any nourishment or food value. Visit pubs and hotels and see the drinking culture, see the 12 and 24 packs of beer as purchased in the off licences or supermarkets, often hoisted on a person's shoulder. This is how we lugged bags of cement or potatoes on our shoulders in the past.*

To one like myself, seemingly there are too few like minded, it is baffling to say the least why the ingredients of all the foods, much of them colour, additive, sweetened and filled with preservative are not printed, framed and displayed in every outlet where alcohol, 'food' or 'drinks are sold or available.

It is ridiculous that the ingredients have by law to be displayed on food and fizzy drinks and not on alcohol beverages.

Take into consideration what I have just told about the type of fast, processed, adulterated and additive-filled foods and drinks the majority are using. Consider the health damage and injury being done to the system. As I have stated, the food and nourishment value is often nil.

I have referred to alcohol and the sad fact that here too is one of the greatest evils in our midst. The drinking culture which has had gigantic growth in recent years, allied to the easy availability of both illegal and legal, harmful and dangerous drugs is just the height of idiocy. The harm being done, and how seemingly foolish and thoughtless people allow these to enter the most intricate and so easily damaged system in the world, is beyond understanding. The mind-set of so many, that when ill, the doctor 'will cure me', cannot be ignored where alcohol or drugs are being swallowed. See the queue up at A & E Departments at our hospitals late at night or very early in the morning, especially at weekends, when most should be resting. Add to this the legalised drugs prescribed so needlessly by the medical profession. Think of the mixture that can end up in the stomach. Those who treat their bodies like this need more than education. They must be made to realise the folly of their ways.

Many people living on their own, whether male or female, young and those not so young, do not feed themselves properly. They become run down and unwell, attending the doctor for more and more prescribed medication. Yes drugs and more drugs. Never is a word asked about lifestyle or what the patient needs as proper nutrition or how he or she exists. A big majority are undernourished".

As an eighties years young man, I have over the past few years discussed with friends this terrible thing which is suicide. Many of them, like myself, knew what it was to have no money. We made our own entertainment. Despite the bleak outlook none of us contemplated suicide. Why? All are in agreement that we ate plain, wholesome, natural food, certainly nothing fancy, all properly cooked, whatever about the way it was presented. We had little if any money for alcohol. There were no street peddled drugs. We drank water, took exercise and had a good sleep pattern. Most of us had to be fit for the games or athletics, also in order to be on time for work next day. Because of all this we were more healthy in body and therefore in mind. It should also be remembered that few, if any, went to the doctor. Anti-depressants and chemical drugs, which are now offered like sweets, were only prescribed in highly serious cases. Very little other than Beecham's powders and pills, Rennies or Aspro, was available over the counter in those days. Few needed medication. Pure food was the medicine.

I fully realise that not all will enjoy good or better health. There will be some who will not respond to any treatment. This is obvious, as daily I see the many who have allowed themselves to become very ill in both mind and body. Some will do nothing to retract or undo the illness other than visit a doctor, where they too will do little to help the patient, although professing to do so by issuing a prescription. There are those who refuse to accept advice, so living out lives which could have improved immensely by a change of lifestyle. The positive side of all this is to talk with the many who have been helped back to better health, by helping themselves, when accepting the advice given to change their way of living, to live life naturally. This advice is handed out daily by way of my writings, talks on radio or elsewhere.

Nobody will convince me or change my mind that one of the chief if not the main reasons for resorting to suicide is because of what is being taken into the all-intricate human body. I make no apologies for repetition as I try to get the message to all who are interested in good health. Part of that theme is that *'The fuel you put into the engine determines its performance'*. This is why it is terribly ironic that in one of the most important areas of life so many disregard this sound judgement. It involves feeding the human body properly, which when healthy leads to a sound mind and a buzz – shall we say a zest for living. Suicide would be far from the thoughts of very many, if all of this advice was accepted. My slogan

'WE ARE AS WE EAT, DRINK, SLEEP AND EXERCISE' was never more relevant than in undertaking the rehabilitation of our people where the mind-set and lifestyle of men, women and children should change. Until this is done, the health problems which have accumulated and built up over the past 15 to 20 years, aided and abetted by the chemical drugs-manufacturing industry and the medical profession, will remain or grow. They will increase as new diseases, like the misleading scam which is high cholesterol, are thought out and promoted. See *Cholesterol* also *Statins* captions

Our Sickness Industry and all concerned with what is now the biggest enterprise in the country are going down the wrong road. The vast majority of those who are ill do not require medication to solve health problems of mind and body. All that is needed is education about prevention of sickness and disease also about how to lead happier, healthier and enjoyable lives. Those who are healthy or reasonably so can learn too, in case that in the future they too might go down the road of ill-health. Much of this can be summed up in three words *'Prevention of Illness'*.

Hopefully in years to come, we can look back and see Suicide as a past light. That is, if those employed by the general public within the Sickness Industry see their folly and accept the advice of one of the greatest medical persons ever. This was **Sir William Osler,** who died aged 70 in 1919; he was a humanist and classical scholar, a wonderful physician and scientist. He was outspoken of his beliefs that the art of healing knew no frontiers, alternative or orthodox. He had many honours bestowed on him for his medical works. His interests in the welfare and health of all is remembered by his words *"One of the first duties of the physician is to educate the people not to take medicine"*. If only every doctor would give serious consideration to this advice before prescribing, at the same time telling the patient to go and change the diet and lifestyle, what a vast difference it would make to the health of those who seek medical aid. I repeat *"There probably has never been a period in human history when the value of pure and natural foods or drinks, including additive free nutritional diet and the health improving factors set out in this book, was more essential than now"*. **A healthy body leads to a healthy mind which can only lead to very much less thoughts about SUICIDE.** Turn to *We are a Sick and Malnourished nation* caption.

CHEWING GUM AND THE CONSEQUENCES

Two years ago, a man, seeking advice, visited me. He was unwell. Having smoked for many years he had bronchial troubles.

For about five or six years he had been taking medication as prescribed by the doctor. He told me **"I don't get any better, the breathing and coughing just gets worse"**. He had at that time a terrible gasping with a kind of whistling sound. He appeared very distressed. He asked if I could help him.

On being questioned he described his Diet, which was terrible. His daughter with whom he resided cooked the meals. Much of it was off the shelf, fast or junk foods. There was little natural, other than vegetables, which from what he said were eaten about twice weekly. The microwave was used for much of the cooking, as was the frying pan. The type of fast food eaten, also the preparation and cooking, could only lead to ill health. I advised him about the need for pure natural unadulterated foods, giving him a copy of my leaflet on Diet, which can be used to help regain better health. He was told to visit the health food shop and obtain a natural Multivitamin also Lobelia tablets and Thyme drops. Stressed was the need to change intake of processed additive-filled meals being eaten. Given to him was a list of what to eat and drink also the many unhealthy foods to omit from his diet.

During the time he was with me, I could see the incessant chewing of gum. In days long gone, the chewing of tobacco was a filthy habit. It resulted in much spitting and also ill health. Chewing gum cannot be looked upon any more favourably.

Having partaken of a good meal of home made soup, fish, vegetables, potatoes and then fresh fruit salad, prepared by my wife, I brought the subject of the chewing of gum into the conversation. Our friend told of how he chewed gum nearly always. On being asked had he some with him, four or five packets were produced from different pockets. With great difficulty I read out the ingredients from the packet. He was no different to the vast majority spoken with or questioned about additives, in what is either eaten or understood about them. He was not aware of what was being chewed or ingested. It was just chewing gum to him. To any person interested in feeling well, it can only be regarded as obnoxious, certainly no aid to bronchial or any other health problems.

When I see sports personalities, people in the public eye, or indeed any person chewing gum, I cringe. The chewing gum contains, as indeed do most of these gum-based confectionery like, over sweetened products, assorted flavourings such as spearmint or indeed whatever flavour is required. All are man-made, as are the other things with the odd exception. Included with additives which do not have to be listed are; Isomalt,

Manniton, Aspartame, Acesulfame K, Gum base, Flavourings, Humectant, Glycerine, Thickeners, Gum Arabic, Titanium Dioxide, Carnuba wax glazing agent, Antioxidant, Butylated Hydroxyanisole, also contained is a source of Phenylalanine, which on its own can be dangerous. So can Aspartame and the Carnuba Wax. The latter can cause skin irritation. What the whole combination does long term to the intestines, the stomach, is anybody's guess.

Since then the person referred to has visited on and off and has told me that after accepting my advice the diet was changed. From the health food store, the Multivitamins and Lobelia were obtained, also the Thyme drops. He said *"I threw all the Chewing Gum in the fire and I am not sorry"* – his exact words. The change in this person's health and outlook is highly noticeable. He is now enjoying life. His bronchial tubes seem to be much better, although he did say *"I have my Lobelia tablets with me and if I start to wheeze I take one. They are wonderful".* Without being asked he said**, *"That Chewing Gum got to me, it nearly killed me. I would not have known about all those 'dubious' additives if you had not told me".***

Here again is evidence of the need to read the labels fully. Here I must say that to read the extremely small print on the chewing gum wrapper is well nigh impossible, the words being almost illegible. This is another ploy by the manufacturers to keep people ignorant of the contents.

Further advice to him was to leave what he called 'dubious' things on the shelf. If all did this the money orientated manufacturers and those who sell their unnatural products would get the message of that wise ruler, **Abraham Lincoln**, spoken almost 150 years ago, when he said, *"You can fool all the people some of the time, some of the people all of the time, but you can't fool all of the people all of the time!"*

Chewing Gum is unhealthy, unsightly and to be avoided. Those who chew gum are just like the many who put rubbish into their bodies. They don't care and amazingly seem unaware that they may be doing serious harm to their future health.

The filthy habit of chewing gum, then spitting out or throwing on the pavement is to be abhorred. Apart from being unsightly there is the cost of removal by the Local Authority or other. Chewing gum accounts for one third of all our litter, being the single biggest litter item by far.

Singapore is the most infamously intolerant place in the world, when it comes to chewing gum. Back in the 1980's, when people were still chewing it there, they didn't just drop it on the ground but carried out acts of public vandalism, placing gum in mailboxes, so that letters stuck together, in keyholes, over lift buttons, and on the seats of buses.

A proposal was made to ban gum as early as 1983, but no action was taken. In 1987, Singapore's new metro system, built at a cost of $5 billion, started operating. The vandals began to target the metro, sticking gum on the floor sensors of trains thus preventing doors opening at stations. As a result, frustrated passengers were unable to get on or off, with the entire system sometimes temporarily slowed down. In 1992 chewing gum was banned. It was no longer sold anywhere in the city, and anyone found smuggling it in was publicly named. A first-time offender had to pay a fine of $1,000 (€485), while repeat offenders got fines of $2,000 and were given corrective work orders, which usually involved cleaning the streets and wearing a high-visibility jacket. The media were invited along to report on the public punishment of the shamed offenders.

Five years ago, the ban was revised. The sale of gum with 'health benefits' – chiefly nicotine gum – was permitted. Nicotine gum is only on sale in pharmacies and is only sold to those who produce Government issued IDs. If pharmacists are discovered selling gum without having checked the ID, they risk a fine of $3,000 and a two-year jail term. Singapore does not have a chewing gum littering problem.

THE SICK MINDS OF THE LITTER LOUTS

Here is food for thought, because if one cares about the environment then the clear examples set by the litter-louts are cause for depression to those who are considerate. Careering along the roadway in the tin box on four wheels, the motor vehicle, the driver will seldom notice the rubbish. I suggest they park up, and walk out of our towns and villages. View the road verges, some of them partly overgrown with foliage. See the piles of crisp bags, luzcozade, coke and other plastic bottles, the beer and fizzy drinks cans, coffee, milk, or the various containers and cups, also the cardboard and plastic trays. See the other various types of packaging discarded. Most of the wrappers and containers are from 'foods' and 'drinks'. Here is further food for thought because it gives a clear picture of what the drivers or passengers are taking into the body. Lucozade, coke, yop, lager, red bull, crisp bags, mars and snickers packaging are in the top 10 which litter the roadsides. The burger and fast food trays are in abundance.

Put it another way – '*There is no thought given to the additive-filled, sweetened, so-called foods and drink, being devoured, as the litter louts travel or drive, eating or drinking at the same time . Much of this 'deleterious' stuff is turning the users into obese, unhealthy and undernourished citizens. Education by the Sickness Industry and throughout our schools and colleges is urgently required. Parents of our young people need to learn and pass on the advice to their families, that much of what is being ate and drank is 'rubbish' food or drink, being terribly 'unhealthy.'* The mindless and cynical people who discard the containers can rightly be called 'ignorant yobbos'. One cannot help but notice the disposal of nappies, perhaps germ laden, or the piles of cigarettes butts emptied from the ashtrays of cars. *These nappies are known as disposable but they were certainly never meant to be left as litter*! It is not to be wondered at that Ireland is the most littered country in Europe. What I write about has been witnessed by myself, working with the many civic minded volunteers who work in groups annually, as a clean up of the verges of all roads within our parish boundary is carried out. If only the drivers and their passengers had consideration for others it would make life easier for all who abhor the litter.

Many years ago, when living in England, I read a compendium of books titled '**The Social History of Britain**'. In it they referred to the filthy Irish living there in the 1800's. I resented this and still do but maybe they were right about some. In other countries one sees the signs '**Please take your litter home**'. The vast majority do so. Perhaps the word '**please**' may help to convey the message that littering anywhere is not acceptable. It should be on large, easily read signs in many locations around the country. **All, young and old, must learn to be litter conscious**.

TOAST

Here is one of the most useless, unhealthy and bowel binding things ever eaten. It is a big help to stopping diarrhoea. This gives an idea of what it does to the system. Almost daily when I interview or speak with people who are ill, run down, lethargic, depressed or with other ailments, they tell me of how they have tea and toast for the breakfast. It never occurs to them that the nutrition and food value of toast is nil, as it binds up the bowel system. Here is processed food at its worst, to be avoided, unless with diarrhoea. A proper breakfast, without toast, is as medicine. Toast is rubbish and certainly not food. It should not be eaten at breakfast time or indeed with any other meal.

TEA

There are teabags and tea leaves. Have you ever opened a tea bag to find that there are no tea leaves, just dust. The invention of the teabag was a boon for the tea industry. It resulted in their being able to utilise the waste. Tea leaves make nice tea. The teabag contents are the leftovers at the packaging stage. Good quality loose tea leaves are recommended for a nice cup of weak tea taken about every two hours. This is natural and health giving.

SALT—THE DANGERS OF

Salt, like sugar, is in almost all made-up foods. Both are evils of better health. We need little salt but no sugar. Unless we are extremely disciplined, the intake of salt is too high. Its over-use leads to high blood pressure levels and the dangers of heart attack or stroke. The six grammes daily salt intake recommended by the Food Safety Authority is well in excess of a healthy level. What can be called 'hidden salts' is the reason one must be careful about salt intake. Breakfast cereals and bread are examples of this. Much of off the shelf salads, soups and sandwiches are over salted. Instead of the labels telling us about health benefits, it should be mandatory to put health warnings on many ingredient labels.

The British Heart Foundation policy office tells us **"Salt is a hidden killer, which can lurk in the unlikeliest of food, but it is hard to distinguish healthy from unhealthy at a glance".** Again I pass on the advice **"If in doubt, leave out, do without".** Surveys reveal up to four times the recommended levels of salt for children in fast foods. This gives them a 'taste' for salt, something that continues with young people, as they grow older. It is used by food manufactures for that very reason. Yes, to give children a taste for salt so that by eating the falsely flavoured foods, the inclination is to eat more. Babies and children are building up future health problems such as heart disease, strokes and renal damage, with kidneys and water retention problems arising. A diet high in salt could affect the intelligence, according to recent research. It seems that raised blood pressure resulting from high salt levels may harm memory, reasoning power and attention span. In recent years, I find that if there is salt in foods which are served in restaurants or hotels the taste is very obvious. Is this because I have become anti-salt and do not use the substance. I have refused to eat and have sent back overly salted food when dining out. This does not happen at home because of non-use of the silent killer, which is salt.

There is no need for salt in either cooking or on the table, because we take it into the body from much else which is eaten.

TABHAIR AIRE DUIT FHÉIN – LOOK AFTER YOURSELF

Why wait for the Health Service Executive, why wait for somebody to do something about our health? Why not do something ourselves? I did and it has been marvellous looking after myself, with no need for chemical pills or medicines. There are many who do likewise, using only natural non-processed foods and drinks, taking exercise, also getting sufficient and proper sleep. Over the years, I have been able to come off all drug medications. I must repeat, that like so much in life, '**Our health is our own responsibility**'. One can safely say it is a cheap care or onus in life. *It would serve all well to practice and follow the dictum or meaning of the well know Gaelic saying, as one takes leave of another, – 'Tabhair aire duit fhéin'.* The realisation will come, if one looks after what is often referred to as number one, that every day can be a better day, that every day one arises in the morning is the first day of the rest of one's life, with much to look forward to.

Ireland and the U.K. rank at the bottom of the list of some 20 developed countries in the number of preventable deaths in any one year. Only Portugal and the United States are below them. When one considers the amount of money poured into the American health industry, they should certainly be ashamed of themselves.

Disease and sickness prevention is certainly better than any cure. Try telling this to the medics who run the Health Services of the developed nations. They do not wish to know, as they promote the chemical and unnatural pills and potions, which help keep the wheels of the Sickness Industry oiled. As if to say to the Sickness Industry gurus *'You have got it wrong'*, we now find that health insurance companies are offering regular gym users up to 50% off premiums, with reports that some of them are offering reductions on proof of eating healthy foods, including fruit and vegetables. The majority of these clients will have to be health conscious. How this will be enforced or proved is difficult to perceive. I wonder will all participating have to keep their food and gym receipts or show proof of visiting the health food store for additive free food and drink?

With the Government, through the Sickness Industry, not prepared to set example regarding prevention of illness, at least the insurance companies are doing something to make the public aware of what is good for their well being. They realise that the prevention of illness is the answer. The insured persons are also protecting their no claims bonus, as well as experiencing a feel good factor. They realise that practicing the slogan ' **WE ARE AS WE EAT, DRINK, SLEEP AND EXERCISE**' is a big money saver regarding resultant better health and the saving on insurance payments.

THE COMPUTER GIVES MUCH NATURAL FOOD FOR THOUGHT

Wonderful allies in the world of natural remedies, medicine, food, drink and resultant better lifestyle are to be found on the Internet. I highly recommend Mercola.com, H.S.I. Daily Health, Natural News (insider@naturalnews.com), Total Health Breakthroughs, or Dr John Briffa (john@drbriffa.com). There may be others, but those mentioned are at the top of my list. They are highly informative, using layman's language, not being alarmist or unnerving, just giving us facts. At the same time it is advisable to read between the lines. Perhaps I should not say this but I don't take it all as 'gospel'! However, if in doubt all can be checked from other sources.

Standing up to the hype of the medical and pharmaceutical industry, who have billions to spend on propaganda and advertising promotion of their chemical drugs, also the food and drinks conglomerates, requires huge research and thought. Much information and news, which makes for some excellent natural health articles, is given by those mentioned.

HEALTHY BODY WEIGHT

HOW TO LOSE WEIGHT SLOWLY, FEEL GOOD AND HAVE MUCH ENERGY.

As one who is slim, trim and with much energy, whose weight has not changed minus one or two pounds over the past 35 years, I set out this simple natural way to maintain ideal weight. It is also a recipe for better health and how to attain and maintain acceptable weight for height and bone structure. I have not got the time or inclination to promote this formula or programme commercially. For the past five or six years I have given it out freely, at talks, symposiums and with books sold. The results have been dramatic.

The plan is implemented naturally, no need to cut down on food, provided the said food is fat-free, additive, colour and sugar free, but rather being nutritious. There is no need to accept the hype of the 'Slimming Industry'. Whatever happened to the much lauded and written about 'Atkins Diet' and many other money-making publications of slimming brouhaha? There's no need to cut down if pure and natural portions are served.

Figures show that last year over £22 million sterling was spent in the U.K. on slimming and diet books. Total sales of slimming literature are not available for Ireland, but one has only to look at the array of printed matter on the subject to realise that slimming and dieting is of major interest. Added to this are the metres of columns in the media, covering the subject.

Those who decide to journey on a slimming or weight reducing course are offered, almost always, a *'Sure and Certain Formula'*. This can include *'crash'* and *'yo yo'* diets, often with abstention from food which contains the all so vital proteins, carbohydrates, vitamins, etc., necessary for good health. Not so with my highly successful recommendation. I stand to gain nothing monetary wise from my advice as I set out this entirely natural way of losing weight, at the same time leading to one feeling good. If I can help somebody it results in much satisfaction.

Frequently prescribed by those who promote the slimming and weight loss concept or notion, including members of the medical profession, who should know better, are the doubtful and perhaps harmful chemical drugs which the commercially focused drug companies now tout and publicise. These include: Xenical, Reductil, Acomplia and several other branded made up chemicals. Amongst their make up is orlistat, sibutramine and rimonabant. The latter is unnatural and frightening in that it curbs the appetite. This is far removed from the teaching of the father of modern medicine. **Hippocrates** proclaimed something, which if adhered to now, would save our nation hundreds of millions monetarily. He had this to say ***"Let medicine be your food, and food be your medicine".*** This is mentioned more than once in this book but I do so again to help get the message home to all interested.

Practically all of the weight reducing drugs are dubious, with adverse effects typically apparent during use, even over a short time. All should give serious thought to the long-term consequences of putting anything chemical, including these so called 'aids' into the body. The long-term implications could be devastating. Similarly with many food additives, few realise the 'dangers' of using proprietary branded products, which have little, if any, history of proper use before being put on the market. Here again, as in so many previous incidents, the gullible, unsuspecting and trusting public, the users, are being treated as guinea pigs. Indeed the use of these chemicals, when combined with certain diets, then stopped because of lack of discipline, will-power or perhaps side effects, can result in a huge increase of weight.

*My simple plan, which has worked for thousands, myself included,
is an enjoyable way to lose weight, which has helped many.
It is set out here:*

1. **Drink 6-8 glasses of pure water daily**. Pure water is to the body both medicine and food, playing a vital role within the system. Very often one is actually thirsty when feeling hungry. This occurs in hot working conditions or when overtired. Many think that alcohol is a thirst quencher. It may be short-term, but if one is dehydrated the alcohol can do serious harm. The same can be said of fizzy and additive-filled drinks. Drinking these liquids gives very serious food for thought.

Only recently has it become obvious that drinking from plastic bottles can be dangerous, even toxic. Bisphenol A, which is used in the make-up of semi-rigid plastic, has been found in liquids contained in plastic bottles or containers. The chemical has been linked to the obesity epidemic we now have. We are told it is responsible for other health problems, especially if the liquid becomes warm or heated. Foods or liquids from plastic containers used in microwaves should be avoided. See *Bisphenol A* caption.

2. Eat regular meals of pure and additive free food. Breakfast is the most important meal of the day. Porridge is pure and natural, being extremely health giving. Study the ingredients labels of the food you eat or buy. No fries or fatty foods. No chips, crisps, fast foods, sugar or salt, confectionery, sugars or other sweeteners. Almost all pizzas, quiches, probiotics and yoghurts contain additives and are therefore unnatural. Use only the natural, which will be non-processed and free from artificial ingredients. Margarines are out. Use butter sparingly. Eat at regular times and if you must snack, use nuts, fruit such as apples cut into thin slices, or try raw vegetables, which are really nutritious. Fingers of brown bread are health giving. Vegetables should be steamed, not boiled.

Visit your local Health Food Store and ask about the pure natural foods available from their shelves. They have very much which is good, also being nutritious.

3. Simple exercise, such as walking, is very beneficial – a must. It is an excellent way to attain better well-being, including proper healthy body weight. Aim for at least half to one hour or more of simple exercise daily, including stretching when warm.

4. Regular sleep and sleep pattern is as medicine. It is not realised that insufficient rest or irregular sleep pattern is often responsible for much of the illness people bring on themselves, including being overweight. This is especially so for young people.

5. Eat plenty of fruit and vegetables. A liquidiser or blender is a must in every kitchen, being far superior to a juicer, because one gets from the full fruit or vegetable the necessary fibres. It can be used to produce extremely healthy drinks and 'smoothies', also for grinding nuts and seeds. These can be mixed with muesli or porridge at breakfast time or taken with salads or main meals.

6. Have meat, fish, salads or egg dishes every fourth day.

Wonderful aids to the above suggestions, which all lead to reduction of weight and resultant better health, are to use,
Lecithin granules. Take a level dessertspoonful twice daily with liquid. Do not mix with hot foods or drinks. Mixing with a little water in a glass or cup is an easy way to take them.
Take one dessertspoonful of Safflower Oil, (virgin cold pressed) night and morning.
Take two teaspoons of pure honey mixed with a similar amount of Aspell's or Martlett's Cider Vinegar in warm water or use 'Honegar' as directed. Honegar has the correct mix of honey and cider vinegar. Take twice daily.
Use 'Go-Cal', as directed on the container. It is entirely natural and far removed from the chemical aids already referred to. **Here is the key to control of and to help the working of the other things mentioned in this advice. This is the vital component amongst all suggested here to attain Healthy Body Weight.**

All of these purely natural products are available from your local Health Food Store.
I have had wonderful reports, feedback, letters and phone calls from many grateful people. So many say *'How much better they feel and how much they enjoy having lots of energy."* I realise it is a wonderful and healthy way to attain proper body weight and have been lambasted by many for not having promoted it fully.
Examples of weight loss over three months have ranged from 12 to 17 lbs (5 to 8 kg.), with up to 35 to 61 lbs (15 to 28 kg) after eight months. One man lost 5 stone (32 kg approx.) over a two-year period. He too was full of praise for the advice given in my brochure, which is as set

out here. He said to myself and some friends when he visited us *"I'm 60 but I now feel like a young fellow"*. I repeat, "Losing weight slowly, as set out here, is the secret for being slimmer, trimmer and more brimful of energy. '*Super diets are a myth.*'

My advice as given here, which has helped thousands to lose weight and keep to a healthy body weight, leads to better health, with extra energy, no need to cut down on natural, nutritious, additive free food. This is a miracle aid to lowering weight if followed diligently. When the required amount is lost just leave out the '**Go Cal**'. Keep to the diet of pure natural foods, with no fast or processed so called foods. There is no need to cut down on natural, nutritious, additive free food. Eat right to feel right by just following my recommendations for a *HEALTHY BODY WEIGHT.*

EXPERTS

Someone in the business sphere said recently *"If each day you spend an extra hour on your chosen subject, you will be a national expert in that field in five years or less."* I have spent over 45 years studying the natural way of attaining better health and I am far from being an expert. I have learned much and I have helped thousands to better health but I am still learning.

Daily, I wonder more and more at the attitude of those who run our Sickness Industry, as they go down the road of treatment of illness by drugs and chemicals. Regularly I see and hear of the results of change of lifestyle from those who have turned to following my advice.

Can those concerned with the health of the nation not take time to see their folly? Is it that the national 'experts' within the medical profession, who run and damn badly preside over the health requirements of the people, have tunnel vision as they help the giant pharma drugs industry to stack up huge profits for the shareholders? Is it that their business instincts tells them that by changing the lifestyle of their patients, they will be working themselves out of a job? With the extreme exception, they certainly will not advise use of natural foods, change of diet and lifestyle or the use of natural remedies where required. All too many have become national 'experts' in their chosen fields, yes, all over a short period of time.

They should learn to open the gate and step out of their field now and again. They should take an honest look at their work, as people tend to become sicker, as the Sickness Industry of which they are part, becomes bigger and more unmanageable.

'Experts' in any profession should be viewed with caution. Very often what they say should be taken with a pinch of salt, to put it metaphorically. Very often what they present as knowledge or reason is just short sightedness. John Maynard Keynes (1883-1946) summed it up correctly when he said, *"There are those who don't know and there are those who don't know that they don't know"*. These words could be used to describe many so-called 'experts' , including those attached to our Sickness Industry.

WHAT FRIENDS ARE FOR

Friendship consists in forgetting about what one gives and remembering what one receives. To talk with and confide with a friend is one of our greatest aids to feeling better. Take time to visit your friends and spend time with them. They may not always be there. Invite them to visit you. Often a cup of tea is as nectar, helping to relieve tension problems and much worry, which are all too often unnecessary. Shared with a friend or friends it is even better. Almost always when I attend a funeral, speaking with friends, acquaintances or others, I remark, *"It is a fact that we deem ourselves to be too busy to visit many we would like to, the excuse used being that we do not have the time, still we can make time to attend funerals."*

Visit your friends before it is too late. A lady said to me recently *"We should be careful of each other. We should be kind – while there is still time."* Talking with a friend is often a cure or an aid to relief of depression, stress and many of the trials of life. To talk is good, to listen is even better, sometimes. All should remember the words of Ralph Waldo Emerson (1803-1882), the American lecturer and poet, *"The only way to have a friend is to be one."* Think on these words. Sometimes it is difficult to develop or court friendship because the person is hard to get-to-know. These kind of people can turn out to be true friends. Many do not have friends because they do not go out of their way to seek them.

FAVOURITE REMEDIES OF A DEAR FRIEND

My very good friend Clair Whitty has submitted, at my request, a list of her favourite remedies. This extremely well learned person has studied alternative and natural remedies for many years. Clair is a 'Bach' Flower registered Practitioner Product Advisor at the excellent **'Only Natural'** Health Store in Wexford. Clair tells of how before joining **'Only Natural'** she hardly knew that a health store existed. Now, many years of working there has taught the good lady much. Told is the story of how **"Once I opened the door of complementary medicine I knew it would never be closed."**

In our discussions, many stories have unfolded about the uses of natural remedies and supplements, including the experiences of both our families and others. Like myself, Clair has listened to heart-rending stories about the use and overuse of chemical drugs. She tells of the vast numbers who do not understand the vital need to put into practice, the understanding and use of the slogans, *'WE ARE AS WE EAT, DRINK, SLEEP, EXERCISE'* also *'A CHANGE OF LIFESTYLE WORKS WONDERS'*.

The reading of the ingredients labels is also included in the advice given. Another subject dwelt on is the question of fats. Many dwell on this issue, telling us of their harm, but we are seldom told of the body's need for certain fats. Clair advises that **"We have to get back as close as we can to Nature, to foods that we prepare and cook ourselves."** Other advice given is to **"Please read the food labels"**, then asking yourself, **"How far away from the field is this product?"**, **"How many man-made ingredients are in this make-up?"**, **"How much salt or sugar does it contain?"**, **"Do you really want all of these additives going into your system?"** **"Would you put inferior oils or fuels into the engine of your motor vehicle?"**.

Clair continues: "In the Health Food Store we see so many conditions that are related to inadequate diet, often with excessive additives, many of which are just fillers, perhaps with a deficiency of quality nutrients. When I talk to someone, it isn't just what supplement to take, it is also about how they feel emotionally, how their diet is and if they are getting sufficient sleep, also if exercising. If one comes into the Health Store, for example because they can't sleep, in my opinion there is no point in giving them a sleep remedy if the cause is drinking caffeine before retiring to bed. Simply stopping the caffeine might be the solution. Discussion is carried out before I decide on what remedy to go with. Here are my favourite remedies which have been constant over the years."

FIRST AID BOX
(Inverted Commas show the brand names)

Acidophilus Capsules
Arnica Gel 'Bioforce'
Arnica Tablets 'Weleda'
Echinacea 'Bioforce'
Nux vom 'Weleda'
'Bach' Rescue Remedy cream
Tea Tree oil
'Bach' White Chestnut Flower remedy

Aloe Vera Gel 'Optima'
Arnica Cream 'Weleda'
Echinacea Drops 'Viridian'
Lavender Oil
'Bach' Rescue Remedy drops
Tea Tree cream
White Willow 'Viridian' capsules

SUPPLEMENTS

Essential Fatty Acids
Rhodiola
Super F 'Naturalife'
Good Multivitamin, high in 'B' Vitamins

Garlic capsules 'Hofels'
Spirulina 'Synergy'
Wart Stick 'Arkopharma'
Vitamin D3

Conditions

Aches and Pains: *Arnica Gel is as good as Ibuprofen*
Essential Fatty acids high in Omega 3
Arnica tablets

If with Arthritic condition there is a need to discuss diet, digestive health and supplements like Glucosamine Sulphate, Celadrin, Turmeric, Boswellia, White Willow Bark or Devil's Claw. White Willow Bark is the chief remedy for pain. The great thing about these remedies is that there are no side-effects, except of course if on medication from the doctor. There is a need to check this out.

BRUISES   *Lavender Oil, rubbed on neat*
Arnica Cream
Arnica Tablets to prevent bruising

BLOATING   *Probiotics, Super F, or watch diet and how you eat.*

BURNS - MINOR   *Aloe Vera Gel mixed with some Lavender.*
Apply plenty of cold water.
Take 'Bach' Rescue Remedy for the shock.

COLDS   *Echinacea*
Garlic capsules, especially if with excess mucous.

CONSTIPATION   *Probiotics. Choose a good brand to suit your age. Super F is an exceptionally good fibre source.*

CONCENTRATION   *Essential Fatty Acids high in Omega 3. At the same time ascertain that you have sufficient Omega 6 in the system. 'Bach' Rescue Remedy if panicky or cannot focus because of stress.*

Rhodiola for memory, motivation, concentration and recall. Rhodiola is a wonderful aid to better health.

Spirulina – Synergy brand, to keep energy levels up.

DIAHORREA   *Probiotics. Choose a good brand for your age.*

EARACHE – MILD   *Lavender Oil rubbed in behind the ear.*

ENERGY   *Synergy brand Spirulina which is good for Iron, B Vitamins and as a source of protein Essential Fatty Acids. Rhodiola if with mood low or lacking in motivation.*

HANGOVER   *Nux Vom or Milk Thistle. Drink copious amounts of water.*

HEADACHES   *Lavender Oil rubbed into temples. I haven't taken an Anadin for perhaps fourteen years. I used to take them regularly. White Willow capsules, an exceptional pain reliever, can be used for any pain. White Chestnut, if brought on by worry or thoughts swirling in the head. It is vitally important to take steps to correct if with high Blood Pressure.*

INSECT BITES *Lavender Oil, Tea Tree Oil, Rescue Remedy Cream or Drops bites, applied to the irritation.*
For prevention of insect bites take Thiamin, which is Vitamin 'B1', for some three to four weeks before going on holiday.

IRRITABLE BOWEL SYNDROME *Probiotics or Super F, also there is a need to look at stress levels, diet and emotional needs.*

JET-LAG *Rhodiola and Travel Essence*

LIBIDO *Rhodiola helps lack of desire and motivation for both male and female. Take essential fatty acids and a good Multivitamin. The base cause must be treated first. Speak with the relevant person in your local health food store. Most are excellent for providing remedies or cures.*

MOOD-LOW *Rhodiola, also Flower Remedies to suit the particular kind of mood, Change of lifestyle is very often all that is needed, also take a multivitamin high in B vitamins.*

NIGHTMARES *'Bach' Rescue Remedy.*

SORE THROAT *Gargle with salt and water, Echinacea or a few drops of Tea Tree oil in warm water. Suck Propolis lozenges. A helpful drink is to use Vogel's Echinacea in warm water. They can be very soothing.*
Apply Lavender oil neat to the sides of the neck for soreness relief.

SLEEP *Put Lavender oil on the pillow or on the temples. The oil can be burned in the room. Take Rescue Remedy if stressed, White Chestnut 'Bach' Flower Remedy if worried or thoughts whirling around in the head. Avoid stimulants like tea or coffee also sugar. Avoid taking multivitamins or supplements late in the day.*

STRESS	*Take 'Bach' Rescue Remedy or Rhodiola if feeling a lack of motivation or energy. Take a multivitamin high in B vitamins.*
SKIN DRY	*Essential Fatty Acids, skin brushing and drink plenty of water.*
SKIN SPOTS	*Lavender, Tea Tree or Rescue Remedy with small amounts applied neat. Take a multivitamin also a 15 mg Zinc/Copper tablet, B vitamins also Silica. Essential Fatty Acids are also necessary. Talk to your local health food store personnel about diet and hormonal issues also regarding skin care products being used.*
SUNBURN	*Aloe Vera Gel, mixing some Lavender oil with the gel is extra soothing. Lavender oils can be applied to temple. Bach' Rescue Remedy can be taken to calm if impatient with the problem.*
TEMPER TANTRUMS	*'Bach' Rescue Remedy.*
THRUSH	*Apply live natural pure yoghurt. Take Probiotics. Avoid all sugars and yeast. Ask for Candida diet sheet in your health store. Apply Vogels Echinacea cream, softened in the hand. Aloe Vera Gel is wonderfully soothing. Wear a pad to protect clothing.*

THRUSH OF THE MOUTH

ADULT	*'Udo's Choice' No. 5 chewable Acidophilus*
INFANT/CHILD	*Udo's Choice Infant or Child Formula. 'Solgar' ABC Acidophilus is excellent too.*
TUMMY BUG OR UPSET STOMACH	*Natural Probiotics*
VAGINAL DRYNESS	*Aloe Vera Gel acts as a good lubricant.*

WARTS	*Wart Stick 'Arkopharma'. Three cloves of Garlic crushed and soaked in olive oil. Wait three days before applying with cotton buds. Milk from the Dandelion stem when in season, or Tea Tree oil applied neat.*
WEIGHT	*Super F before a meal can help one feel full. It also helps to keep the bowel healthy and empty. Read Ronnie Plant's instructions in this book under **Healthy Body Weight** caption. It is extremely successful.*

The above list is a personal list of remedies that have remained constantly in my cupboards or on the shelves over the years, obviously with variations. I sometimes try something new on the market, as those who visit me for advice praise them for their aid to better health. Many do not realise the goodness and help of 'Bach' Flower Remedies of which there are 38 in total. Like many who use them, saying how wonderful they are, I am in complete agreement,

For a small selection of perfectly safe remedies they have many uses amongst them. I will, however, offer a word of caution, **"Herbs are safe if safely used."** You must always tell the health food store staff member if you suffer with a medical condition, if taking any prescribed medicines from the doctor, if you have any food allergies, also if pregnant or trying to conceive.

Enjoy a chemical drug free healthy life and get to know your local health food store personnel. They will be happy to guide you. The above are my own remedies and a good starting point. We are all different, so experiment and see what works best for you and your family.

WHEN IN DOUBT, LEAVE OUT, DO WITHOUT

Where there is controversy, question mark, or the slightest doubt about anything which enters the human body and this includes the contentious prescribed chemical processed drugs, many issued without due thought, my advice is, *IF IN DOUBT, LEAVE OUT, DO WITHOUT.*

This is certainly applicable to many chemical drugs, food additives, colours, and preservatives, so called sweeteners including sugar, also alcohol, coffee and much else additive-filled or anything processed. Who gives thought to the purchase or use of off-the-shelf chemical so called remedies such as painkillers, codeine based drugs, mouth washes, coughs and cold aids, or the vast selection of other legalised drugs available? How many realise or understand the consequences, long or short term, of administering these chemical compounds or stimulants, whether they be for children of any age, teenagers or adults? Yes, remember my repeated slogan **WHEN IN DOUBT, LEAVE OUT, DO WITHOUT.**

PROBIOTIC AND FUNCTIONAL FOODS

No doubt, you too have heard the hype about the goodness of Probiotic or Functional foods, again much of what is offered being foodless. The word *'Functional'*, which means hardwearing, useful or working, is an old word. Probiotics or functional 'foods' are descriptions which have only recently been created. They refer to micro-organisms, which supposedly provide benefits to the stomach, resulting in better health. The majority of things offered as probiotics are far removed from giving better health.

All too often the alleged probiotics are nothing short of a scandal, as the consumption of the fermented products has increased alarmingly. Unless the purchaser is fully aware that what they contain is pure and natural, without a single additive, they are processed, so the advice is to *'Leave them on the shelf.'* Apart from buying a natural health food book or magazine to discover the good of genuine additive free and natural gut health giving probiotics, the only place to look further is at the ingredients labels of the much processed and unnatural food offered as functional. **You may need a magnifying glass to discover what is in yoghurts, low fat spreads, margarines, and many others, which offer additive-containing and almost always far from natural so called probiotics or functional foods**. The money made through the sales of these products for the powerful multi-nationals and other manufacturers, as they seek higher profits for the shareholders, is enormous. Cutting costs, one could add cutting corners, with supposedly healthy giving, manufactured, processed products is one of their chief aims. The all-too-gullible user or person interested in better health should realise that much of the advertising humbug is ridiculous. The reader or viewer all too often laps it up, thinking and believing it to be true.

In front of me is a carton which contained probiotic yoghurt, note the word **'probiotic'**. The hype tells us that it is virtually fat-free and with less than 55 calories per 100 grammes. Few understand what they are purchasing. Ninety-eight per cent of the probiotics, yoghurts or functional foods offered as such, contain additives, are processed and are not natural. These over hyped products are known as pretentious foods.

Visiting one of Ireland's German stores, to queue and note what people purchase as food, which is a hobby of mine, I picked up an eight-pack carton of the 'probiotic' yoghurt referred to. I got hotter under the collar as I read the ingredients. I removed a container to discover there were no ingredients listed. It was only on the outer wrapper of the eight plastic or synthetic tubs or containers. The consumer reads the highlighted words, virtually fat-free probiotic yoghurt. The outer wrapper tells us too, that this junk 'food' contains amongst other things, fructose, glucose syrup, preservative, potassium sorbate, modified maize starch, sweeteners, aspartame, colours and anthocyanins, flavouring, salt, acidity regulator also tri-sodium citrate. Most of these are 'E' numbers.

Aspartame is certainly not to be recommended as far as better health is concerned. The German stores are touted as cheap supermarkets. Many of their products are all too often overly additive-filled. This helps cheapen the 'food' they offer. The trusting and unsuspecting consumer trusts these people as they do other supermarkets. The ingredients labels are ignored. I repeat, it is not to be wondered at that we are a sick and malnourished nation. I should mention here that the supposed probiotic yoghurt referred to was poured down the drain. The cartons were washed and replaced in the outer wrapper. This is now used at my regular talks as I try to convey the message that much of the 'food' offered is rubbish.

Probiotics and functional foods are a clear example of this. Most of them contain additives. Reading the huge amount of 'ballyhoo', as in the advertising of these products, gives one the impression that they are health giving and a truly genuine product in that respect. Additive-containing and processed products are not health giving and to be avoided.

Truly good, additive free and purely natural probiotics, which can be used to keep the gut healthy, are available at the Health Food Store. **'Udo's Super Eight'** is one which immediately comes to mind. It is the king of probiotics, being extremely natural. These stores sell excellent natural products, which are first in the field as probiotics. Like much which has been pure and natural, the commercial bods, the multi-nationals, saw the money spinning potential. The much produced and processed products are just another example of where advertising of additive-filled spreads and allegedly health giving products can brain wash people into believing anything. See *Pretentious Foods* caption.

Some time ago the food and supermarket trade magazine '**Check Out**' wrote, *'Probiotics is an exciting area for the food industry at present.'* It certainly is as they gather in the spend of the easily deceived, foolish customers, who are not aware of what is in the so-called probiotic or additive-containing functional 'foods' being purchased.

RETIREMENT

This word, according to the dictionary, means loneliness, obscurity, privacy, seclusion, solitude, and withdrawal. Just image using the word 'retirement'.

Everybody pictures it as the very opposite to the description given. Forget the word retirement and remember it is like starting into a new job. People are born to work and my advice is **'Never give up.'** Be active. Put the body and mind to use. Too many in their 50's and early 60's have a fixed idea of retirement. They dream of giving up work and sitting back – **'feet up'** so to speak. These words, giving up, sitting back, are to be shunned.

It is hard to believe, but figures show that amongst public and civil servants, teachers or some Government personnel, the average life span or take is two and a half years after retirement. This is incredible but it is no over statement. It is no wonder the Government Pension Scheme is never heard of with regard to being a drain, or with shortage of cash, except when raided by the Government.

Speaking personally, as an octogenarian fellow who punches in a twelve/fourteen hour day, I often wonder how I found time to work. I retired at 66 and went back to work again on being asked. Indeed I went back twice. This was a mistake because later I found many other enjoyable things to do. At aged 75 I was offered a position, with big responsibility, on a huge civil engineering contract, which I declined.

As people get older, they seemingly forget the nine words of my slogan *'WE ARE AS WE EAT, DRINK, SLEEP AND EXERCISE',* often falling into bad health and when it comes to retirement or giving up work, they are unwell – dare I use the word 'banjaxed'.

Many have a line of thought that as they get older, they can ignore the advice about eating nutritious foods, drinking pure water, having proper sleep and sleep pattern, and above all exercise. This is wrong. Walking is one of the greatest aids to better health. Keeping the mind and body active is vitally important. There are various organisations that one can join. I.C.A., Active Retirement Groups, Community helpers, Fundraising, Church organisations and many others are there. They don't seek members, one just volunteers. Writing short stories or articles for magazines is a good therapy. Consider writing a book.

Mícheál Ó Muircheartaigh is an example of keeping active. In his book or speaking recently he tells about age and aging. I agree whole-heartedly because I see it daily in the people I meet or when I give talks throughout the country. He said, *"Ageing is an attitude of mind. I have met people in their 40's and they are old. They think old. They think the world is gone to hell entirely, instead of looking to the positive side".*

Frequently I tell people *"You can't stop getting older, but you can stop getting old."* Get active as far as possible, think natural, be natural, and eat natural foods. I know that all cannot get up and go, but where possible do your best to move about, even if it is only to dangle the legs when sitting on a chair or to do some upper body stretching exercises. **If with a medical condition it is best to consult a doctor before taking serious exercise.**

GRAPES

In the autumn of last year, I picked a bunch of grapes from a friend's glasshouse. The day before I had purchased grapes from the supermarket. They were placed side by side on two dishes. I did this purposely. I had read sometime previously that bought grapes would keep for weeks. Within 10 days the picked or natural grapes were going soft and within another week were inedible. The purchased grapes were left untouched except to examine them from time to time. Some four months later the majority of them could be regarded as eatable. Why? It is a fact that commercially imported grapes are sprayed regularly before and during ripening, perhaps up to 10 times before being picked. Here is further food for thought. Thoroughly wash grapes before eating, or *'If in doubt, leave out, do without.'*

BUTEYKO METHOD OF BREATHING

ITS GOODNESS IN ALLEVIATING AND CURING ILLNESS, ESPECIALLY ASTHMA

The **Buteyko Method** is a programme developed by Russian Respiratory Professor Konstantin Buteyko in the 1950's who discovered that habitually breathing too much causes narrowing of the airways. Factors of modern living such as stress, processed foods and drinks, high temperatures of houses, lack of exercise and public speaking, all serve to increase breathing volume. It involves:

1. Becoming aware of correct and incorrect breathing.
2. Unblocking the nose using a simple breath hold technique.
3. Switching from mouth breathing to nasal breathing permanently.
4. Learning breathing exercises to correct breathing volume.
5. Adopting small lifestyle changes necessary to assist with this, thus commencing the road to full recovery.

What is over-breathing? Clinically, over-breathing is known as hyperventilation. Put simply, it means breathing more air than the body requires. The standard volume of normal breathing for a healthy adult is three to six litres of air per minute. Scientific research conducted by Professor Buteyko over three decades, along with scientific trials at the Mater Hospital in Brisbane in 1995, demonstrated that people with asthma breathe a volume of 10 to 20 litres per minute between attacks, and over 20 litres during an attack. While over breathing is often hidden, it can be recognised by mouth breathing, frequent signs of yawns, having loud breathing during rest, or if there is upper chest breathing.

In the case of an asthmatic, breathing too much causes cooling, drying of the airways and a loss of carbon dioxide. As a result, smooth muscle constricts, inner walls of the airways swell and increased mucus is secreted. It is a combination of these factors that present symptoms such as wheezing, coughing and breathlessness. In addition, an asthmatic may also experience frequent chest infections and colds.

Over-breathing is a habit whereby the body has become accustomed to breathing too much. Like all habits it is one that can be reversed through observation of breathing also practice of simple exercises. Over a period of time through attention to breathing, the volume of air required reduces to more normal amounts, thus allowing the airways to open. **The technique has been subject to five scientific trials in the Western world and is published in a number of Medical Journals.** The most recent paper published, in the New Zealand Medical Journal, concluded that it **'is a safe and efficacious asthma management technique'.**

Buteyko Clinics in Ireland. Patrick McKeown was a chronic asthmatic for many years until he applied this method. After completely reversing his condition and helping others to do so he was convinced that here was an entirely natural and unique way of alleviating or curing asthma. He trained at the Buteyko Clinic of Moscow and is accredited by the late Professor Buteyko. He conducts Asthma Care Clinics throughout Ireland and his books **'Asthma Free Naturally'** and **'Close your Mouth'** are available from most bookstores. **The Buteyko Method** can be taught to all from the age of five years upwards. **Patrick McKeown can be contacted at Freephone 1800 931 935.** See *Bibliography* section regarding his book details.

Those who prescribe the many non-curing chemical drugs as aids to asthma do not entertain the fact that **The Buteyko Method** is a marvellous way to help overcome breathing problems. I see many who now live normal lives after having miserable times. **Money is not in the prescribing of this simple aid by the medics as they conveniently**

ignore the method. Again, it is too natural for them.

As with many other ailments, I often wonder if they are afraid the patient will be cured. A number of people have told of how they were put off attending **Buteyko method** workshops by the medical profession and others, including Asthma Society personnel, saying there is insufficient evidence.   This is utter nonsense, being unacceptable to those who understand and realise the curative properties of Dr. Buteyko's method. The evidence is there as set out. The scientific trials are not acceptable because they are too natural. I repeat, the asthma problem in Ireland is part of the thriving Sickness Industry we have. It must not be interfered with, especially using anything natural, which would not add money to the medicos or drug companies incomes.

I have approached the Asthma Society, only to be given a brush off, cold-shouldered. **Having excellent results published in various medical journals and with recorded experiences of the many who have been cured of asthma, what other evidence is needed?** Turn to *Asthma* caption if further interested.

GOSSIP AND RUMOUR

Rumour and gossip are busy dames
They are at it night and day
dispensing their prescriptions
with clichés like 'they say'
My name is Gossip; I have no respect for justice
I maim without killing, I break hearts and ruin lives
I am cunning and malicious and gather strength with age
The more I am quoted, the more I am believed
My victims are helpless
They cannot protect themselves against me
Because I have no name and no face
To track me down is impossible
The harder you try the more elusive I become
I am nobody's friend
Once I tarnish a reputation it is never the same,
I topple Governments and wreck marriages,
I ruin careers and cause sleepless nights
heartaches and indigestion
I make innocent people cry in their pillows
Even my name *hisses*
I am called Gossip

One of the sayings of some people which really irritates me is the phrase '**They say**'. It means that the person talking to you is not taking responsibility for what they say, putting the blame on unnamed people. The stories vary, but there is consistency in the whispers. Someone needs taking down a peg or two and there are ways to do it. It might be a person, or an institution, a school or a business, but the task in hand is to destroy, by word of mouth and innuendo.

There is great safety in '**They say**,' for no one is identified. They like the anonymity that it offers. Gossip catches people's interests. Just look at the tabloids, chat shows and phone-ins. Gossip happens all the time, but as anyone who has ever been the subject of gossip knows, that doesn't make it right. Some people have nothing better to do than gossip. Maybe they think that it gets them attention or that it's fun to talk about others. They don't realise the hurt that they are causing others.

You may not be able to control the fact that other people gossip about you, Here are some suggestions as to how you can deal with it.

Ignore it when possible. Try to let go of anything not said to your face. If you have a good self-image, you will come to understand that you cannot control the idle talk of others, but you can control the way you choose to respond. Ignoring malicious gossip is often the best response because it deprives those who gossip of what they really want – an angry or upset reaction from you. Remember that gossip is not worthy of the respect your anger would give it.

Correct it when appropriate. Sometimes harmful lies can really do damage and you have to set the record straight but there is no need to talk about it to the whole world. You will keep a rumour alive if you make a big deal out of it. Often you will have to go directly to the source and confront them. This is important. Find the time to talk to that person alone, stick to the facts and talk about how the rumour makes you feel, without condemning the other person or making him or her defensive.

Look for ways to stop the gossip and repair the damage that has been done. It is good to be trusting but it is also wise to be a little bit careful about whom you trust. People earn your trust by showing that you are honest.

Build your self-esteem. If you start to feel down on yourself because of what others might be saying, make a list of all your good qualities. Remember, the tremendous goodness that is within you and let yourself feel good about being who you are. Gossip is evil because it does violence to another human being's character. It is a form of verbal abuse.

Do not be part of starting gossip, spreading it or believing it. Words can hurt as much as physical violence, sometimes more. It takes courage to stand up to gossip but it is worth it. You will find friends who will feel the same way. People who do not believe in gossip often make the best friends.

Before you repeat a story, ask yourself. *" Is it true? Is it harmful? Is it necessary?"* Carefully ask yourself , *"Do I repeat it?"*

My sincere thanks to Rev. Fr. Tom Ryan, P.P. Shannon, for this caption, taken from one of his many excellent homilies.

HEAD LICE WARNING

Parents are warned to avoid the use of many chemical based shampoos and other similar type unnatural treatments for head lice. Some of these toxic solutions are dangerous when used on the head, just as they can cause life long affects. The Health Food Shop promotes natural treatments for head lice which have proved to be excellent where the instructions given are followed diligently. They contain only pure products.   Thiamin (Vitamin B1), taken for three to four weeks, is both the cure and preventative for head lice, just as it is for protection from insect bites, especially if travelling abroad. This warning is given because on several occasions I have seen the terrible results of the use of unnatural treatment.

RESPECT FOR THE BODY

How many can honestly say that they have respect for their bodies, apart from a shower or a bath? How many have three meals daily, meals of simple nutritional, non-processed, additive free food? Do they eat regularly? I make no apologies for repeating that many do not know what they are eating.

How many make a point of taking daily exercise? I mean enjoyable and refreshing activity, including walking or other outdoor pursuit, which means getting to the point of some sweat being raised. **How many respect the body's need for rest, including sufficient and regular sleep?** It is absolutely necessary. How many smoke, drink alcohol and literally abuse the system with no respect for the wonder which is the human torso? How many drink copious amounts of pure water? It is a wonder tonic. Fizzy and so-called drinks are taken without thought given to their ingredients, or the harm they may do, especially long term.

How many realise that there is seldom, if ever, a chemical cure, often being merely a stopper, whether it be pain or otherwise? **The result is that a person's resistance in many instances has done just that – resisted.** Much bacteria is now untreatable by antibiotics. It is obvious that many bugs and micro-organisms are now rampant. They are indeed gaining in strength. Throughout this book the need for change of lifestyle by many is laboured upon and constantly repeated.

If we reverted to the old ways of plain food and pure water, taking sufficient sleep and exercise, our emergency rooms and doctors surgeries would be practically empty. This opinion is not just something from the top of the head. No, I have seen thousands over the years who have returned to good and better health simply by changing the mind-set, **by learning to have respect for their bodies.**

BISPHENOL A

PLASTIC BOTTLES AND CONTAINERS, FOOD TINS AND THE 'DANGERS' OF BISPHENOL A

Bisphenol A (B.P.A.) is a chemical now being looked upon as 'dangerous' to health. We are informed that over two million tonnes of the highly questionable product is used annually. It is in the make-up of plastic, especially plastic containers. It helps to keep them semi rigid and flexible. It is also found in the lining of food cans which contain soups, baked beans and other liquid type foods. For use as a coating on tin cans it is a liquid resin type product before use. Researchers in various parts of the world are now regularly issuing findings which point to the B.P.A. being linked to neurological, heart and other health problems, including birth defects and infertility. We learn of the big cause for concern regarding women's ability to become pregnant, with reproductive health problems being highlighted. *Further food for thought is that Bisphenol A may be one of the chief causes of obesity.* This western world problem of being overweight has only become of epidemic proportions in recent years. All this since the implode in the use of plastic coverings and containers, many filled with liquids, often loaded with sugar, sweeteners or other artificial additives. The whole combination, including the discredited B.P.A., could be the real cause of being over-weight.

A doctor friend, speaking on the telephone from Spain, has reported that a new study showed that Bisphenol A may be linked to type 2 diabetes. He read from a report of trials carried out in Spain, which showed that mouse pancreatic workings were altered by the use of B.P.A. The pancreas produces the all so necessary insulin to help prevent diabetes.

All can't be wrong, as the plastic manufacturers refuse to accept the results, also denying that there is anything unsatisfactory with the containers made from plastic which include B.P.A. in their makeup. **They would, wouldn't they?** There is a call for a ban on plastic bottles and the use of B.P.A. Some baby bottle manufacturers have very quietly, without provenance, removed B.P.A. from the baby milk plastic containers. The European Union (E.U.) is outlawing the manufacture and sale of baby bottles and **other** semi rigid plastic containers. So far we do not know what is meant by the word **OTHER**.

It must be regarded as an admission of guilt, no matter how small, that a chemical the producers claim is perfectly safe, will not be used in future manufacturing of children's plastic bottles. There is grave doubt about the continued use of B.P.A. and until such time as it has been proven to be perfectly safe its use should not be allowed. Here again '*If in doubt, leave out, do without*', by using glass bottles when feeding babies. Indeed this advice should be heeded by all before partaking of any liquids from plastic bottles and containers. It is vital that plastic containers are not used in microwaves. I repeat that there are huge implications to health from the use of the microwave. They should be banned, as Russia has done.

One of the major problems regarding the use of the contents of plastic bottles is that if exposed to warmth or heat, the liquid in the synthetically made-up containers can become contaminated by the controversial and suspect B.P.A. Note the plastic bottles of water, fizzy drinks and other liquids left in motor cars or stacked on shelves. Very often they become warm or hot as the glasshouse effect alteration takes place. It is then that the dangers occur. I tend to wince when I see, as I often do, plastic bottles containing drinks, when left exposed in motor vehicles.

Plastic containers, many of which contain B.P.A. in their make up, are used regularly in microwaves. There is the big hazard of health problems accruing when the plastic is warmed or heated. **We now see Flahavan's Breakfast Oats, which is the doyen of breakfast cereals, placed in thin plastic vessels for use in the microwave as fast food, fast breakfast. These plastic containers DO NOT have the chemical Bisphenol A in their make-up.** Yes, the contents of plastic bottles and lined tins should be rejected until the plastic manufacturers get their act together, **banning the use of B.P.A., as Flahavans have done.** All the studies, which show the dangers of the use of the chemical in plastic, cannot be wrong. It is not as if one body came up with the idea. **There are dozens of reports setting out the hazards of Bisphenol A.**

THE WONDER VITAMIN, WHICH IS VITAMIN D3

I firmly believe that all in our damp, often dull, western isles climate, need to supplement with the wonder vitamin which is Vitamin D3. It is sometimes referred to as the *Sunshine Vitamin.* Frequently we read of doctors saying that there is no need for vitamins, minerals or food supplements because there are sufficient in the diet. It is foolish to make absurd suggestions like this, because all should be aware that our factory made 'food' is often not **FOOD**. Most doctors, like the majority of their patients, do not realise what is, or rather what is not, in much of the foodless food consumed. A properly balanced diet is impossible, unless we are prepared to be extremely diligent, painstaking and careful in what is chosen.

There is no doubting the fact that natural Vitamins, Minerals and Food Supplements, as supplied by the health food store, can be a panacea or remedy, an invaluable aid to cure or prevention of illness, often leading to much better health. It must also be remembered that these aids to better health are certainly no substitute for pure, natural, additive, colour and preservative free food. In plain language taking junk and additive-filled food with supplements is a waste of time and money. Taking the foodless junk, not the supplements, is what leads to ill health.

For many years I have advised and promoted the use of Vitamin D3 simply because we do not get sufficient sunshine. In times past we heard little about protection from the sun's rays. **Now we are told by the health 'experts' that they were wrong in advising people to not allow the sun's rays on their bodies. Again, so much for the so-called experts, who very often advise differently from day to day**. Myself, my friends and very many others lay in the sun, worked, or competed in games, often with burning consequences. Sunscreen creams or lotions were unheard of. We heard little of skin cancer then as of now. *DOES THIS NOT POINT TO THE TYPE OF 'FOODS' NOW BEING CONSUMED, TO THE OVERUSE OF ADDITIVES OR PERHAPS THE CHEMICAL DRUGS OR COSMETICS WHICH CAN EFFECT THE SKIN?*

Some years ago an Australian approached a group of us, as we lay stretched in the sunshine. In his drawling accent he berated us for exposing our skin, telling us of the extremely high incidences of skin cancer in his home country. One of our party immediately said *"Have you ever given thought to the fact that it may be as a result of the chemical additives in all the 'Fosters' lager being drank?"* There wasn't a laugh – just silence. Here indeed is food for thought about the additives in our drugs, food and drink, including alcohol. I am not advocating basking in the sunshine for long periods – if you can find any, but we do need either the suns rays or we must supplement with Vitamin D3. The advice is, **"Use your own discretion."** Even getting sunshine on the body for up to 15 minutes daily will give sufficient Vitamin D3 to the system for some considerable time. This Vitamin, which is so essential for better health, is not made by the body system except when it is exposed to sunlight, now very scarce in our land.

Theoretically we should get sufficient Vitamin D3 by spending a short time in the sun daily. Most people do not get enough, especially in the winter. The result is a Vitamin D3 deficiency in the majority, especially children and older people. The Vitamin is in the top range of medicines or tonics. It is a wonderful preventative against illness. One would have to take large amounts of the fish oils promoted to obtain sufficient requirements of Vitamin D3, therefore supplements are necessary. Even some of them are not strong enough to meet daily requirements. Only recently have we seen or heard increased writings and advice about the need for Vitamin D3, despite the natural food and health fraternity telling of its need, also its goodness, for decades.

Describing Vitamin D3 as a wonder Vitamin is no overstatement. Most people should take it. Setting out its advantages includes many benefits. This Vitamin is essential for healthy bones, slows the advancement of osteoporosis, strengthens the immune system and is both a preventative and an aid for asthma. It aids the absorption of calcium and is essential for avoidance of macular degeneration, being an aid to better eyesight. Deficiency of Vitamin D3 has now been linked to onset of Alzheimer's disease and dementia.

It is a good aid to help achieve proper blood pressure levels. Recent reviews tell us that it *'Can reduce the chances of falls in the elderly'*. It is indeed a must for all, embracing good or better health. We have been told in the past about the good of Vitamin C for colds. It has been left behind by Vitamin D3, which is an outstanding, all round health aid. Is it coincidence, that since we were told from the early 1980's onwards to avoid the sun and cover up, that the incidence of autism has risen dramatically? Can this be attributed to a lack of Vitamin D3 in the body? Can the huge onset of Alzheimer's disease be attributed to the entirely false warning of being told to avoid the sun?

Doctor Richard Mills, research director of the National Autistic Society says, *"There has been speculation about Autism being more common in high-latitude countries that get less sunlight, and a tie-up with rickets has been suggested – observations which support the theory."*

Vitamin D3 is an aid to heart health and circulation, being helpful in the healing of varicose ulcers. Taken in combination with the external use of Manuka honey in the treatment of varicose ulcers, here are two purely natural remedies, which seldom fail. Try telling this to the doctors also the chemical drug-manufacturing companies, only to be laughed at. A woman to whom I prescribed this combination told her doctor. His retort was *"These kind of people don't know what they are talking about."* It worked for this good lady and when 10 weeks later she visited the doctor he had retired. She told me how she was so disappointed because she wanted to show the medic her leg, which was healed in a short time, by the use of Vitamin D3 and honey, after years of useless treatment by him. See *Varicose ulcers* caption

If only the message could be got to those who prescribe sleeping pills, that a Vitamin D3 capsule with one or two teaspoons of honey which has been dissolved in a little warm milk or water, taken at bedtime, is a wonderful aid to a good nights sleep. It is better than and certainly safer than chemical drugs, such as sleeping tablets. The doctor will certainly not recommend natural Vitamin D3. It is not a money-spinner. Again it is too natural.

If one so desires, visit the local Health Food Store and request a good quality natural Vitamin D3, as made by reputable producers of products free from drugs, preservatives, flavours or colours. Solgar, Quest, Lanes or Lifeplan brands come to mind. Their supplements, including Vitamin D3, are excellent. I repeat that **Vitamin D3 is the Number One Vitamin.**

TONICS

Floravital, Floradix, Vitamin D3, Comvita Herbal Elixir or Bio Strath Elixir are magical natural tonics, which can safely be called excellent aids to better health. They should be used regularly in the winter months, if run down or 'feeling under the weather'. Note Brian McNichol's quote given here. One or other of the tonics suggested, used in conjunction with his advice, will help work wonders for one's health, energy and general well being. Kindervital is a very good tonic and pick-me-up for children and teenagers. Some of those mentioned here can also be invaluable for children's health. Your health food store can advise correctly. Apart from these, which I have recommended to thousands with admirable and excellent results, the sound advice of the late Brian Manus McNichol should be practiced. It is, *"The only tonics of any value are a well balanced and adequate diet of natural foods and drinks, sensible habits of behaviour and bowel function, sufficient sleep, exercise and fresh air"*. I agree wholeheartedly with this quote and advice, but in order to be reassured I recommend the use of one of the tonics mentioned, especially in the winter months, to be taken with what Brian sets out.

ROAD SAFETY

WHICH GIVES MUCH FOOD FOR THOUGHT

Daily we hear and read about the carnage on our roads. We have advice about the dangers of speeding, the need for care and common sense. Added to this are the warnings about drinking and driving, also much more. Many are obsessed with the tin box on four wheels. The attitude appears to be that when strapped into the most sought after artifice in the world, all too many feel they have a divine right to the road. Sometimes there is little courtesy or consideration for others.

How many drivers, of any age, take a regular eye-test to ascertain if their sight is good enough to enable them to drive safely? I question people regularly about this and the answers are alarming. Some have never had an eye-test. What drivers do not realise is that if with inferior eyesight, which affects the majority of older people, a pair of glasses can be a major uplift to the mentality. Amongst other things, glasses assist the brain to relax, therefore helping to avoid over-tiredness.

Many years ago I wrote to the Government Minister responsible for road safety, setting out that it would be an excellent idea to send a copy of the '**Rules-of-the-Road'** to every licensed driver, including learner drivers. The reply was political jargon, setting out what they were doing for road safety with no reference whatever to my advice, not even a word of thanks. Years later it was decided to send all drivers a copy of the new and updated version of the '**Rules-of-the-Road',** as set out by the Road Safety Authority. I have questioned quite a number of drivers and have to report that many have not even given it a glance, with the booklets in many instances left unopened from their wrappers. Like the users of drugs, those who drink and drive, those who mix drugs and foods containing additives, those who have not read and re-read the '**Rules-of-the-Road',** all are a menace to both themselves and other road users. Here is certainly food for thought.

The Road Safety Authority Head also the president of the Pharmaceutical Society tell us that there should be greater focus on the dangers of drugs when driving. This is not just illegal or illicit drugs but most important is to recognise the dangers of driving when over the counter or prescription drugs are taken. As with eyesight considerations, how many are aware of how they can be affected by the use of much which is chemical medicine? Over the counter anti-histamines, such as Piriton, codeine containing preparations and many others lessen judgement. **It is worrying when one considers that two tablets of some codeine based drugs can equal the drinking of one and a half pints of beer.** Few, if any, know this.

Prescription drugs, like anti-depressants, anti-anxiety tablets, muscle relaxants and much else, which the general public know nothing about, can potentially impair driving. Many are unaware that the mixing of drugs and alcohol can be lethal. Long-term carry-on like this leads to extreme ill-health, even death. I have spoken with the relevant authorities regarding the need for warning to this effect on all medicines. Nothing has been done, from my observations.

There are many with glasses, which have been prescribed for them because of their need when driving, but they refuse to wear them. When questioned or advised about using them they are often unforthcoming, saying they don't need them. This is going against professional advice. My opinion is that the persons referred to do not give in to the need for the use of spectacles because it would be admitting getting old. It can be put down to pride or vanity, which is a wrong idea.

A report in the Irish Medical Journal tells us that G.Ps. incorrectly believe that newer types of anti-depressants, known as S.S.R.Is., do not effect people's ability to drive. S.S.R.Is. mean Selective Serotonin Reuptake Inhibitors. There is also the question of how some chemical drugs react with certain unnatural food additives, such as 'E's, as listed on the 'food' ingredients labels. I repeat my two mottos, slogans, or call it advice, which are *'When in doubt, leave out, and do without'*, also *'Read the ingredients labels'*, whether food, drink or drugs, leaving the unnatural on the shelf. All should remember that when they drive a vehicle it is no different than having a loaded gun in their possession. *SAFETY IS PARAMOUNT.*

HOSPITAL CAR PARKS

During the past few years we have witnessed big extensions to most of the hospital car parks. Car parking fees have in some cases more than doubled. Apart from the reality of the extra income to the hospital there is an absurd and blatant pointer to the future. *One would imagine that with the huge influx of orthodox or synthetic medication, people would be cured and the need for extra spaces would be unnecessary.* It seems the way of thinking is different. **The blatant pointer is that there is a huge expectancy of future business.** Here is another example of the belief that it is not in the interests of the Sickness Industry to cure. Keep the money-spinner going, make it bigger, help the medical profession get rich as the people get sicker and sicker. **The Sickness Industry is indeed thriving, certainly unnaturally.** I reiterate that the hospital car park extensions are just another indicator. The car park charges are an added perk for the

Sickness Industry as they take in millions annually.

   Nothing surprises me today. One would be inclined to think that as more chemical drugs, medicines and vaccines hit the shelves there would be less sickness. This is not so. The Sickness Industry has other ideas. The whole business continues to mushroom, with extra car parking facilities being provided for those who part with serious money, in order to visit the sick. Here again is further evidence that the Sickness Industry thrives, with selling of sickness extensive, at the expense of the much overburdened tax-payer as it continues to expand.

SELENIUM

HOW TO OBTAIN YOUR DAILY REQUIREMENTS EASILY

Selenium is a vital trace mineral essential for better health. In the past one did not have to worry about being short of the nutrient. Now with modern day farming, particularly with regard to the use of artificial fertilisers, it is not in the soil as of old. Selenium can help prevent cataracts and macular degeneration. It guards against damage done by free radicals including protection against cancer, heart disease and strokes. It works well when taken with the other excellent antioxidants Vitamins E & C. Requirements of this invaluable antioxidant can be obtained by eating four or five Brazil nuts daily. When purchased fresh, place in an airtight container or jar. All nuts lose much of their goodness if allowed to dry out. Brazil nuts are recommended by the writer, who has witnessed the improvement of health and well-being of those who use them.

DOCTORS

Doctors say when they are in doubt
"Of course there's a lot of it about"
Or murmur maybe to one's rage
"You must remember it's your age"
They tell you, looking most profound
"It is something that is going around"
When they say, "A virus has laid you low"
It is an evasive way of saying "I don't know"
When I complained about my hip, the medic told me
" You will have to live with it"
Prescribing pills, on the pain to act
Regardless of the long-term fact
As the tablet makers watch with glee
No thought of the side affects on me
Their coffers filling up apace
All at the expense of the welfare state
(Not forgetting the taxpayer).
They treat you with synthetic pills
Aggravating many ills,
With all things natural being taboo
They wouldn't mention '**change of diet**' to you
There are only some among the lot
Who'll tell you plainly what you've got
I'd willingly lay a liberal bet
I'd be better medicated by the Vet

DOCTORS AND THE MEDICAL PROFESSION

I am not anti-doctor, just vitriolic in my condemnations of the way many of them operate. I am most certainly against their almost snobby attitude, their often cold, almost callous nature, their all too liberal dispensing, their grab all attitude. Their cash till is their prescription pad, the result being that there is all too much over prescribing. In my humble estimation the majority of doctors are despicable in the way they manage or carry out their business.

Their profession, once regarded alongside divinity and law as being highly respected, can be likened to 'pickpockets', as they extract their gains from the all too gullible public. At least the doctor does provide a service of sorts. Doctor friends I have are very often in agreement with much of what I say, even though we agree to differ from time to time.

First of all let me ask the medical profession *"Why are you so besotted with the idea that chemical pills and so-called medicines are necessary"? "Why do you seldom, if ever, mention or suggest change of lifestyle, diet, or natural way of living"?* The patients in many cases could also be asked these questions. Instilled into the minds of all too many are the thoughts that there are pills for all ills.

We learn of G.Ps. coming under increasing pressure from their patients to prescribe drugs or medicines. Many of these people are not even ill. The propaganda about the swine and other so-called flus, which gripped those who can be regarded as pill poppers, has helped lead to the attitude. All should be aware that the only people to benefit from all this ballyhoo are the mighty chemical drug manufacturers and their pushers, the doctors.

Now that doctors can advertise their services as part of the sickness industry, they can sell more sickness. This leads one to ask the questions, *"Will this mean a keen rivalry where charges will be reduced, or will there be competition?"* I doubt it. *"Will The Competition Authority seek out, as they do in business, that there is not a cartel in operation?"* Again, I doubt it.

Printed up within all hospitals, surgeries or where the Sickness Industry operates should be the words, *'CHANGE YOUR LIFESTYLE AND ENJOY BETTER HEALTH'.* Also they might consider other advice, such as, *"The doctors of the future will give no medicines, but will interest her or his patients in the care of the human frame, with a proper diet, in the cause and prevention of disease."* Thomas A. Edison (1847-1931) or **"Let food be thy medicine, let medicine be thy food."** Hippocrates. (c460-c375)

Both of these eminent men referred to, lived many centuries apart, but their messages are the same. Try telling this to doctors, only to be laughed at, even though **Hippocrates** is regarded as the father of modern medicine. Try telling this to the administrators or managers of what we call the Health Service Executive, which in reality is the **sick** Sickness Industry.

If you wish to read more about the two biggest and most inefficient industries in both Ireland and the UK see *Health Service Executive/Sickness Industry* caption

Nutrition should be the first thing checked by doctors before recommending anything. They should pay attention to well-being at the outset. Now it is nothing but an after-thought, seldom if ever discussed. **The system we now have should be changed to where doctors are paid according to how well their patients are, how little money they cost the state or the patient.**

Daily I speak with and interview people who are sick. Also spoken with are many who have been to the doctor because they felt a bit down in themselves. They are not sick, just feeling depressed, very often tired, just seeking a word of assurance. This is not forthcoming, because seldom will a medic bother or take time, even for a few minutes or more, to speak casually with a patient, discussing food, drink, sleep pattern or if taking exercise. The vast majority of G.Ps. prescribe drugs and more of the same. Many people tell me of how their lives have been ruined by the use of medication. As one who will not use chemical drugs I can empathize with them. I have helped many to come off drugs, especially those who have been told they had diabetes, arthritis, and many other ailments including what is perhaps the most difficult of all, depression. I could relay volumes about this.

One person whom I tried to help was on 19, yes, 19 various items of drugs. Imagine what a combination like this would do to the partaker. Don't tell me one was not interfering with or reacting with another. Apart from this she was grossly overweight. This helpless person was beyond my remit. The lady had gone too far before seeking natural help. We hear of people who have sought the help of homeopaths or alternative medicine practitioners. They tell of how they were of no use to them. The don't tell the reason why. They had gone down the road of chemical drugs and could not be treated successfully. They had gone too far. The lady referred to was one of these people and has told somebody that "He was of no use", or words to that affect. She was of course referring to myself. Being on so many drugs, taken daily, I cannot see how anybody would have been of any help to her. I gave serious thought as to how this lady could be helped, but it was a hopeless case. I decided not to even consider to help the 'créatúr'. She was another unfortunate person who had being led down the wrong road by the medical profession.

Some time ago a woman whom I met in the past telephoned me. The person told of how she had attended one of my talks and had taken my advice about the uses of natural foods and natural way of living, putting some of it into practice. Some weeks before speaking with me she told of how she had visited her doctor for a full check-up, which she said I had advised all to have annually. The lady doctor informed my friend that her blood sugar levels were awry, advising her to come back in four to six weeks. Nothing else was suggested, such as change of lifestyle or a little advice given about diet or exercise. The appointment was duly kept. There was a male doctor this time. Apparently he was very abrupt or dogmatic. On taking a sample his retort was, ***"You have got diabetes, I am putting you on medication"***. This is my friend's description of the interview. All this had to be paid for of course.

When I questioned this nice person, it was to discover that she exercised daily, had given up smoking and followed a couple of other things suggested at my lecture. Her lifestyle was still appalling and far more needed to be changed. At her own request and almost beseeching me to give her further advice, which I agreed to do, she travelled over 140 miles to visit me. We spent over two hours discussing and deciding what could be done to attain better health. Eight weeks later this person went for a blood test for diabetes to be told she was OKAY. No medication had been taken as prescribed for her by the seemingly arrogant medic.

She did not need drugs. She should not have been prescribed them in the first instance. A complete change of lifestyle was all that was required. Daily there are thousands of people being diagnosed incorrectly. It is an undeniable fact that the prescription pad is being grossly over used in the **selling of sickness** in order to obtain money. The word OKAY, which I have referred to, was like music to Marie's ears. To realise or hear more about this kind of carry on, see *Diabetes* caption

It would appear as coincidence, but soon after this episode, we were informed of trials carried out over some years, which bore out all that is wrong about the treatment, physically, financially and otherwise of the lady I write about and indeed all too many patients. The trials referred to were carried out by three doctors over a period and their conclusions were, **"If the doctors, who like their associates   mentioned here, did their business properly, some seven out of ten persons diagnosed in the first instance as having diabetes would need no medication."**

All the patients needed was advice to change their lifestyles. This is what can be termed **Prevention**, which as already referred to, is to most doctors an unknown or abhorrent word. In a sentence it comes down to the simple fact that diabetes drugs are being prescribed and given too soon. It is obvious to all, except the medical gurus, whom I have already stated have drug tunnel vision, that lifestyle change management, if given a chance, is the answer to the diabetes epidemic with which we are supposedly plagued. Indeed it is the answer to better health, very often bringing freedom from drugs and synthetic medication. The researchers found that many diagnosed were actually on two drugs within the first few weeks of being told they had type 2 diabetes.

*In short, 700 people out of every 1000, supposedly with diabetes, did not have it before being put on drugs .*What was necessary to be well, meant just a change of lifestyle.

The complete and disgraceful overuse of the prescription pad is scandalous. Who does anything about this? We get the answer to this question all too often – '**NOBODY'**. I repeat myself when I say that the prescription pads are like the cash tills of old which used to jingle when the total amount was placed in the drawer. It is like having a licence to print money, **as sickness is being sold.**

At least one leading psychiatrist had the courage and honesty to say, *"By over diagnosing and over treating we are robbing people of their own innate coping skills."*

As already stated, doctors freely admit to prescribing antibiotics where they are unnecessary. Many give the excuse that they feel pressurised to give prescriptions. Surely these learned people have minds of their own, knowing the difference between right and wrong. None admit to sensing the lure of payment for another cash till and lucrative transaction.

A couple of years ago the British Government launched a national campaign to remind doctors and patients of the potentially lethal consequences of prescribing antibiotics when they are not necessary. The National Health Service in the U.K. said advertisements would appear in national newspapers, magazines and that posters would be placed in G.P's. surgeries, also pharmacies. The Chief Medical Officer said, *"Family doctors are wrongly prescribing antibiotics to treat minor ailments such as coughs, colds and sore throats, in a third of all cases".* It appears that very little happened in Ireland except the usual bleating, despite the Irish Medical Journal findings being almost identical to that of their British counterparts. **Who did anything about the findings? Did the admonition or advice given, if any, fall on deaf ears?**

A Citizens Information Services report tells us of a case where a person paid a €50 fee for a five minute consultation, €75 for a blood test, and another €35 for a renewal prescription. There are many who cannot afford to visit the doctor, with patients putting off seeking care and advice. Here is further evidence of the carry on of 'pickpockets'

"It is nothing short of scandalous that a doctor can take a sample of blood from little more than a pinprick, or carry out a urine test, deciding in an instant that a person has diabetes." It is totally wrong, being unacceptable, that at the whim of one person, someone who is in full health can be put on medication, which is supposed to be taken for the rest of his or her life. **There should be two, perhaps three opinions sought, before condemning a healthy person to a lifetime of being a drug user.** Some words of advice about changing the mode of living, eating, drinking and sleeping habits also the need for exercise, might be all that is required, at the same time telling the person to return in six weeks for examination. In the majority of cases the once border line cases of diabetes would be non-existent.

A lady told me of how her 79 year old mother was on an Immune

System Treatment, having been bad for over two years. A doctor in the quest for money – there cannot be any other excuse – had advised and given the elderly lady the flu jab. The poor woman has had a terrible time and is now most unwell. **Will the doctor be taken to task for prescribing vaccination when it should not be given where there is a weak, or in this case, an extremely delicate immune system. Who will interfere or do anything? The answer again and again is 'NOBODY'.**

Another caller seeking advice told me about how her husband, who had never been ill in his life, visited the doctor for a check-up. Again this was done on my advice. He was **sold sickness**, being told the cliché, the drivel, *"YOUR CHOLESTEROL IS HIGH."* The man was put on Lipitor, which is a well known brand name for one of the various statin drugs which are all too haphazardly prescribed now. Here again the patient suffered terrible side effects. He had chest, bone, muscle and other pains. She told me of how it was only then when she remembered my advice to avoid statins like the plague, that she destroyed them. The great **'Cholesterol Con'** was being tried on again. This healthy man was able to come off statins. Now, some 12 months later, he is feeling good. I have heard many similar reports.

My advice again is *"Give very serious thought to taking statins. Apart from anything else, they are a scam, a fraud."* I reiterate that this cholesterol storyline is another invented sickness which the drug-manufacturing companies have put in place for the medical profession, as they resort to further **selling of sickness**.

Keep your blood pressure levels correct by diligently following my slogan **WE ARE AS EAT, DRINK, SLEEP AND EXERCISE.** With the use of natural aids such as Lecithin, Hawthorn, Rutin and a good Multivitamin you are on the way to good and better health. This is sound and sincere advice to avoid strokes, heart attacks and very many things which can be triggered off by high blood pressure. All too often strokes can be fatal. See *Blood Pressure* caption

Over a period I have compiled a list of people, all of whom were told they had diabetes. They simply changed their diet to natural nutritious food and fruit also drinking pure water. They take exercise and watch their sleep pattern. The suggestion to eat at regular times and to allow one hour for the main meal has been accepted. Some of them have demanded appointments with diabetes consultants and tell me of what must be standard practice, this is to keep appointments, have tests, then drink an amount of lucozade. **After a lapse of a few hours, they had further tests for diabetes. All had the 'all clear' given.**

One must presume that the sugars in the yellowish drink had not in these instances defeated or interfered with the insulin in the body. The well prepared patients, had simply, by change of lifestyle, shown that as healthy people they would not be browbeat into using diabetes drugs. They tell of how their health, especially energy levels, have improved immensely and of how they feel so much better. All this can be attributed to the change of lifestyle and mode of living. It is not to be wondered at that diabetes is of epidemic proportions. If the medics have '**Their way and say**' it will be unmanageable in the future.

As I have asserted, 700 out of every 1,000 who are diagnosed with the ailment could be told that they do not have anything wrong, if the doctors would only see the light, the truth and most importantly '*BE HONEST WITH THEIR PATIENTS*'.

I repeat, many people just need advising about lifestyle and manner of living. It is time the Sickness Industry realised, or better still the general public, that one's health is one's own responsibility, and to advise accordingly.

A gentleman who came to me last year, had been prescribed a patch for arthritis by his doctor. This person suffered terrible side effects and had unnecessary pain brought on. He had not been told about the greatest help known to alleviate, avoid or to be rid of arthritis or gout. It is proper, nutritious diet of additive free foods and drinks. This can be aided immensely by taking a joint complex tablet of Glucosamine, Magnesium, Calcium, and Boron as sold by the Health Food Stores. The Arthritis Diet advising 'What to Eat, What Not to Eat', is set out in my encyclopaedia **'Health is Wealth.** '

In my opinion and talking to the many who visit me, or those whom I speak with at my talks, it is obvious that doctors are not honest with people when it comes to the serious matter of drugs side effects. Very often they are fobbed off, being told *"It is your age",* or even going so far as to say that it is imaginary, or of little consequence, and not to worry about the all too often horrible feelings or pain.

There are many stories, which I have recorded, on being told regularly regarding the prescribing and over prescribing of drugs. A doctor friend tells of how he frequently sees patients discharged from hospitals who are on more than 10 different medications. He tells of the subtle way drugs are added to the *'prescribing pool'* and become commonly used. This is even though these drugs may offer no real advantage over existing cheaper or generic medication.

Typical of the way the Sickness Industry is run in Ireland, almost all education for prescribers is funded by the pharma-drugs industry. At the same time many national colleges of medical specialities, also some so-called charities and others of which there are many, rely on the help of mostly unsuited or what should be referred to as unacceptable sponsorship, to run their medically and drug orientated activities. This is looked on as an integral part of the Sickness Industry. There is the huge question of drug-manufacturing companies having what can only be termed 'an unhealthy influence' over G Ps.

A doctor relative gave me some eye opening information and there is not a doubt but a far too cosy relationship exists between all too many within the medical profession as far as drugs are concerned. We have the Irish Medicines Board, The Medical Council, also the doctors Trade Union which is the dictatorial, autocratic, powerful Irish Medical Organisation, (I.M.O.), with numerous spawned committees, who apparently act only in the interests of their members. Most work in collaboration with drug companies.

The cholesterol gimmick referred to is one of the biggest deceptive schemes within the sickness industry, being perpetrated by the drug companies, aided monstrously by the medical profession. This is the production, prescribing and retailing of statins for the supposed correction of a non-existing disease, known as cholesterol. Yes, it is not a disease, being merely a symptom. I repeat, "Nobody dies from cholesterol symptoms". The galling and annoying part of this ridiculous set up is that our G.Ps. have been sucked into the hype and propaganda of what is a totally unnecessary promotion. This is a huge money-spinner for the medical profession, the pharmacists, but above all for the drug-manufacturing companies, benefiting nobody else. Some doctors are now telling us that those as young as 35 should be put permanently on these cholesterol lowering drugs. In America the medicos are advocating that children down to four years of age be given the statins. Here are more examples of *selling sickness*.

One can ask the question, *"What is the world coming to?"* when we consider the upsurge in the taking of medicines such as statins and the thousands of other useless chemical drugs which has only built up over the past 25 years. It is a worrying revelation. Before this sequence of events we were a very much healthier nation. This is sufficient proof that the chemical drug industry, aided by the doctors, has built the Sickness Industry we now have into a get rich business, all at the expense of the tax-payer and a stupid Government, along with the extremely gullible patients who trust and accept the advice of the medical profession. How foolish can people become? If you wish to learn more about this waste of time and money on what can rightly be regarded as a burgeoning con or scam turn to *Cholesterol* also *Statin* captions.

The word '**big bucked**', which I have used to describe many doctors, is not a strong enough word to describe what may be a 'criminal' tendency by some of them. Some years ago there was this huge question of payment to doctors who had made false claims for deceased patients. The sums involved were between six and €10 million. This is taxpayer's money, obtained by some doctors surreptitiously. Many of the medical cardholders on their books, and for whom they made the fictitious claims, were deceased. This money cannot be regarded as an over-payment. What happened can only be termed as dishonesty and fraud. If this very serious matter, of what must be regarded as stealing, was perpetrated by a layperson or other body they would presumably have been prosecuted, with every likelihood of ending up with a criminal record, perhaps jailed.

What happened in this case? I doubt if anybody knows. It appears at the time of writing, several years after the deception, that it has been brushed under the carpet, forgotten about. I have written numerous letters asking what was the outcome of the matter. Copies of this correspondence are held on file. In the hope of receiving a reply, some of these letters were sent by registered post to those supposedly in charge of the day-to-day running of the Sickness Industry, The Health Service Executive, including the Minister for Health.

I did not have the courtesy of a reply, except one, and that from the Health Spokesman for the Opposition Party in the Dáil, which at the time was Fine Gael.

Remember this deceitful and swindling episode was discovered several years beforehand. Here is his reply, *"The issue you raised regarding the nine millions spent on over payment of doctors has not been resolved. The figure is being disputed by the Irish Medical Organisation (I.M.O.) and I believe the H.S.E. is also in the process of looking at how this debacle happened in the first place. When I asked and enquired into the issue, the Health Service Executive was no more informed than what I have already outlined, Yours Sincerely."* First, note the words 'over payment', which is a politician's and the doctor's way of construing this very serious carry on. In this instance it is a case of 'thievery'. Like many other highly serious or alarming episodes which occur in governing, where there is often gross mismanagement and deception, this 'fraud' will be conveniently forgotten about. Again who does anything about it? The answer is '**NOBODY**'. The doctors can keep the looted loot.

Some years ago the I.M.O. offices were raided. It transpired that the I.M.O. had an action taken against them, in other words they were prosecuted, for allegedly fixing the fees of GP's. charges to life assurance companies for medical reports. Another part of the allegations was that the I.M.O. or its members, the doctors, threatened to withdraw their services if the life assurance companies did not agree to accede to the demand for proposed increase in fees. Several years later we learned that the High

Court received from the I.M.O's. legal representative a file setting out the settlement. **No details have been given – all are secreted away.** We learn that costs of the Competition Authority who took the action against the I.M.O. were understood to be in excess of €60,000. If this lot ran their business properly these exorbitant expenses would not occur. The I.M.O. agreed to pay this amount. **If the organisation was innocent, would they agree to pay this sum?** Just as with so much of their scheming, the quest and greed for money can be related in dozens of the episodes or stories emanating from the Sickness Industry. Here too this affair was hushed up.

Having a hearing problem, which came from working in confined spaces when I was younger, where there was unbearable noise, I attended the doctor. An appointment was then made at one of our biggest hospitals, which I duly kept. A five-minute examination by a consultant resulted in my being given a prescription in a sealed envelope. Although I did not know it at the time this was for something to soften the wax, which the medico said was in my ear. Another appointment was made at the time.

On visiting the chemist next day there was a queue, which I joined. The temptation to speak out could not be resisted. In a loud voice I said, *"The Sickness Industry is certainly thriving. Just look at the queue for chemical drugs."* Not one person smiled or made comment. They probably thought who is this pariah or loud mouthed person.

Sometime later my prescription was handed to the pharmacist. Having looked at it and in order to be heard over the heads of the many standing around she loudly said, *"You will have to take this to the supermarket"* I said, *"Why?"* By this time some were laughing. The answer was *"It is for olive oil."* I cannot put here my retort because I was no way diplomatic, but it was to this effect, *"Do you mean to tell me I travelled over 240 miles to be given a prescription for olive oil? Why did my doctor not instruct me regarding wax softening and removal when I visited him on the first occasion? Won't I look a right fool when handing this in to the supermarket, telling the assistant it is a doctor's prescription?"* Here again there was much laughter.

From the Health Food Store I obtained cold pressed olive oil, which was heated and used over a period of days. I travelled a round trip of 480 miles to keep my next two appointments, when they worked on my ear and I presume removed the wax, or some of it. Each time I was told that I would hear from them. Some weeks later I got a notice of a new appointment to visit the same consultant. I was not examined by him, being spoken with by a different assistant on each visit. Why I was sent for a fourth time I do not know, but the answer was "There is nothing we can do for you". I said, *"The supermarket 'drug' did not work even though I travelled almost 900 miles in total!"*

Many have told me of how they have been given future appointments, often duplicated or triplicated, with no reason for these consultations. My experiences, as recorded here, are an illustration of the many ways the consultants and doctors operate. If the patient is covered by health insurance it is like a bonanza to them, as they arrange appointment after appointment, knowing they are on a guaranteed transaction or dole out. If you wish to read more, see *Consultant's Money Saga* caption.

Last year my eye became blood-shot and got progressively worse over a few days. Constant stream of advice to me from friends, my wife and others, was to visit the doctor. This I did not do because I regard the majority as being pill pushers and drug orientated. This annoys me because we are responsible for our own health. I have diversified as I too often do. To get back to my blood-shot eye and not visiting the doctor, I decided to visit my optician, whose first question was, *"Did you have a fright recently"*. I told of how I was nearly knocked down by a car the previous week, with the vehicle stopping within a few inches of me. It was a dull, overcast, damp day, and the driver was wearing sunglasses. She opened the window saying, *"I am sorry but I did not see you"*. My answer was, *"If you took your sunglasses off you would be able to see better. Sunglasses are for the sunshine, it is certainly not shining today"*. My legs felt like jelly from the fright received. The optician explained that I had Sub-Conjuntival Haemorrhage. The lady told me that as people get older, the delicate membrane that covers the front of the eye and lines the inner part of the eyelids, becomes thin and weak, breaking easily, especially if shocked, as I was.

The advice given was that it was nothing to worry about, that it would clear up in a few days. **No money would be accepted by the lady optician for the advice given.** This is very different to where one visits the doctor, where the attitude is that of giving a prescription and seeking payment.

A week or two later I visited a farmer friend in a neighbouring county. He had a really bad blood-shot eye. He too had a bad fright a few days previous to my visit. I asked had he done anything about it. He had visited the doctor the previous day, was asked little, certainly not about having a fright and was prescribed drugs.

The total cost of the visit to the doctor and chemist was over €100. My describing many of the medico's as 'pickpockets' to state the role they play in extracting money from those supposedly ill, a big majority being healthy, is no exaggeration. This episode is a clear example of my referring to many doctors as being 'pickpockets'.

The call on my G.P. for an eye-test for drivers licence application, resulting in signature and official stamp on the application form, all of which took five minutes at the most, resulted in a charge of €20. When I questioned this cost, for just a few minutes of his time, he immediately said, *"I will check your blood pressure while you are here"* My indignant reply was, *"I don't wish to have my blood pressure checked, I do that myself"*. One can only presume that he made this offer to defend himself against what I thought was a blatant charge. When you consider what the consultants can earn, the €20 charge was miniscule in his eyes, but certainly not in mine, or that of the majority on whom they depend for a living.

Recently a young mother visited me, seeking advice about natural remedies also how to attain better health for her family. Her words were, *"I am peed off with doctors. All they seem to want is money"*. She explained how she had taken her child to the G.P. some days before, where the child was examined for just a few minutes. He said it was nothing serious, giving instructions to keep the patient warm. On being given some tablets by the medico, the lady proceeded to pay the demand, which was €60. Not being satisfied, a few hours later a second opinion was sought, when croup was diagnosed, this consultation costing €50 . Croup can be a very serious ailment if not treated quickly and properly. On being asked did she not report the doctor the reply was, *"What is the point, I'd get nowhere."* Many have said similarly. Even if a complaint was made, nothing would come of it, as is usual with so much within the Health Service Executive. People have to die first. The report, criticism or grievance would be referred to themselves, the Medical Council, made up of the medical profession. I repeat, "One professional, as I well know, whether doctor or other, will never let another down".

When the Minister for Health took steps to regulate the profession, by introducing a lay majority to bring some form of discipline to their cosy cartel, the Association of General Practitioners and the Medical Council Membership Support Committee were **'spitting fire.'**

The latter mentioned support committee said the new act to appoint a lay majority to regulate their profession was, *"Rail-roading them into acceptance, being utterly insensitive and insulting"*. The medics are employed and paid by the Government with taxpayer's money. Up to now they are responsible to nobody but themselves and their own professional bodies, committees, sub-committees and councils. Here is a cosy cartel in the country as it milks the Government and public. Try changing their format, as things get worse instead of better. Who will act on this? The answer again is '**NOBODY**'. The weak kneed Government we have, frequently, all too often, moves to the verge to make important decisions only to pull back, usually because of lobbying or persuasion by the party or body likely to be brought under control. One of the biggest ailments within the Sickness Industry is that of procrastination.

Many who have private health insurance have told me of their experiences when with pain, ache or some kind of illness. They visit the private hospital or clinic, sometimes kept in for tests, often sent home, with appointment after appointment being made with the '*POOR*' consultants or doctors. In the majority of cases nothing was found to be wrong with the patient. I often think and ask myself **"Would the medics have pursued the matter so vigorously if they did not have private health cover"?**

Here again is a depiction of the money-spinner, which is the Health Service Executive/Sickness Industry, and how the consultants obtain their money.

The attitude of the doctor's trade union, The Irish Medical Organisation, sets a classic or standard way of notion or aim for its members – the medical profession.

Here is a pronouncement issued by that organisation some years ago, with their line of thought unaltered, even worse today. This body, as already mentioned, is the doctor's trade union.

We have identified the number of proposals, which, if implemented, would facilitate the Government in its task of improving the overall quality and efficiency of the Health Service Executive, and improve health outcomes for the people. These include:

♦ *An accelerated building programme of public nursing home beds.*

♦ *An increase to 15,000 public acute hospital beds.*

♦ *An accelerated expansion of appropriately staffed consultants, physician-led AMUs and additional A & E consultants.*

♦ *A €2 increase on a packet of twenty cigarettes, leading to a decrease in tobacco consumption, improving cardio vascular health and lessening development of tobacco related cancers.*

One can safely ask the Irish Medical Organisation, have they taken leave of their senses issuing this kind of baloney? Where was the money for all this supposed to come from? They too think the Health Service Executive, which is the Sickness Industry, has a bottomless pocket. About the only sensible piece in their proposals is the last paragraph. Sadly any increase in the price of cigarettes will not deter most smokers because of their addiction. As is usual, there is not one word about prevention of illness, diet or lifestyle changes needed, exclusion of alcohol or need for pure water, exercise, or how to feel and be better, with little, if any, expense. No, the end product, their bottom line, is clearly obvious. This is the greed, the greed for money. They are blind to the obvious, dim-witted in their chemical, pill, tablets and drugs obsessiveness. I repeat again, our health and keeping us unhealthy is an industry, with continual **selling of sickness**.

When I give talks around the country, with the subject built around my slogans, *'WE ARE AS WE EAT, DRINK, SLEEP AND EXERCISE',* or **'A CHANGE OF LIFESTYLE WORKS WONDERS',** very often it is put to me that people are living longer now. They certainly are, but there are many factors which easily outweigh the use or value of the medical profession and the drugs industry.

Vastly improved sanitation and housing, little manual or extremely hard work, with few working in wet or terrible weather conditions, wall to wall carpeting, light and heat at the flick of a switch, central heating, transport, and other modern aids are a huge factor as far as longevity is concerned. The vast majority of the drugs on offer, if not all of them, whether prescribed or off the shelf from the chemist, supermarket or filling station, are of no use. Many of them do more harm than good. Some may be stoppers of pain, but none of them cure anybody.

There is too a very big question remaining unanswered. Many are living longer, but at what cost? Visit the many nursing homes and institutions where elderly people are being nursed or cared for. All too many have little or no quality of life. How often do we hear, on being told of a death, *"Oh sure, they are better off now".* Turn to *Elderly People – How they are being 'Maltreated'* caption.

Tables setting out requirements for entrance exams to the various professions, which are far and away higher than in the past, show that extremely high marks are required to allow one study medicine. It would be interesting to know who sets out the required entrance points needed. It seems little thought is given to the thinking, personality or traits of those who wish to be doctors. The result is that all too many act in a haughty or business like manner, being far too formal, appearing as uncaring.

Most of the doctors of some years ago, many with a much lower standard of education in facing life, but gifted as G.Ps., were brilliant. They had ample time to give to their patients, often sitting down with them to discuss their problems. Recently a team study showed that *'Practitioners who attempted to form a warm and friendly relationship with their patients, and reassured them that they would soon be better, were found to be more effective than practitioners who kept their consultations impersonal, formal and uncertain'.*

In the past, not so many years ago, before the doctors became obsessed with the present-day thinking of the enormous value of over use of the prescription pad, quick turnaround and how much they can extract from the patient or the Health Service Executive, the medics had an amount of time for all. There was a personal touch as they spoke casually with the patient. They understood then that the mind as well as the body very often needed help. Sadly, there is no time for this method of treatment nowadays.

When with imaginary ailments, when words of encouragement would act better than drugs or medicines, there is a need for a psychological approach to the patient. It is sometimes all that is needed. If with ailment, seldom if ever nowadays does one visit a doctor and not come away without a prescription or some form of medication. They will not miss a sale, to add to their daily tally.

Recently there was a letter in a national newspaper, suggesting that doctors, on examining a patient, should issue written reports. Two days later a reply from a G.P. was printed. The medico stated, *"On an average day, I consult with about 50 patients, either in person or on the telephone"*. If one works this out, allowing for the doctor to work a nine hour day, taking no time for meal breaks, also allowing for the entry and exit times of the patients, plus issuing of prescriptions, he would have approximately four to five minutes with each.

Need one dwell further on this kind of treatment. There would certainly be no time for the personal, warm or friendly relationship suggested as being necessary. At €50 to €60 as charged for a visit in Ireland this man was certainly milking a cash cow. It was like a goldmine. This set up makes it obvious why so few patients are cured as a result of their visit to the doctor. Their in and out treatment points to the conveyor belt system mentioned.

As I stated at the outset of this caption on doctors and the medical profession, I am not anti-doctor, only anti the way all too many of them manipulate and run the Sickness Industry, which of course includes the patients. There are many doctors I have met, visited, or am friendly with. Some are close friends and what they do or don't do is not my affair. There are some good but all too many not so good. The way of operating of a big majority of them is not sincere, as they supposedly act for the betterment of their patients. Their line of thought leaves much to be desired. To put this into context, or way of looking at it, one need look no further than a former Health Service Executive boss, a Professor. He was paid well over €400,000 for the previous year and had the brass neck to say that he could earn a lot more if he had stayed in medicine. One can only presume he meant that if he had stayed as a doctor or consultant.

Nicholas Culpeper, the 17th century herbalist, was in frequent conflict with the counterparts of the Irish Medical Organisation and the British Medical Association when he referred to them as *"A proud, insulting, domineering and narrow-minded lot"*. It seems that a majority have passed the unseemly attitude down over the years.

TILLING THE SOIL

Anyone who has not gardened or tilled the soil in some way, does not realise what they have missed. One gets out of a garden, small-holding or farm, by tilling or sowing, the reward of enjoyable work. It is one of nature's greatest therapies.

THE GREATEST DANGER TO OUR HEALTH

Daily we are told of the dangers of cancer, heart disease, stroke, obesity and much more. Every autumn and at the beginning of winter we are warned of the pandemic flu which we are still waiting for, after many years of listening to the propaganda and ballyhoo which is similarly continuous year after year. We are offered the flu jab, which to me is an affront, an insult.

The greatest danger to the health of all, young and old, is a *LACK OF EXERCISE*, combined with what is being put into the human body by way of inferior food and drink. It is a type of pure laziness which can be looked upon as endemic. We see a few lines now and again in the media about the need to be active. I have yet to hear of a doctor sitting down with a patient or patients and questioning them about their lifestyle, especially exercise or the lack of it. Take just one of the hundreds of ailments which benefit enormously from regular exercise, which is a wonderful aid. That is depression. Turn to *Depression* caption for further facts or briefing.

Walking daily is one of the best ways of taking exercise. There are many other ways of exercising. Walking if depressed is a marvellous tonic.

I don't just mean going for a saunter. There is more to walking than just that. It is after a good brisk walk that one feels so much better. As written elsewhere, there are many who are unable to do so but if one was to sit on the edge of a chair and dangle the legs, put the arms up and try and take a little bit of exercise in the chair, every little helps. There is an old slogan, which I use frequently, especially at my talks, *"Do your best, and if you can't do your best, do the best you can"*.

Depression is at the top of the G.P.'s. lists of ailments, with many people having this problem. The majority tell pitiful stories about how the doctors have put them or their kin on pills, one can say for life, with never a question or word about lifestyle, which means exercise, sleep and proper diet. The prescribers, the medics, are condemning the sufferer to a life of hell. It is all too obvious that the patients are being used financially as well as being sold down the river. It is a fact that no drugs will cure depression, so what is the point of prescribing them. Without doubt and I have proved it thousands of times, the greatest evil to our health is **lack of exercise, combined with the use of unnatural, processed, additive-filled fast foods and drinks.** I have proved it because I have changed peoples attitude to life, changed their lifestyles. After only a few weeks there is a vast difference in their mindset, outlook and their health problems. After some months this turns into a revelation. Pills are not the solution.

Exercise is one of our greatest medicines and tonics. I know there are many who wish to be active, such as the infirm or disabled, but as I have said they can only do their best in whatever way possible. There are all too many who could take exercise but don't. In almost all too many instances it is down to laziness. An example of this is that there is a 'state of the art' gymnasium provided in Dáil Éireann for those who supposedly govern us. It cost over €250,000 to build and has annual running costs of €40,000. Last year it was used on average only eleven times weekly, one presumes by politicians. **What an example this is to raise the minds of all about the extreme need for exercise.**

As I have said at the outset the greatest danger to our health is lack of exercise.

LIFESTYLE

A healthier lifestyle need not be hard work. See LIFESTYLE caption

GINGER

The wonder of this herb root is untold. It is an aid to better circulation, cold feet and hands, appetite loss, and prevention of colds and flus. It helps to stop vomiting and nausea. It is of immense help when taken after surgery or chemotherapy. Ginger can be obtained from the health food store in capsule or tablet form, which makes for easy carrying and taking. It is also available as ground or powdered ginger. It is a very good preventative of travel sickness. Take two or three capsules before commencing the journey and one or two later, if desired. Like thousands whom I have recommended ginger to, I take a half teaspoon daily, mixing it with porridge at breakfast time. This is a huge aid to keeping blood sugar levels correct as is a level teaspoon of ground cinnamon. If pregnant, consult a doctor before taking ginger. It must not be taken if with kidney problems.

ECONOMY AND THE WEATHER

When I was a small boy I listened to my parents and others as they discussed the economy of the country. Things always appeared to be bad. Times have not changed in this respect. When I was a young person, and until middle age I never gave serious thought to the main topics of conversation, the economy and the weather. I did as I have advised others to do. *'Take one day at a time, walking and talking with GOD and all will be well.'* Only today, a friend said to me after I had spoken these words that she used similar advice in her daily life. It is the guidance of Saint Augustine; *"Trust the past to GOD'S mercy, the present to GOD'S love and the future to GOD'S providence."*

INFLUENZAS (FLUS) –

THE SUPREME DECEPTION

With acres of media space taken up with the flus that never have been, who wishes to hear more. There is still much flu for thought! Some, indeed many, have explaining to do about the so-called flu fiascos, especially the one referred to as the swine flu.

There have been so many claims and counter claims, so much propaganda and lies, that it is obvious that we will never know the real truth about the money-spinning deception. If the avian flu (H5N1) was a huge con, then the swine flu (H1M1) has to be ranked as one of the greatest deceptions of all time. The Governments and Health Authorities of the world were sold an enormous costly hoax. They listened to the World Health Organisation (W.H.O.), the medical profession, the drug companies and to all too many who make up the Sickness Industry.

In front of me is evidence that from at least 15 years beforehand there was a slow but uncanny build up to this explosion of hype, spin off and prevarication which related to the swine flu, which in the end grew into a pandemic that never was.

The W.H.O. were the protagonists in the drive to promote the use of and purchase of Tamiflu, Celvapan, Relenza and other vaccines.

Millions of chickens and other birds were slaughtered because of the avian flu. Not long ago, and many years too late, we were informed that scientists had discovered that the birds were not responsible for the outbreak in any manner.

The poultry industry suffered huge disruption and massive losses as a consequence of the lies. While there is no risk in eating pork, bacon, other pig meat, or chicken, if properly prepared or cooked, the question can be asked, *"Why use the birds and pigs to describe the flus"?* It is most unfair to those who earn a crust in rearing them or promoting their sale.

We heard many warnings about the 'Spanish flu' of 1918, of how the bird and swine flu could be equally serious. The pig or 'Spanish flu' had nothing to do with Spain. It may not have been flu, being bacterial pneumonia. Indeed it may have been man made, deliberate, but that is a story for another time. There were crude forms of vaccinations then, as used by the armed forces. Aspirin, which when used overly much can cause severe internal bleeding, may have been the main cause of many of the millions dying. The aspirin when made up then, was done in a crass manner, with no proper controls in place.

I have referred to the hectares of newspaper space devoted to the nonsense about the swine flu pandemic. For years I have had daily access to almost all of the Irish and U.K. papers including the tabloids. Because they are so depressing, giving us only the bad news and what suits them, I don't read them anymore. The swine flu baloney put me off them completely. Night and day the 'news' increased peoples anxiety about the swine flu. Never a sceptical word about the mighty con being maintained. *'Woman dies from Swine Flu'*, **was headlined in the** *'Irish Times'*, **as if no one else in the country had died that day.** Those who did die in almost all, if not all cases, had an underlying illness, which was usually the cause of death.

The t.v. teletext is now used instead. The news, sport and weather are looked at in that order. Only the news headlines which are of interest are read. At the flick of a button the head is uncluttered.

Reading the newspaper health supplements frequently raised my blood pressure. Journalists, those allied to the Sickness Industry, often promote chemical pills and medicines. Seldom, if ever, was there a word about the need for proper natural food and drinks or how sleep and exercise are our greatest medicines and preventions of ill-health, including flu. None of these medical hacks appear to have heard of or know anything about Vitamin D3, which can be of wonderful benefit to one's health. I repeat, **"Prevention is a forgotten idea by those interested in promoting legalised drugs."**

As set out, the build up of the flu propaganda has seen growing publicity over many years. Several years ago we saw headlined in *'The Irish Times'* health supplement, then a broadsheet, *'Flu pandemic is inevitable, experts warn'.* It told us in the wording beneath that the *'Pandemic could result in 2,000,000 people in the Republic being infected and some 53,000 deaths'.* This to me is irresponsible journalism, like much else frightening as written by health journalists. I often wonder if some of them are hand in glove with the drug industry or the medical profession.

Some years ago a leading article in the same paper was way off the mark, highlighting and telling us, amongst other worrying health aspects, that *'The rate of infection will speed up considerably with a likely risk developing between the spread of H1M1 (swine flu) virus and the rate of inoculation of the population with an effective vaccine'.* *'The Irish Independent'* told us that the swine flu would infect one third of the global population. A heading told us *'Coroners are preparing for impact of swine flu'.* We are still waiting, knowing it was all a con, but to many it was extremely frightening.

Whole pages were devoted to what was continually referred to as the pandemic. We were told about the second wave of flu when the first wave had not even arrived, and it never did. The opposition party politicians were spouting, *'State faces swine flu pandemic,,* words from Fine Gael, (F.G.). We had the usual drivel from a doctor from the same party telling us that the H.S.E's. campaign was a shambles. What has been done to un-shamble it? Again the answer is '**NOTHING**'. More faultfinding.

At the turn of the century there was a headline in *'The Irish Independent'* *'Tests of flu outbreak is nothing to be sneezed at'.* It said underneath *'A flu pandemic – an epidemic on a total scale is due to hit Ireland. It is not a case of if, said the experts, but when'.* The writer did not tell us **When** it would be due! No, the chemical drugs industry and the medics were cranking it up, stepping up the pressure.

Even business firms and many other types of business were caught up in the farce. Many of them spent an unwarranted amount of money taking steps to be prepared for the still awaited pandemic. The H.S.E. warned businesses to plan for absenteeism due to the H1M1 pandemic. Much more waffle was directed towards them as to what they might do. The statement issued told of how the pandemic was *'Currently gaining a foothold in this country and it will be a number of weeks before it is widespread'.* Before that we heard about chicken-flu, bird-flu, avian-flu, all similar of course, which like the over-hyped warnings about the swine flu were unjustified, causing worry and distress to many.

I could quote from dozens more headings, which I have accumulated by way of old newspapers, collected or sent me by friends in Ireland and the U.K., over the past half century. Many of them are ridiculous. They make people afraid for the future. Very often what is printed are the ideas of people with one-track minds. Good news, it appears, does not sell newspapers. They like to pontificate on certain things, which are as fixed ideas to them. Much of this has been done over the past 25 years, as all of the time the Sickness Industry we now have was being built up. We had a huge growth in influenza propaganda during this time.

Highlighting the words epidemic and pandemic must have worried some on reading or hearing the various news predictions. I have asked many people what is the difference between the two words. Only two could explain the variance, indeed I was not too sure myself. An epidemic is a concentrated incidence of a virus within a limited region of the community. A pandemic is a widespread and concentrated occurrence of the virus, spanning several regions of the world. As already stated, we have not had either epidemic or pandemic. So much for the swine flu promoters!

The Council of Europe issued a scathing report on how The World Health Organisation (W.H.O.) performed during the varied flu outbreak. According to the Council, the organisation had wasted public money and raised unjustified scares about the health risks involved. The Council also raised concerns about the involvement of the pharmaceutical drugs industry, when choices were made and money was spent.

The report's contention, that the industry may have influenced the W.H.O., is backed up by an investigation published by the British Medical Journal and the Bureau of Investigative Journalism.

The investigations said, amongst many other serious things, that some scientists advising the W.H.O. had done paid work for pharmaceutical chemical drug-manufacturing firms.

Both reports also highlighted the fact that the W.H.O. had refused to publish the names and declarations of interest of members of its emergency committee, and European advisory bodies, directly involved in recommendations on the so called pandemic.

Imagine the cost of the swine flu debacle to the H.S.E., the N.H.S. and the extremely overburdened taxpayer. Pages were taken in national and other newspapers setting out information about swine flu vaccination and the action to be taken. Posters and much printed jargon were distributed. Much was prepared and posted to all households throughout the country. At the behest of so-called experts millions of vaccines were purchased and stock-piled. Additional nurses were trained to deal with swine flu vaccinations. We were told that the number of intensive care beds would double. Millions of masks were ordered. In supermarkets, hardware stores and D.I.Y. stores, even in the filling stations, pre-packed disinfectants and other somewhat similar products were displayed for sale.

The frenzy whipped up by the W.H.O., The Sickness Industry, the media, also the H.S.E. and N.H.S. statements, was to lead to a windfall for the all powerful drug-manufacturing companies and many within the medical profession. **Here the business of organised *SELLING OF SICKNESS* was seen at its zenith.**

The drug companies, such as Roche, Glaxo Smith Kline (G.S.K.) and Baxters, makers of Tamiflu, Relenza and Celvapan were riding on the crest of the wave. Several years ago we learned of G.S.K. being in talks with the W.H.O. about a proposal for a subsidised mass vaccination programme against avian flu for developing countries. With all the hype about the swine flu pandemic they now had the situation they had dreamed up. As a doctor friend said to me *"The pharmaceutical drugs industry, with public health officials and the media acting as a mass marketing team, pulled off one of the biggest profiteering schemes in the history of the world. The swine flu hoax, 'swindle', perpetuated on an international level, added and generated unheard of profits from a non existent pandemic".* It did just that.

The stories and facts which emerged after the global hoax or 'fraud', fuelled by the W.H.O., the powerful drugs industry, the Sickness Industry, which includes almost all health professions and their cohorts, would be the basis for a thriller. The fact that much less than one sixth of the vaccines were used stands out conspicuously in this scandalous hoax, which as already stated, had been planned and worked on by the drug companies for many years. The billions involved were colossal. The release of the figures, showing the sums involved to pay for the unwanted drugs, are only minimal when other costs are considered. When the sums paid for administration, distribution and redistribution, prescribing, purchasing from pharmacies, as in Ireland, retrieving because of non use, storing and re-storing, destroying or getting rid of unwanted vaccines, are all added to the initial outlay, the total is astronomical. *'Who pays for all of this'?* The taxpayer is left to bear the burden to pay for the 'thievery'. It has been nothing less. The idea of giving the unwanted vaccines, which are perishable, over a period to the third world countries, was put forward. **They were wise enough to tell the givers to keep them.** These are well past their use by date now so the general public will never know the outcome. In America, enormous amounts of stockpiled vaccines were destroyed. It had been proved that they neither prevented nor cured illness, with only a very small minority accepting this kind of vaccine, almost all of which was untested, having been fast-tracked.

Many of the Governments, including Ireland, gave immunity from claims to the vaccine manufactures, this to include side effects or even fatalities. Who in their proper mind would accept the chemicals? The W.H.O., which is at the apex of the Sickness Industry, made proper fools of all who were foolish enough to listen to their spiel.

The *'Daily Telegraph'* **told us of Glaxo Smith Kline being set for a boost of $600 million, having received orders for 128 million doses of the swine flu vaccine. <u>This was only at the beginning of supplying the jabs.</u> The article stated that orders from many governments had been taken. During the height of the propaganda, the story of a vaccine shortage was fabricated and broadcast. One does not have to guess who was behind this. It is not the first time this kind of thing has happened. In 2004 when President George W. Bush was in power, one of his henchmen, Donald H. Rumsfield, was Defence Secretary. Before this Rumsfield had been Chairman of Gilead Science Inc. who developed and patented Tamiflu. His Assistant Secretary for Health Affairs issued a directive to the effect that supply was extremely limited worldwide, and its use will be prioritised. This made a huge contribution to the resultant panic buying of Tamiflu by Governments around the world. There is no way to describe this other** than CONNIVING.

The galling part of all this is that the strain of flu we had was no worse than the usual type of seasonal flu experienced annually. In fact the realisation is that it was one of the mildest ever.

An ironical situation arose where Baxter International, a health care outfit, sent seasonal flu vaccine to Austria. It was then distributed to the Czech Republic, Slovenia and Germany. This was, we are told, all in the name of research. It was found that Baxter's had released contaminated flu virus material which contained live H5M1 (avian flu) viruses. This only came to light when the firm in the Czech Republic inoculated ferrets with the vaccine and they died. It was supposedly an error on Baxter's part. Just imagine the catastrophic consequences if this chemical had been promoted or allowed into the mainstream medicine run. Baxter's were in no way forthcoming or helpful.

The W.H.O. were supposedly monitoring all of this. As is usual, where the Sickness Industry is concerned, when something occurs, even serious or deadly, who does anything? The answer again is **'NOBODY'**. Big business is protected, more especially if it is a lucrative drug making combine. Baxter's Celvaplan flu vaccine is sold in Ireland. Who in their sane senses would prescribe it? Indeed the same question could be asked about Tamiflu or any vaccine jabs.

Many who had severe or lingering colds were given the jab, despite advice to doctors to the contrary. Tamiflu or the other flu vaccines were not tested on people with illnesses other than the flu. Indeed many of them were not tested on people with the so-called swine flu. Their effectiveness, or perhaps harm, has not been analysed on those with heart disease, lung or bronchial problems, diabetes, kidney or other serious ailments. Nobody knows the significance of treating or perhaps the dire consequences when with other illnesses, whether serious or not. The many vaccinated who have had adverse reaction will never be told or know of the long term consequences. I repeat, **"When in doubt, leave out, do without"**.

In 2006 the *'British Medical Journal'* concluded that *"The evidence shows that flu vaccines have little or no effect"*. Other eminent doctors tell us similarly. The trusted publication *'The Lancet'*, urged *extreme caution in the use of vaccines because of their fast tracking"*.

Many of those who had been vaccinated and became infected by the flu, which was seasonal and not the swine flu, were extremely ill. When, in the past, one caught a flu or heavy cold the remedy was to go to bed, pull the curtains, and stay there for five or six days. It worked well when given good food or liquid as medicine. All this and little expense compared to the moneyed Sickness promotions we now have, shows up the nonsensical situation the majority have been led into. Some of the vaccines caused terrible side and after effects as have many of those administered over the years. I have yet to meet one who was not effected after having the jab, some seriously.

As already stated, the biggest culprit in all of this swine flu shambles is the World Health Organisation (W.H.O). Even they admit to allowing live flu virus into the population through the use of synthetic or trial vaccines. According to their website, *"Such advanced studies can greatly expedite regulatory approval".* Fast tracking is a way to describe this carry on. I wonder how many people have been badly effected as a result of this?

The Organisation declared and upped the global swine fever pandemic level to six, which is the highest phase. **The W.H.O. issued various statements, such as how the flu virus is likely to keep spreading rapidly, within countries and throughout the world.** This is the same W.H.O. who admitted they squandered billions on false **AIDS** scares. The B.B.C. in their news programme informed us, and I quote: *"W.H.O. DEFENDS ITS SWINE FLU WARNING".* They defended their handling of the swine flu episode after the Council of Europe cast doubt on its actions. Their denials and unconvincing excuses were what we have come to expect from this organisation, which is made up of public servants, who like so many within the Sickness Industry are apparently answerable to nobody.

I repeat, countries rushed to order hundreds of thousands, even millions, of vaccine doses when the pandemic was declared, with the virus proving to be relatively mild. The W.H.O's. links to drug-manufacturing and distributing companies were questioned at a hearing by the Council of Europe Health Committee.

A W.H.O. *Flu expert* denied there had been an improper influence from drug-manufacturing companies. **He would, wouldn't he?** When a pandemic was declared most European countries changed their health priorities to accommodate thousands of expected patients, including spending billions of euro or dollars on vaccines to be used against swine flu. Allegations from politicians and the media about links with drug companies prompted an internal review at the W.H.O. and the Council of European hearings.

Later we learn that Dr. Wolfgang Woodard, of the same World Health Organisation, claimed the swine flu outbreak was a *'False pandemic',* orchestrated and driven by drug-manufacturing companies, which stood to make billions from the hyped up propaganda generated and which still does to a large extent.

Whether Dr. Wolfgang is a spokesman for the W.H.O., or not, then the independent experts who will review how the H1M1 so-called pandemic has been handled, should arrange for many at the W.H.O. to be prosecuted. This will not happen. I repeat, *"One professional will not let another one down. They are a breed apart".* Like so much within the Sickness Industry the question can be asked *'What will happen'?* The answer again is *'NOTHING'.* It will all blow over, dying a natural death. All concerned will be tried and defended by themselves. The bods who run the W.H.O. do not have to worry about where the next salary cheque will come from. No, it comes from the Governments who squander taxpayer's money.

Would any privately owned business or shareholder company, if responsible for the health of all, allow money to be misused as they have done and continue to do so? The answer is **NO**, because if they did those at the top would be fired, or to put it nicely, made redundant. The privately owned companies could not turn for a bail out to the Government for taxpayer's money as these un-business-like public employees do.

What has happened to the vast stockpiles of the flu vaccines that nobody wants? Have they ended up in landfill sites to poison us further? Will there be a liquidator's sale? Remember this stuff is perishable. It has a use by date.

There must be many whose egos have been dented after these farcical episodes. They are the 'fools' who work cohesively within the W.H.O., the Sickness Industry and also the many Governments who threw away millions in the rush to stockpile swine flu vaccines. As related, the big beneficiaries were the pharma drug-manufacturing industry conglomerates as they laughingly deposited their gains. The shareholders are delighted.

When it comes to the doctors, the purveyors of the Sickness Industry, they too must be giving thought to the fact that the majority were not convinced by all the brain washing, ballyhoo, and selling to the public of vaccines. Some people saw it all as the 'sham' it has been.

Dr. James Lee Fanu in his ***Doctor's Diary*** in the *'Daily Telegraph'* sums up the mood of the people, many of whom are turning away from the many chemical medications which are being prescribed. He writes, *'Looking back over the past twelve months, there are signs of a popular rebellion against the 'experts' and their scare-mongering tactics in persuading us to take drugs we neither need or want. The fiasco of the swine flu vaccines and statins prescribing are a case in point'.*

Highlighted at this time, in a review, was the fact that the flu jab may be a waste of time to the elderly. There was *'poor'* evidence that it effectively prevented the illness. One bod, a Professor, a Director of

99

Immunisation at the Irish Department of Health, said, *"The review offered no new evidence"*. Does this mean he knows this evidence is true? Does this mean that he will give up his cosy job of Director of Immunisation? Are we to take it that in his estimation the report of the highly recognised research groups, from which the report originated is foolish? Like most medics he is cynical of the truth or anything natural.

Many have told me of how they had been telephoned on up to as many as six occasions by people who were associated with the Health Service Executive/Sickness Industry. These sensible people, including those with families, had not availed of the vaccination push. One lady told of how when spoken to on the telephone she felt intimidated, as if being bullied into having the family vaccinated. Here are further cases of the huge industry *selling sickness*. The fear of being left with millions of vaccines on their hands was a driving force in the efforts to sell their jabs.

I received from the Health Service Executive a letter and also two printed circulars, setting out that aged 65 and over, the swine flu stopped with me. All were in both the Irish and English language. I wrote a very diplomatic letter to the doctor who signed it. If I needed medication I would seek it. I will not be **sold sickness** as this sales doctor was doing.

In their rush to extract the last penny or euro there were many who were diagnosed with flu, very often only having a head cold. Britain's Health Protection Agency (H.P.A.) disclosed that only one in five people who were diagnosed with swine flu actually had the ailment and that four-fifths were instructed to take Tamiflu unnecessarily. The Government Agency reported that after approximately one million jabs of Tamiflu had been prescribed, more than 800,000 of these were not necessary.

These alarming figures only came to light after the H.P.A. took swabs from patients. This meant that over three quarters of a million had to stay at home needlessly and in isolation, in the false belief that they had swine flu. These 'patients' were lied to by the doctors whose prescription pads, allied to their greed for money, were the key objects, further indication of the 'pick-pocketing' referred to.

The doctors, who diagnosed them incorrectly, will continue to draw their huge earnings, nobody will discipline them. Who does anything about this fiasco? Again the answer is '**NOBODY**'. Here again is an outrageous example of *selling sickness*. This is just one incidence of what can rightly be termed skulduggery. There must be many, many more cases where there is no Health Protection Agency to catch out the wily doctors who have prescribed Tamiflu, Relenza and other vaccines.

Passing through my local town I saw large signs, with direction arrows, pointing prospective and over trusting clients to the Vaccination

Clinic, as stated in big letters over the arrows. I wonder how many were wrongly diagnosed in those clinics. In the majority of cases there is nobody to check on or put a brake on these *sickness-selling* medics, especially in Ireland, who as I have mentioned more than once, can be compared to 'pickpockets', except that the medics extract the money legally.

We do have in Ireland what is called the Health Promotion Surveillance Centre (H.P.S.C.). This is run by 41 staff, including doctors, consultants, also microbiologists, surveillance scientists and others, all allied to the medical profession. As is mentioned elsewhere one profession will not let another down. Will any of this lot set out to track down doctors whether prescribing incorrectly or overly so?

To put into perspective the scenario of the swine flu fiasco, here are further examples of the type of cross-purpose advice given. The W.H.O. informed us **"That healthy people with mild symptoms of swine flu need not be vaccinated. Most people will make a full recovery within a week"**, they added. Other sources dictated that **"Drugs should be given to all those complaining of flu like illnesses regardless of the severity of their condition"**. The instruction to give the anti-viral to children was outlandish because of the warnings against its use for young persons.

One of these 'experts', with which we are plagued, an international one at that, had the audacity to tell us that *"Irish children are being put at serious risk because we have the lowest rate of child influenza vaccination in European countries"*. All this after researchers from Oxford University had warned that children should not be given Tamiflu or other vaccines because their harm outweighed the benefits. **I accept this as a warning to forget about vaccination.** Deaths from the flu were highlighted frequently. As already referred to, the figures were well below the winter average, with death in almost all cases, being from an underlying cause.

If these supposedly learned people are at cross purposes with one another, as is frequently the case with prescribing of much synthetic chemical medicines or drugs, then all are faced with huge dilemma or conflict. It must be understood that much scare mongering is endemic in all routine infant vaccinations. In our family and in the families who think likewise the slogan *"WHEN IN DOUBT, LEAVE OUT, DO WITHOUT"* is practised. **No vaccine is safe.** Now in our 80's, my wife and myself ask the question, **"How did we and our extended families manage throughout our lives without the use of VACCINES?"**

HARMFUL - CHEMICAL - SYNTHETIC DRUGS

Have you heard of, been prescribed or used any of the following, some of them now banned, as are others frequently? Mesulid, Avandia, Champix, Celebrex, Seroxat, or Cox 2 Inhibitors of which Vioxx, also a banned drug, was one of them. Questions are being asked about Fosamax, Gardasil and Lamisil.

There are many, many other branded names of pharma drugs, which could be added to this list. These are just some of the prescribed pills or medicines which come to mind which have caused 'harm', or with much doubt about their safety when used. If you have not taken or used those mentioned you are amongst the lucky people to have escaped the terrible side effects or long or short-term consequences of taking them. These are the kind of chemical medicines which should not have been allowed on the market until there was not the slightest doubt about their safety, whatever about their ability. Human beings are being used as guinea pigs, all in the pursuit of money for the chemical drug producers, the medical profession and the pharmacies.

A doctor relative told me *"When manufacturers realise that peoples honesty and honour are number one, then all benefit".* Sadly this is not how the legalised drug and medicine barons, or indeed their shareholders see it. Money and profits are the *god*. Profit, not safety, is their way of thinking. If it were not so then we would not have the scares and withdrawals of drugs or so-called medicines we hear or read about regularly. The studies and trials of some drugs are a disgrace, bringing more scandals to add to all the other embarrassments being brought on the chemical drugs manufacturers. In the vast majority of cases these very worrying facts are kept concealed or hidden from the public.

The scandal of Vioxx was headlined for quiet a period of time. Thousands of claims are with the legal profession, with actions being taken against the mighty Merck & Co. because of the alleged harm done to the human body. There have been reports of many deaths from Vioxx and it is a scandal that the drug was ever allowed to be used before it had been proven fully to be safe. It is clearly evident that people must die before the pulling of dangerous drugs from the market, as the health and lives of people are experimented with.

At the time of the Vioxx withdrawal we were informed that the Irish Medicines Board (I.M.B.) were surprised by the speed of the decision by Merck & Co. to withdraw it. A spokeswoman, a doctor, said, *"You don't take a knee-jerk reaction to pull a drug".* This is nothing short of idiotic balderdash from a medic. It was known for some years that the drug was dangerous, with many, all too many, suffering cardiac problems, including heart attacks, strokes, and irregular heartbeat, other circulation problems, even fatalities. **There is a vast amount of evidence now to show that Vioxx should have been pulled from the market for up to four years before it was.** If the I.M.B. members had studied and accepted the evidence, which accumulated over the years, there would not have been the Vioxx reactions patients suffered from.

It makes one fear for the health of all, where professionals like this are apparently living in a climate of near reverence for the medical drugs being produced, as if they are goodly. As mentioned elsewhere in this book *"The relationship between the drug companies and those who prescribe their chemicals, all too often dangerous, is too close an affinity"*. The same I.M.B. in the past has stated that they were looking into this. It is like much in the Sickness Industry. There is much looking into, talk and promises, but there is very little being achieved. '**NOBODY**' quietly looks on, but not into, dangerous and perhaps long term 'killer' drugs, being prescribed.

There are all too many drugs on the market, which are not safe. With Vioxx it was the long-term consequences which were the undoing of Merck & Company's charade regarding another of their 'dangerous' drugs. Of the drugs, which I have listed, the facts are that Mesulid was withdrawn as was another drug, Roaccutane. Champix has resulted in terrible side effects. Celebrex is similar but more especially when taken for an extended period. Fosamax and Gardasil have nothing good to be said about them. The promotion of Avandia and related drugs has been disgraceful. It appears that the mighty legalised drug manufacturers, call them drug pushers, put profits for their shareholders before people's welfare or even their lives. The manufacturers of Avandia, Glaxo Smith Kline (G.K.S.), are an example of this. It was known for years that it had many associated risks but G.K.S. continued promoting and marketing the chemical drug. In my humble opinion no drugs are worth the risk of taking simply because there are too many unanswered questions.

Fosamax is an osteoporosis drug which has been linked to an extremely serious condition known as Osteonecrosis of the jaw. Many on Fosamax have had broken bones or fractures, for no apparent reason. In this book there is a diagram of a bone. Bone is another wonder, and the bones of the body give much food for thought. To think the drug pushers would sell or prescribe something that interferes with any part of the body can only be viewed as murderous. The pharmaceutical drug-manufacturing industry gets away with this. See **Bones—The Body Skeleton—A Marvel** caption.

There is the odd fine for a criminal offence, which is seldom. To these conglomerates this is miniscule when compared with the billions of euro or pounds they gross. Now that laws have been enacted whereby whistleblowers will be generously compensated, if they can provide evidence of corrupt or nefarious conduct in industry, we may see changes in the future. The lure of big money is a huge incentive 'to spill the beans'. I repeat my advice, as given to the many who have asked for help to be more healthy, *'If in doubt, leave out, do without.'*

Lamisil has received much adverse criticism. This anti-fungal drug or cream is a prime example of the scary difference between the conventional so-called remedy and a natural alternative such as Allergenics Non Steroidal Cream. As an anti-fungal, the latter, obtainable from the health food store or some chemists, is a wonderful aid.

There is another remedy, the best one for fungal problems. It is the world's greatest medicine. It is good, pure nutritious foods and drinks, all to be yeast free. Again I make no apologies for repeating a clear and concise fact.

Some of the harmful drugs pulled over the years include Baycol, supposedly for cholesterol lowering. Mesulid, Aulin and Mesine, all Nimesulide containing drugs were linked to liver failure. It took years for the licensing authorities to withdraw them, or to make up their minds, despite very much evidence being available about their dangers. A dubious product for weight loss, Reductil, was withdrawn over heart risk. Another weight loss drug Accomplia (rimonabant) which was linked to depression, was banned. Some of these drugs were said to cause psychiatric disorders including anxiety and sleep problems.

The person who directs Irelands largest public weight management clinic said, *"I was disappointed when Acomplia was withdrawn because it was a new kind of anti-obesity medication"*. He set out how it had been properly tested or evaluated. If it has been, then either he is a fool or the makers of these dubious weight loss products, like Reductil or Acomplia, takes the general public who purchase their drugs to be fools.

There are very many other 'dangerous' drugs which have been withdrawn, but space does not permit their inclusion. The printers tell me, "There comes a time to draw the line, if you wish to include all which makes up the book, *Selling Sickness!"*

Frequently we hear or read of the dangers of the contraceptive pill. Women should give much thought to the use of this form of contraception. The first of many questions I would ask is *"Why the increase of cervical cancer or breast cancer?"* The same question can be asked about obesity, where the contraceptive pill also comes under scrutiny.

One has only to look at the Thalidomide infamy to realise the lengths to which both the drug producers and the Governments have gone, in order to cover up this terrible tragedy. Here was and indeed is a lesson on how to procrastinate. The saga has gone on for so long that if it is extended for some years more there will not be any survivors. This terrible drug was produced and prescribed for morning sickness. As with other dangerous drugs, although warned of the harm, the Government failed to ban Thalidomide. The whole sad saga has had kilometres of columns written about it.

Road accident deaths are highlighted frequently but only seldom is reference made that synthetic drugs kill more people than ever before. I don't mean illegal drugs. Prescription drugs and over doses of over the counter medicines kill more than ever. Like much in the Sickness Industry in Ireland and the U.K. we are kept in the dark. I repeat, and make no apologies for doing so *"One professional will never let another down"*. This includes many professions other than the medics. This is an unwritten tradition. This is despite the fact that accidents, over dosing or fatalities are supposed to be recorded. This is also in relation to side effects. These degrees or rules are only partially obeyed, very often never.

I have stood and addressed thousands in both Ireland and the U.K. about the subject of how harmful and dangerous drugs have been prescribed over the years. I have written much on the same subject. Not one person has ever challenged me or told me *"I am wrong"*. The Sickness Industry, which comprises the Health Service Executive of Ireland, the National Health Service U.K., the doctors, consultants and other professionals, is part of a multi billion set up. The pharma drug industry, which is unafraid to talk down to Governments, is a huge part of this commercial enterprise.

Mention or speak about natural remedies, natural vitamins or food supplements to those within the Sickness Industry, only to be given a vacant stare or even laughed at. Tell them about herbal or homeopathic treatment, all of which work, most of which are cures, and be given the cold shoulder. The multinational drug conglomerates who manufacture, promote and sell chemical drugs, is a multi billion euro or pound industry whose main interest is profit, **MONEY**. I reiterate my conviction or belief, with many in agreement, that our health is near the bottom of their files, if there at all, as far as they are concerned

Try telling that lot, or our Government, about a nutritional

push towards good or better health. We know it will save billions by practicing my nine words which I repeatedly use, and they are, *'WE ARE AS WE EAT, DRINK, SLEEP AND EXERCISE'* or use the shorter version *'CHANGE YOUR LIFESTYLE'*. No, they would rather keep on allowing prescribing, making people use harmful, some of them dangerous drugs, but at what cost to the so silent taxpayer, as the Sickness Industry enlarges and expands. They are obsessed with the idea, even though drugs don't cure. I say again and again, indeed I scream out "Who will put a stop or a huge brake on this nonsensical carry-on?" I reiterate, it is stupid, absurd, crazy and just cannot continue.

ARE YOU BLESSED?

If you woke up this morning with more health than sickness, you are more blessed than the millions who will not survive this week. If you have never experienced the danger of battle, the loneliness of imprisonment or the pangs of starvation, you are ahead of many millions throughout the world. If you attend church, without fear of harassment, arrest, torture or death, you are more blessed than almost three billion people in the world. If you have sufficient food, clothes and a roof over your head you are richer than three quarters of the world's population. If your parents are married, still alive and living together, you are very rare among the children of today's world. If you can hold your head up with a smile on your face and are truly thankful, you are blessed, because many can, but most do not. If you could hold someone's hand, hug them or touch them on the shoulder, you are blessed because you can offer GOD'S healing touch. If you can read this reflective offering, then you are more blessed that over two billion people who cannot read anything at all. You are indeed blessed in many ways you will never, never know.

Taken from 'The Word for Today'. See *Bibliography* section

BELIEF

G.K.Chesterton (1874-1936) *said,* **"When people stop believing in GOD, they just do not believe in nothing, they believe in anything.**"

MANY COMPLAIN AND DO NOTHING

It is very obvious that the people of our nation have lost their sense of outrage when it comes to taking action. All too many complain and do nothing.

I am not contemplating anarchy or lawlessness. An example of the people taking on the dictators, in what is supposed to be a democracy, is the attitude and get-up-and-go of our older people. When the Government of the day said *"We intend to cut out the medical cards for the majority"* we old fogies said *"No you don't"*. We won the battle.

The people of Ireland said *"NO"* to the Lisbon Treaty, in other words *"NO"* to Europe, simply because they felt they were being dictated to. These Eurocrats, nameless and faceless, formulate and dictate policy, all too much of it unacceptable. Very often we can ask ourselves, *"Are we being ruled by the E.U., where much is rubber stamped without the M.E.P. having said yea or nay. Why are we being dictated to by two Governments?"* This is certainly not democracy, as we knew it.

Like the older generation, we have no option other than to assert some of our authority. We must regain that sense of outrage so obvious in past generations and organise ourselves to act on Henry Ford's maxim, *"Don't find fault, find a remedy"*, instead of doing nothing.

ASTHMA AND ITS TREATEMENT

What are now known as The Diabetes Federation of Ireland, The Irish Heart Foundation and The Asthma Society of Ireland had humble origins. All were started in a private house, a family home. Three or four people decided to do something about the asthma problem they had, as did a similar number of families of persons with diabetes or heart problems. Cystic Fibrosis Association, Down Syndrome Ireland and many other health related registered charities started somewhat similarly. Some of the founders I knew personally, all those years ago. **Now many of these organisations, which have changed dramatically, can be looked upon as a cog in the almighty big circle or wheel which is the Sickness Industry.** This has been built up, only in recent years, by the drug-manufacturing companies, aided by the medical profession. To understand more about what I mean, but before doing so read further for more explanation, then turn to *Diabetes* caption.

These charitable organisations, including the Asthma Society, have been hijacked, infiltrated, by the representatives of the various drug companies and the medics, whose sole interest is monetary. They are businesses from which the chemical manufacturers benefit, as do the medical profession. Being charities any more is open to question because if business enters a charitable organisation it is no longer legally looked upon as being charitable. Many of them are headed by doctors or other members of the medical profession, whether on committees or otherwise. Visit their meetings or annual general meetings, as I have done, both in Ireland and the U.K. See the various trade stands or other methods used to indoctrinate the public into believing that there are pills and medicines for all ills, including asthma. Astra Zeneca, Merck Sharp and Dohme, Novartis and Teva Pharmaceuticals are prominent. So also are many others as referred to in *Diabetes* caption.

The Asthma Society issue a magazine titled *'Asthma News'*. To strengthen my views of the predominance of medical drugs and those who manufacture and dispense them, it is interesting to read the various articles in the periodical. Here is one, *'Our job is to translate and research laboratory findings in the field of asthma and develop them into new and better treatment. This opportunity also contributes hugely to the training of Irish doctors and scientists in research techniques, not only relevant to asthma but to all diseases'*. In the magazine there was a piece headed *Ireland leads way in finding asthma cures'*. It tells of how €600,000 had been awarded as a grant to Connolly Hospital in Dublin for research into asthma and its treatment. Here is another cash cow for the medical profession. It begs the questions *"Will anything natural be researched?"* Will they look into the importance of proper breathing by asthmatics? Will they highlight the fact that the use of Paracetamol and other chemical drugs or so called medicines, prescribed or off the shelf, given to young children, have been linked to increased rates of asthma?

All parents and those responsible for children's upbringing, this to include their health, should be aware of the dangers of giving them any chemical drugs, except in extreme cases. We learn that young children who spend more than two hours a day watching television are at an increased risk of developing asthma. This finding does not bode too well for future generations. See *Child and Infant Health* caption.

On the outside of the latest copy of *'Asthma News'*, just received, is the large lettered hype *'THE ROAD TO CONTROL, LET YOUR PHARMACIST GUIDE YOU IN THE RIGHT DIRECTION.'*

Inside the journal is the following *'INTERNATIONAL EXPERIENCE HAS SHOWN THAT WITH AN EMPHASIS ON EDUCATION AND SELF MANAGEMENT, ASTHMA CARE CAN BE GREATLY IMPROVED.'* This must involve a range of health care professionals including G.Ps., hospital specialists, nurses and pharmacists. Here is more publicity for the drug companies and medics as further illness is being sold by the Sickness Industry. Nowhere in the copies of *'Asthma News'* was there a word about nature's great aid to asthma, one that has left many who have found out about it not needing medicine, inhalers or other drug aids, indeed very often cured. This is the ***Buteyko Method,*** which is explained under that caption in this book.

With the exception of an extremely small piece there was nothing to be found about diet, need for lifestyle change, types of foods or drinks taken, or need for exercise and proper sleep pattern. There was nothing about anything natural such as pure additive free foods or drink. Many food additives are affecting us, especially those with asthma. Those with the illness or those who look after children and teenagers with the problem, should read the ingredients labels, avoiding foods or drinks which are processed, unnatural and with additives.

It is advisable to avoid swimming in public or chlorinated pools. **None are aware of what toxic or other chemicals are in the waters. Chlorine is an enemy of good health including breathing and asthma problems. Fluoride is even worse. Who would consider bathing in waters contaminated with sweat or urine, mixed with the various disinfectants used? Chlorine is often added in excess to already fluoridated water.**

All on the medical side concerned with sickness or illness appear to have a one-track mind - that of drugs and medicines. Nowhere do we see a word about attaining better health by natural means, including the use of supplements where necessary, but most of all the need for Vitamin D3 if with asthma. Vitamin D3 is a wonder, a very necessary supplement, to be taken daily. See ***Vitamin D3*** caption

Recently I spoke with a representative of the Asthma Society. This person definitely had tunnel vision way of thinking. The uses of nebulisers, drugs or inhalers were the norm for asthma treatment as far as she was concerned. When I asked if she heard of the Buteyko Method treatment by way of proper and controlled breathing I sensed a kind of annoyance in the answer. It was to the effect that there is insufficient evidence. All this despite wonderful findings being published in five medical journals. I asked her could I bring a number of people to visit, all of whom had been cured of asthma by use of the Buteyko Method. She gave me a haughty stare, and certainly did not give me a definite yes or no. It makes me feel like throwing my hands up in the air saying, ***"What the hell do these people need to convince them that the vast majority go down the wrong road of treatment.?"*** The evidence is there.

The Medical Journal reports are extremely favourable and there are many who can verify as to the excellent results and goodness of the Buteyko Method. Few, if any, who have gained relief or been cured by using this method go back to the Asthma Society, the doctors, or whoever has treated them with drugs or by chemical aids. They are better and feel there is no obligation to tell these people that they are now free from Asthma, needing no more help from the medics. The Asthma Society was not responsible for helping them to good health. Proper breathing, such as that practiced by Patrick McKeown, was the 'cure'.

The question can be asked, *"How can sufficient evidence be gained to convince the sceptics that the Buteyko Method, if put into practice, is a winner, a wonderful aid to Asthmatics"?* Turn to **Buteyko** Caption

It is evident that the medical representatives who represent the Asthma Society, just as others of them attached to many of the charities or groups linked to health associations, do not wish anything natural to be used. There is no money in it for them. I retell my belief, *"It is not in their interests to cure people".*

In my encyclopaedia, '**Health is Wealth**', there is an article headed the Buteyko Method. Thousands of copies of the book have been sold and as a result of this I had many replies, including letters of thanks, e-mails, cards and telephone calls praising the Buteyko Breathing Method. One man came over 120 miles to visit me, just to say 'Thank You', although we did take the party to see part of the lovely South East. This includes one of Ireland's gems, which is Kennedy Park Arboretum. He told of how himself and his niece were both cured. Many had similar stories. Recently a woman visited me, bringing her teenage daughter. Again I was thanked and told of the marvellous recovery of the young lady. She too explained of the benefits of the Buteyko Method for asthma sufferers. Almost daily, people who have regained good or better health by use of natural remedies or methods say, *"What a pity I did not know about this years ago".* This is often mentioned regarding what has been said about the Buteyko Method. I put this on paper for the benefit of those who suffer, very often unnecessarily.

I have no monetary or other interest in promoting this discipline, no more than I have financial interest in anything I write about or say. I just wish to help people. As the wonderful **Androzzos** put it in their hit song of 1945, *" If I can help somebody as I pass along, then my living shall not be in vain. "* I would not have thought about passing on the information and praising the good of the Buteyko Method had it not been for a lady and her son visiting me today – just to say "Thank You".

Many have mentioned Patrick McKeown of Asthma Care Ireland, who is fully qualified in the use of the Buteyko Method. I have been to some of his clinics, which are held all over Ireland and Europe and I was highly impressed.

He explains about the need to breath through the nose, also saying, *"To put it simply, over breathing through your mouth creates a cycle by taking cold, dry and dirty air into your lungs, and when you breath out you get rid of too much carbon dioxide which your body should use to dilate the smooth muscles of your airways. This further restricts the nasal passages, forcing one to breath more through the mouth and so a vicious circle continues. It is like a chicken and egg situation, does the asthma cause the over breathing, or does the over breathing cause the asthma?"*

We are told there is no cure for asthma. This is totally incorrect. One can safely refer to it as a lie. I've seen many who have been cured by Patrick McKeown's methods. To prove my assumption I can refer to my daughter who spent months in hospital with asthma, as a youngster. We moved about 100 miles when I relocated to new employment. The asthma disappeared, never to return. So it is with the Buteyko Method, where the majority who use it have gained relief and cure. **It is highly obvious that the treatment of asthma by the medics has been built up so that it is another large cog in the Sickness Industry we have.** Reference regarding how to contact Patrick McKeown of Asthma Ireland is given in *Buteyko Method of Breathing and Asthma Care* caption.

BONES—THE BODY SKELETON—A MARVEL

Just as so many give little or no thought to what is put into the body, so it is with care of the bones. All should realise that bone is an engineering masterpiece of comprehensive, tensile and elastic strength. As the human body is a marvel, so too is bone.

The human skeleton consists of approximately 206 bones and 68 joints. For instance, there are 26 bones in each foot and about the same number in each hand.

When one considers that the average person may in a lifetime walk the equivalent of two and a half times around the world, the pounding the bones take is phenomenal.

Bone is an essential part of countless living organisms. It is dynamic, being able to repair itself, respond to hormones that effects its growth and development, and even play a key role in the manufacture of blood cells. Like muscle, it slowly grows stronger as the load on it increases. **Hence, athletes have much heavier and stronger bones than do so-called 'couch potatoes'.**

Bone is composed of collagen fibres, containing salts such as calcium carbonate and calcium phosphate. To add wonder to wonder the outer shell or covering is made up of and grows in parallel layers. See

111

diagram of **Bone Structure**, which for easy viewing is enlarged.

The enormous numbers of what look like honeycomb pattern are inter-connecting spaces, all containing marrow. To keep bones strong and healthy one must eat, drink, sleep and exercise properly. Looking after the body in a proper manner ensures that one will have healthy bones. See **Calcium** caption, which includes advice on how to care for the bones also helping to prevent osteoporosis. See *Bibliography* section.

Some of this information has been extracted from the religious and informative magazine 'AWAKE', distributed free by volunteers who are Jehovah's Witness members'.

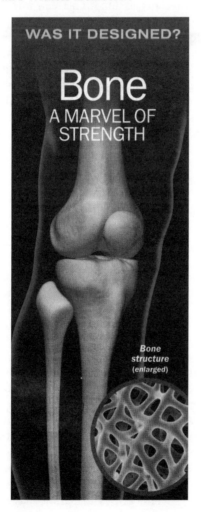

WAS IT DESIGNED?

Bone
A MARVEL OF STRENGTH

Bone structure
(enlarged)

What do you think?
Is bone a product of chance?
Or was it designed?

Don't tell me there isn't a
GOD.

EAT WELL ON A LIMITED BUDGET

Whether there be recession, depression, regression or whatever setback, financially or otherwise, one must at all times eat. Frequently we hear of how those not so well off, or the lower paid, eat what can be an inferior or non-sustaining diet also being more likely to drink alcohol or smoke. I know from my visits to homes or speaking with many, even those who can afford to eat well, that much fast, processed, additive-filled, so called foods and unhealthy drinks, are purchased and consumed. Much of it deserves to be classed as garbage, not to be taken as food or drink. How many realise this or understand about what they purchase as food or drink? In this respect, also with regard to smoking or consuming alcohol, many have got their priorities altogether wrong.

How many understand that 'food' from the microwave is to be avoided if they wish for nourishment? I repeat, **"How many give thought to what is taken into the human system, or who bothers to read the ingredients labels to learn about the non-sustaining additives which are used in the make up and processing of much of the food, often foodless, being purchased?"**

Professor Alan Maryon-Davies, president of the Faculty of Health said, **"There is a public perception that a healthy diet was an expensive diet. This is not so. There is much which is reasonably priced, which can be eaten, and which is valuable as regards better health".**

When younger, my wife and I did not have much money as we started out in married life. We were like Dwight Eisenhower, one time army General and later President of America, who when being interviewed by the media, on being asked, "Mr Eisenhower, we understand you came from a poor family?" replied, "No, we were not poor, it was just that we had no money!".

We reared our family and all eat well. In order to do so we budgeted weekly, buying not what we wanted, only what we needed. Potatoes, carrots, turnips, onions, cabbages and certain other vegetables are not excessively priced. Neither are certain fruits, such as pineapples, bananas, apples and some other kinds of health benefiting horticultural produce. Frozen vegetables are excellent value for money. It is not appreciated that they can be much fresher than vegetables which have been prepared or harvested for some time. Vegetables usually go direct from the producer to be frozen and packaged, with little delay in between. Many are under the impression that some of the goodness is lost in the freezing process. This is a wrong line of thought or notion.

Porridge oats is the cheapest and best value breakfast cereal. It is highly nutritious, full of goodness, being purely natural. It is not flavoured or with sugar or other additives, as are the majority of the fancy packaged breakfast cereals. Minced meat can be excellent value. It can be used in shepherd or cottage pies or can be used separately with vegetables, including potatoes. Burgers filled with a mixture of left over mashed potatoes, mince and sliced onions, can be delicious. Stewing meat is not expensive when compared with other cuts. Using a pressure cooker is a quick way to cook, especially for stews, with an assortment of vegetables included. Little meat is needed. Casserole dishes are easy to cook. Salads for main meal or as side salads are easy and quick to prepare. Onions, beetroot, grated vegetables such as carrot, cabbage and turnip, with corned beef, chicken or ham, combine to make nutritious salad meals. Serving fruit, such as pineapple, helps make the salad meals tasty. Cold mashed potatoes made up from left-overs, mixed with onion, chives, parsley and or chopped celery, mixed with a natural salad cream, as available in the health food shop is a good homemade coleslaw.

There are some simple recipes set out in this book, *Selling Sickness!* See *Recipes* caption.

There is the perception that potatoes are fattening. This is false. Colcannon is a simple meal to prepare. Most people are of the opinion that meat should be eaten regularly. I know many who never eat meat. They are healthy, living on inexpensive but extremely good natural food, all of which gives a varied and well balanced diet. If not eating meat it is very necessary to take Vitamin B12, obtainable from the health food store as a food supplement, in order to prevent pernicious anaemia.

Certain brands of tinned beans contain much which is good. Milk puddings are simple to prepare and cook. Sago, tapioca, semolina or the really health giving flaked brown rice, can all be cooked on the hob or hotplate of cookers. All can be nutritious. Given here is a minute selection of good pure natural foods which come to mind as being reasonably cheap and of good value. Searching the shelves, learning about what is non-processed and additive free, then with a little thought and some planning, one can be set up to lead a much easier life in the future. When shopping for food it should be remembered that what appears to be cheap, especially if processed and factory made, will have little goodness or food value. Health-wise, cheap can turn out to be expensive in the long term. *If one shops carefully there is no reason why one cannot have a nutritious, varied and well balanced diet, even if on a limited budget.*

NAGGING

A nagging person is one of the crowning works of the devil

THE SICKNESS INDUSTRY, WHICH IS KNOWN
AS THE HEALTH SERVICE

The biggest and worst run industries in Ireland and the U.K., which have not taken very many years to develop, have sprung up, mushroomed and now flourish as the Sickness Industry. There are certainly no healthy signs for those outside the industry, including the taxpayer, with hundreds of millions being creamed off by others.

The Sickness Industry in its present configuration consists of the Irish Health Service Executive (H.S.E.), the U.K. National Health Service (N.H.S.) as well as the private hospitals, clinics and the many nursing homes, which come under their remit or umbrella. These are at the heart of the sickness business which embraces the Pharmaceutical Multinationals, Doctors, Consultants, Psychiatrists, Psychologists, Anaesthetists, and other allied professionals. Add to these the Hospitals, Surgeries, Chemists or Pharmacies, Health Centres, Health Insurance Companies and the many thousands employed therein. Private enterprises, such as the Blackrock, Galway, Whitfield at Waterford, Cork Medical Centre, Mount Carmel group and various other fee-paying hospitals or clinics, turn over and make millions at the expense of those unlucky enough to have health problems.

Regularly we hear of health speculators having been either granted, been refused, or seeking planning permission for further private hospitals or nursing homes. The Sickness Industry is ever expanding, as all foolishly allow this to continue.

The H.S.E. is the largest employer in Ireland, as is the N.H.S. in the U.K. The pharmaceutical drug and chemical medicine industry, including the chemists or pharmacies, have much to do with the other groups mentioned and without them the Sickness Industry would not function. Hence, their inclusion in the group which makes up the carousel.

Much has been and continues to be written about the H.S.E. and the N.H.S. There is seldom a day when there is not something headlined about some facet of the Health Services, whether it be in the newspapers or on T.V. I have files which include newspaper clippings also the wording of T.V. articles. These go back many years. They set out the gripes, complaints, faultfinding, costs, withdrawal or side effects of drugs, some of them dangerous, overspending, scandalous wasting of the taxpayers money and very much else relating to health.

The N.H.S. of the U.K., the old health boards which were the forerunner of the H.S.E. in Ireland, and the drug conglomerates are all mentioned. It is not my intention to dwell on this, which is like water gone down the pipe or under the bridge. **Suffice to say that things have got** bigger, but not better, with very much of the Sickness Industry as we now see it, uncontrollable. One can honestly say, that with approximately 109,000 personnel and a budget between €13 and €14 billion, the returns from the H.S.E. by way of service are minimal, miserable and totally unacceptable. The budget figure in 1997 was a mere €3.7 billion. Since then money has been poured into the Health Service/Sickness Industry as if it came from a bottomless pit. This is tax-payers money. It has become a cash cow for many who are part of the money squandering business.

Here are examples. There are dozens of others, which could be set down if space permitted. **It transpires that the taxpayers had to fork out €45 million to pay legal fees to barristers and solicitors.** Despite being asked, the HSE refused to furnish details of the top 10 solicitors and barristers it paid and for what purposes. They were most uncooperative. The taxpayers pay out huge amounts of money and are then more or less told "Go to Hell" if they make enquiries themselves or ask some bureaucrats or others in authority to do so. The infuriating part is that the Sickness Industry keeps growing, as the nation gets sicker, with insurance companies paying out huge money against claims for treatment. There must come a time in the near future when the whole build-up of the Sickness Industry which we have, will come tumbling down. It can be likened to a 'house of cards'.

Recently a dispute arose when an internal audit uncovered serious irregularities in what was referred to as a partnership body for the Health Service/Sickness Industry, which received more than €41 million over the previous 10 years. Note the word **SERIOUS.** The body referred to is known as the Health Service National Partnership Forum (HSNPF), which consists of 24 members. This is just another of the all too many costly branches, circles, set-ups, call them cliques if you wish, all spawned off from the sick Sickness Industry. The latter mentioned industry pays dearly for all of this. *The main points resulting from the audit show that the HSNPF ignored the rules, when paying out €1 million for one programme.* When something like this occurs or pertaining to the Health Service most people do not show or express surprise anymore. It is as if €1 million to the Sickness Industry we are burdened with is a triviality. To return to the other salient and what are extremely worrying points in relation to the taxpayers, *we learn that large, very large, amounts were given to Trade Unions by the HSNPF. There is the matter of how funds of well over €1.25 million were spent on a programme or scheme to improve Human Resources; of about €12,000 spent annually on credit cards, mostly self certified or unauthorised; of over 20 foreign trips undertaken; of no evidence of any documentation in relation to the* *hiring of consultants, also much more. The auditors expressed much concern about the Human Resources scheme and how it was handled.*

As with the millions paid to the doctors when thy made spurious claims for payment for services rendered to deceased patients, it will be very interesting to see the result of all this mismanagement. The outcome of the HSNPF handing out money as if it was confetti will be like much other narrative, some of it soap opera material, which emerges regularly from the Health Service/Sickness Industry, where **Ms 'NOBODY'** does nothing, as referred to frequently in this book, *Selling Sickness!*

Alleged nepotism within the Sickness Industry, better known as the Health Service, reared its head when there were reports of relatives of some senior personnel being employed for what are referred to as 'summer jobs'. Apparently the correct procedures for recruiting were by-passed. These positions paid at a rate equivalent to between €20,000 to €30,000 per annum, according to what the work entailed. Not bad for a 'summer job!' It would be interesting to hear if any references or C.V.s were needed. As witnessed down the years, **'It's not what you know, but who you know, that matters'.** Here again **NOBODY** does anything to expose to the taxpayer what might be relevant regarding the claimed favouritism. It will all be 'Widgeried', swept under the carpet.

In recent years many public and private hospitals, health centres, nursing homes and other health facility buildings have emerged. We have seen the building and extending of hospitals with enlargement of car parking facilities at many of these places. All of this points to the expectation of more sickness with the enlargement of the Sickness Industry. I repeat **"It will not be feasible in the future to have funding as it is now carried out."**

If the highly paid bods who run these organisations and institutions are in the business of curing people then questions must be asked of them. It is obvious that healing and cure, also ensuring better health, is not in their vocabulary. It would not be in their interests. They just appear to play at it as they extort money for their efforts of keeping people on the Sickness Industry conveyor system. The whole set-up, which has been and is enlarging all of the time, is daunting. It is a mighty disgrace as things spiral further out of control. I repeat again and again that prevention is a word seemingly unheard of within the realms of the Sickness Industry

In 2005 when the Health Boards, as we knew them, were dissolved, we were told of their inefficiency. There were allegedly obstacles, much of which could be improved on. They were certainly no worse than the set up we have now. Money was not then squandered as like now, where it is treated without consideration of how much is being misused, frittered away. A few years later there was another change of direction. The H.S.E. admitted that a mistake had been made, the new idea being to appoint regional directors. Since the formation of the H.S.E. the aim seems to be to milk the cash cow dry. Regional directors and jobs for the boys and girls have varying ways of dubbing things as steps in that direction.

The Sickness and Drugs Industries have led us to the position where the H.S.E. cannot continue to function as of now, being completely out of control, spending and otherwise. Spending over 10% of the total Government income on health alone is unsustainable. It will only lead to bankruptcy of the nation, if allowed to continue as at present, with huge costs climbing all of the time. I repeat, it is out of control, being totally absurd.

We learn that the ageing population will increase so much in the future that the Health Service Executive requirements by 2050 will be double what it is now. A symposium, in Dublin, on the subject of growing old, came to this conclusion. They did not give a figure and it would be interesting to know what figure is being doubled. There is no need for comparison because if the Sickness Industry is allowed to carry on as of now, with no reduction in costs, only rising sickness figures, the end of the Health Service Executive/Sickness Industry is nigh. Speaking with my friends, all agree that there will be no health service by then unless there is an entirely different approach to treatment, this to include the running of the Health Service Executive and the money leaking Sickness Industry. They too will be bankrupt, having helped enormously to liquidate the exchequer funds.

A large book could be written giving facts and figures, also setting out the lunacy that afflicts those who man and run the Sickness Industry. I just give brief facts. We are informed that there will be cuts of over €700 million within the set-up. It remains to be seen if this is carried out. Of course if there is little money left in the seemingly bottomless pocket, from which is paid out the enormous amounts to keep the carousel working, the proposed reductions might be much bigger. The fact that a redundancy package offered had only low take-up will not help the H.S.E's. finances. Anyway, not many, except in certain circumstances, would consider leaving secure and well paid jobs, as provided within the Sickness Industry.

At time of writing, in the N.H.S. (U.K.) there are over 1.25 million employed as against 980,000 some five years previous. Between the years 2000 and 2010 the annual budget went from £60 billion to between £102 and £103 billion, a 70% rise. This is for a population of approximately 61 million. In Ireland the budgetary figure for the H.S.E. is around €14 billion euro for a population of approximately 4.1 million. In the U.K., where treatment is free to all, the cost on average

works out at a figure of approx. £1670 per person regardless of whether sick or not. In Ireland even if the service, as in the U.K., was free, which it is not, the cost of treatment to all is an astronomical €3400 per person

Looking at these figures and taking into consideration the fact that health care in the U.K. is free for all, also allowing for the difference in the money rate of exchange, it is highly obvious that the Irish Health Service is costing extremely much more than that of the U.K.

Because of the use of medical cards in Ireland and the charges paid by those without them, who have no claims to free or part free medication, the H.S.E. in Ireland could be costing well over three times that of the N.H.S. in the UK. It is almost unbelievable that when one takes the figures given here, then working out the cost per person, (i.e. every man, woman and child in the U.K. and Ireland), the variance in the sickness treatment cost is scandalous. It is obvious that nobody becomes shocked when it comes to charges or money squandering within the Sickness Industry in Ireland. Even the tax-payers, who eventually end up paying these overwhelming costs, remain silent.

On the basis of calculation, which is almost impossible because of the circumstances whereby the majority do not have free treatment in Ireland as in the U.K., the figure I give for Irish costs is extremely conservative, **at the same time being outlandish. They are doubly so when it is realised that well over 50% of patients in Ireland pay for their treatment. All who have reason to use the Sickness Industry are being exploited in many ways. The pathetic figures of the cost of treatment to all is confirmation, if that is needed, that those in charge of the Health Service Executive/Sickness Industry in Ireland have lost all control of leadership and managing. It is obvious that their influence over governance of money, colossal amounts, has evaporated. One cannot be blamed for using the cliché 'RIP OFF IRELAND'.**

From my experience of living in both Ireland and the U.K., the N.H.S., despite all the criticism in Britain, is streamlined compared to Ireland. When the administration costs are compared it gives much room for thought. Some 27% of the Irish budget spend is on administration as against a figure of just over 14% in the U.K. Why? Don't ask me, ask the seemingly clueless Health Service Executive leaders. No doubt they will come up with a glib-worded reply.

Many years ago a friend said to me, when we were in the upper storey of a hospital, as he pointed to the walkway between three separate parts of the institution, **"Come and look at all these people walking, carrying wads of paper. Walking like that makes one look really busy"**.

Just imagine the billions, yes billions, which could be saved annually if we could follow the U.K. standards. This is a glaring example of the bungling and incompetence in the way the Health Service Executive is run in Ireland. I don't blame the man wholly but when Professor Drumm took over the running of the Service things were bad but when he left they were much worse. The various Government Health Ministers which we have been saddled with over the past 17 years, have without exception, been incompetent and bungling bureaucrats.

Who does anything about this incompetence? The answer, as is so often the case, where our Government and The Sickness Industry are concerned, is *'NOBODY'*. Despite so much which has been and continues to be said or done, often reported with large headlines, all remain quiet. The taxpayer forks out without any action being taken. I reiterate *"Our sense of outrage is quenched compared to times past. Voices will not be heard."*

Some years ago the then Minister for Health told us that the regulatory bodies which would in future adjudicate on the fitness of all healthcare professionals, including doctors, nurses, pharmacists, social workers and other grades would be made up mainly of lay people. At the same time we were informed that the Minister was of the opinion that people would have more confidence in a system where there is a majority of lay participation. What happened? The Minister backed down after much whining and wringing of hands. Another case of the employees dictating to the weak kneed employer, the Government.

One constantly hears of the unions interfering in the affairs of the H.S.E. We saw headings such as *'Crunch time for the H.S.E'.. 'Costs saving talks with unions'. 'Unions call for extra funds for Health Services'. 'Our unions call for end of cutbacks'. 'Union official denounces the H.S.E. over therapy posts ruling'.* This does not happen to nearly the same degree in Britain. In times when all should try to live within their means they should stop whining, stand back and look at the cash cow and bonanza they have in the H.S.E. Their approach is often pitiful to behold. They should also adopt some common sense, realising the present set up cannot exist for the future.

In this book, *Selling Sickness!*, I endeavour to show the carry on, the conniving, the scheming and money obtaining methods used throughout much of the Sickness and parts of the Food Industries, those which supposedly improve health. I repeat "I could write books on the subject." I will rest my case. Maybe you the reader will stand up and shout *"ENOUGH IS ENOUGH, AS I AM DOING"*.

Again I quote Henry Ford's maxim *'Don't find fault, find a remedy'*. All too many whinge, moan and complain, doing nothing to find the remedy.

The remedy for reducing dramatically the embarrassment which is the Sickness Industry we now have, and to improve the health of all, rests in our own hands. We hold the key to better well-being through change of lifestyle and mode of living, at the same time saving the taxpayer billions.

It is only over the past 25 years, because of the hype of the drug companies and their servants, the medical profession, that we have been swamped, overwhelmed, with drugs. **The mighty Pfizers and their promotion of the 'dangerous' side effects giving Statins is an example.** Elsewhere in this book is set out the scandal of putting healthy people on Statins to treat a non-existent disease, only conveniently thought up in recent years. It is called cholesterol. Drugs have not been responsible for people living longer, there is much more to that, as described amongst these pages. See *Statins* also *Cholesterol* captions.

The answer, the principal remedy for many suffering from ill-health or feeling unwell, is so simple, it is ludicrous that people have not recognised its value. It costs little except discipline. I repeat, reiterate, making no apologies for doing so, that we are as *'We eat, drink, sleep and exercise'*.

Again I reiterate, *"A lifestyle change to include pure natural additive free food and drink, little or no alcohol, no caffeine, sugar or sugary products, everything to be good, nourishing and sustaining, is a major or often complete part of the answer. Learning to read the ingredients labels on the food or much of the foodless food we are offered should be a compulsory requirement. Exercise and proper sleep and sleep pattern must be added. The other requisite is discipline. If all practiced the nine words of my slogan, the thriving Sickness Industry would be killed off, hospitals and surgeries would be closing daily"*. I know, I have seen all of this work for thousands, including myself, now in my 80's.

We learn that diabetes and its treatment is a €1 billion drain on the Health Service Executive. Both the blood and urine test methods of diagnosing are a caper, very often being misleading. The doctors are costing the state billions by not advising those diagnosed with diabetes to change their lifestyle completely or enormously and to return in six to eight weeks for check up. Here too there should be a second or even third opinion. **To learn that almost three quarters of those with diabetes do not have it when it is diagnosed** see under *Diabetes* caption

If evidence is needed about anything I write about, feel free to speak with me, or some of those whom I have helped to offload and rid themselves of the need for synthetic drug and medicine treatment.

Our Government, the Health Service Executive and all concerned with the Sickness Industry must make vital changes in their approach to safeguard the well-being and health of the people. What is needed is a huge turn towards health education and **PREVENTION** of illness. Their approach to what I suggest will not take place. They are imbued with the idea of wooing and cultivating a close relationship with the almighty drug industry, which is one of the chief mainstays of the economy of the country. **They will not rock the foundation of what is the Sickness Industry.**

To help substantiate what I have stated, again I ask a simple question? Why has the Government kept secret the already prepared **National Policy on Nutrition,** which was promised for publication in 2005 and then by different politicians in successive years? Now we are told, *There was no reality behind any of these dates".* To put it bluntly, some of the politicians, those whom we perceive as governing, have been telling us lies. It is not to be wondered at that so many of them are regarded as being devious, untrustworthy, and wily. I have some idea of what was within the pages of the National Policy document which I keep harping about. The people who compiled it had the sense to advise huge dietary changes, because so much of what is offered as food can be termed *'RUBBISH'.* In this respect no word strong enough can be used here to describe the Health Service Executive, now the Sickness Industry, and those who profess to run it. **'Nobody'** is evident throughout the whole organisation. 'Nobody' accepts responsibility for anything there except picking up the pay cheque or salary. Turn to *National Policy of Nutrition* Caption

The fat cats of our Government are like the fat cats of the H.S.E.

They are all '**Ms. NOBODYS**'. They do little or nothing to properly correct, rule or govern, particularly the Health Service/Sickness Industry they have been responsible for burdening the taxpayer with.

THE PROBLEMS OF LIFE

There are few if any homes where it can honestly be said, "We have no problems". To use a cliché – 'It is a fact of life'. Many imagine or think they have problems until they hear those of others, then realising that theirs are trivial, minuscule.

STATINS
THE SHAM OF LOWERING CHOLESTEROL

When you read under the *Cholesterol* caption in this book, set out is much which is unknown to many, much about one of the grossly over-hyped, nonsensical ideas, which the Sickness Industry has domineered most people into believing. This is because of the huge financial rewards for both the major drug companies and those who prescribe or sell their statins. When I give talks to various groups, organisations, at corporate health gatherings or other symposiums, the realisation is there that the majority are taken in by the propaganda of the drug conglomerates, with the question asked all too regularly *"How do I lower my cholesterol"?* My answer to this is *"Don't bother about your cholesterol, concentrate on normalising your blood pressure".*

Up to 25 years ago the word cholesterol was almost unheard of. **Then suddenly the drug companies latched on to it as they invented another sickness.** Perhaps I digress because I set out to explain about statins. It appears there is much explaining to be done. So many including my good wife, who is well-versed in the natural way of living, have asked, *"What are statins? Why are they used"?* I am not surprised there is little known about them or their gross over prescribing and use, because the medical profession certainly will not explain.

Statins are a cholesterol-lowering drug that includes Lovastatin, Pravastatin, Rosuvastatin, Simvastatin and others. **They are promoted and prescribed under various branded trade names in what must be regarded as a highly organised but utter CON.** As chemical drugs they are supposed to lower the lipoproteins, the supposedly bad ones, which we are told reduce the risk of heart disease. Atorvastatin is sold as Lipitor and manufactured by Pfizers. Cerivastatin was Bayer's product and also known as Bacol or Lipobay. This was a disaster, having to be recalled and with claims totalling millions now in the hands of the legal profession. No doubt they will procrastinate, as is usual where claims are made for side effects, fatalities or whatever. Very much harm has been caused to a vast number of people, the majority of them healthy beforehand, who have been prescribed statins.   Lipitor from Pfizers is the one hugely prescribed. There are many others, which are sold in various countries, under varied brand names, for what is the biggest selling drug in the world

We hear of side-effects, of the dangers of taking statins or of mixing with other drugs. Loss of memory occurs frequently. Warnings of harm to the liver, bones, joints, and much else are given, also about driving when under the influence of these chemical made statins. Machinery drivers and operators are especially at risk. Of course this is relevant to many other drugs. If taking statins it is not advisable to take fruit juices or fruit drinks, especially if made from berries.

It should be added that bone and muscle pains, some unbearable, are being reported daily as further side effects. The doctors are not co-operative when it comes to decrying the use of statins. Why should they? It makes millions for them as they prescribe the various brands of statins. They are helped, no doubt by the advertising and propaganda hype of the drug-manufacturing companies, who also promote the education of and one can safely add, the indoctrination of doctors.

Consider the sales of statins in billions of euro, pounds, dollars or other currencies. It is perplexing.

Reflect on the extra and little heard of huge costs, where the G.Ps. and pharmacists come into our lives, when money assimilation is considered. These include: examinations, cholesterols tests, prescribing, sales, etc. Cholesterol and statins are to be taken as one to describe a single item in the billions of euro or pounds poured into the black hole, which is the Health Service Executive or Sickness Industry.

What should be an extremely worrying feature is that a Heart Protection Study published in 2004 gives us to understand that all should be on statins, irrespective of whether we have high or low cholesterol levels. In other words if we are well, we are to be made sick. Now, years later, the idea is that children from the age of four should be drawn into the net as more and more medical bods recommend the use of statins.

The same scientists who carried out the studies into this scenario and who supposedly carried out tests, which have led us, probably deliberately, to believe them, studied a majority of older people. There were no tests done on the young and not so young, such as those in their

30's and 40's. By doing this they were able to tell us that the use of statins can lower cholesterol effectively whatever the age.

The American Government is now entering into the fray, with numbers of Congressmen putting forward the same idea as the Heart Protection Study group. With billions being spent on health lobbying, perhaps Dr. Rath, the natural health pioneer, is not wrong in his assumption that, *"Where some Governments and the mighty Drug Industry is concerned it will soon be a case of 'Who rules'."* One could ask, *"Is the tail wagging the dog?"*. All of this carry-on points to vested interests, with the healthy but all too trusting public, being the target. The Sickness Industry aim, with money being the number one factor, means the health of all is given little, if any, thought.

We now learn that a British plan envisages a screening of *all* adults aged 40 to 60, offering statins to those considered to have a 20% risk of developing heart disease over the following decade. The new recommendations come from Britain's National Institute for Health and Clinical Excellence. This body is run by the medical profession, who in turn advise The National Health Service which is the hub of The Sickness Industry in the U.K. More about this under *Cholesterol* caption.

Dr. Declan Sugrue, Consultant Cardiologist at the Mater Hospital, Dublin, says, *"There is a valid economic argument for introducing screening and prescribing statins to cut risks in stroke and heart attacks. The general trend in medicine over the past 30 to 40 years is for early detection and screening rather than treating advanced disease"*. The really galling part of all this is that statins do not prevent heart attacks, I repeat, *"THE TAKING OF STATINS DOES NOT PREVENT HEART ATTACKS OR STROKES"*.

Have these supposedly learned people not heard of prevention? It is very apparent that it does not suit them to prevent illness, including the elimination of cholesterol by change of lifestyle. Their past ideas do not seem to have got us very far as people continue to get sicker and sicker and our hospitals fuller and fuller.

A recent study published in The British Medical Journal tells a completely different story. *'For every heart attack prevented by the statin drug, two or more suffered liver damage, kidney failure, cataracts, extreme muscle weakness also bone and muscle pain as a result of taking the drug.'* **It is apparent that statin drugs harm far more people than they help.**

Statin drugs in the opinion of many, including a huge number of doctors, are useless. If the truth about statins were openly known, the drugs would not be prescribed to anyone. The drug companies would be sued for billions of dollars for false advertising and marketing manipulations. I repeat my thoughts when I say that doctors who recommend statin drugs are selling a non-existent illness. In so doing they can certainly be looked upon as being 'pickpockets', which I have mentioned on more than one occasion elsewhere in this book, *Selling Sickness.*

Again, and I know I keep on about the fact that there is not a word about diet, change of lifestyle, exercise or the natural way of cure, but it is a fact. There is little debate of the use and over use of statins. **Why?** Despite their harmful side effects, when it comes to getting the message across, pro and anti, the pro's with a capital P, meaning the drug-manufacturing industry, are on an unlimited budget to propagandise, advertise and promote drugs such as statins. The gullible person, the patient, is completely at the mercy of the benefiting, monetary gaining adviser – the G.P., and of course the drug-manufacturing companies.

The whole scenario with regard to statins could be regarded as a joke by any health conscience, intelligent person, if it was not so terribly serious. Above all it is another ploy to line the pockets of those under the umbrella of the Sickness Industry.

We now learn that children may be exploited, simply to extend pharmaceutical patents. The makers of Lipitor are allegedly likely to promote a chewable form of the statin drug, which will be just like 'sweets'. The people who may allow this to happen in the Sickness Industry must be out of their minds if they agree a really immoral arrangement like this to be encouraged.

Watching the blood pressure, keeping its levels right by leading a proper lifestyle, that which I harp or keep on about throughout these pages, then one is 80% of the way to good or better health. Statins are being prescribed for healthy people, to be taken indefinitely, one can say for life, if fool enough to listen to the medico, the G.P. Like diagnosing diabetes, we have the nonsensical situation where at the doctor's whim, following the taking of a very small amount of blood or a urine sample, they can bluntly tell one *"You have diabetes"* or *"Your cholesterol is high".* As I have said elsewhere this is totally unacceptable. Any person who accepts silly and meaningless advice to take statins is foolish to the extreme. I repeat, **"Healthy people are being sentenced to a life of illness by accepting and using prescriptions for Statins."** Even the wrapper on the drug tells us they don't prevent heart attacks.

I reiterate, *"To be sensible one needs to look after the blood pressure. This is very often easily done by a simple change of lifestyle, taking pure additive free, non-processed foods and drinks, exercising and with proper sleep and sleep pattern."* Statins give much food for thought. To those like myself who live by the advice given here, they are to be avoided at all cost.

When you the reader of this book, have read, studied and absorbed what is set out under both Cholesterol and Statins captions, I respectfully suggest that you form your own conclusions about what I have termed the Statins and Cholesterol humbug or scam. Turn to *Cholesterol* also *Blood Pressure* captions.

HAPPINESS

Happiness does not come from having much but from being attached to little. We are often told that money can't buy happiness. Of course it can, spend it on others.

DIABETES

ITS DIAGNOSIS AND TREATMENT BY DRUGS IS UTTERLY UNACCEPTABLE.

What is Diabetes? Many don't know why this health problem arises. They are sent on their journey through life, by the doctors, when diagnosed with the disease, all too quickly being put on drugs for life. The medic will explain little, certainly not why diabetes occurs or how it can be prevented, avoided or even reversed.

To put it in simple words, diabetes is a disease in which blood glucose levels are above normal. Most of the food we eat is turned into glucose or sugar for our bodies to use as energy. The pancreas, an organ or gland that lies behind the stomach, makes the hormone called insulin which helps glucose enter into the cells of our bodies. When one has diabetes, the body either doesn't make enough insulin or can't use its own insulin as well as it should. This causes sugar to build up in the blood. When blood sugar levels are too high the body is unable to cope with or use it properly.

We are afflicted with what is supposedly an epidemic of ever-growing proportions of diabetes type one and type two. All that is written in these pages regarding proper lifestyle and mode of living can help one live with, reverse or be free from type two diabetes. Type one is much more difficult to deal with.

Type one diabetes is an autoimmune condition. People with it must inject insulin. Inferior diet and especially the taking into the body of sugar and sweetened 'foods' and 'drinks' can lead to diabetes. All of this type of health harming stuff is to be avoided if with the disorder, whether types one or two. Despite being told to the contrary a sensible diet of natural, additive and sugar free, non-processed, pure foods and drinks can help immensely if one is with type one diabetes.

Type two diabetes is a metabolic condition. This means that there are both synthetic and destructive reactions within the body regarding manufacture of proteins and fats, also the breakdown of sugars which release large amounts of energy. Here again the evils of sugar and sweetened products are highlighted.

Diabetes in middle age, or when older, is becoming an increasing health problem. No matter what the age, if all followed my advice, diabetes can be prevented, reversed or even cured. Diabetes is now supposedly endemic, due mostly to the lifestyle of so many who are diagnosed as being with the disorder, also by the over and wrong diagnosing by the medical profession. **It is not right that a prick that allows a small amount of blood to be taken for testing by a doctor is accepted as the answer when it shows positive, as is a urine sample. There should be one or perhaps two other opinions sought before coming to a conclusion.** The consumption of sugars, certainly one of the most harmful things eaten, taken into the body as sustenance, also confectionery, sugary products, including sweets and chocolate, fast foods and so much more which contains sugar, even in minimal amounts, has seen diabetes spread alarmingly. Fizzy, so-called energy and other processed, sweetened and additive-filled drinks, are enemies of good health, especially diabetes. Turn to *Sugar and Sugars* caption to learn more about what is terribly adverse and injurious to one's health

If lifestyle issues are not addressed, those with diabetes can go on to develop many complications. These include heart disease, circulation problems, kidney disease, nerve disorders, foot and leg ulcerations, even blindness.

Obesity or being over-weight, which has always been associated with people in middle age, very often leading to diabetes, is now soaring in children and young people. We learn that 80% of people in Ireland with diabetes are overweight. Never was there a need for prevention of diabetes and indeed all illness so relevant as of now, but certainly not by use of chemical drugs as prescribed by the medics. See *Healthy Body Weight* caption.

An old saying, learned as a boy, was that '*Diligence calls for self-discipline*'. One must be motivated, alert and following the slogan through earnestly. **Ill health and obesity are a result of being undisciplined**.

Just stop and think that in Ireland over 10% of the Health Service budget is spent on treating diabetes. Doctors have warned that, *"With our western lifestyle and our aging population the prevalence of diabetes will continue to increase"*. What an attitude the medical profession have. If they were honest with patients, with proper and sensible advice given, there would be very much less diabetes.

It is all very well to say that our Government should advise the people about lifestyle changes. Isn't this what our G.Ps. and consultants are paid for, but sad to say, they are not prepared to do so? After all they are supposedly responsible for the health of all. Not long ago, I read in a long-winded article, facts and figures which were set out about diabetes, including the cry for more money and funding to help the *'poor'* G.Ps. What brass neck they have!

Recently, at a corporate health function, at the usual Question and Answer session, I was asked, *"What causes diabetes?"* The answer or main reason is set out and often repeated in this caption. In a condensed form this is what I told the group, *"As the use of three things, which certainly look incompatible, grew, the illness grew too. The three things mentioned are the inordinate over production and taking of sugar into the body including everything which contains sugar and sweeteners".* *Sugar sales grew by over 800% between 1900 and 2000. Then there is the easy to possess tin box on four wheels, the motor vehicle. This has led to gross negligence of our health because the majority who use this form of transport take little, if any, exercise. The harm of television cannot be highlighted sufficiently. It affects mind and body in a huge way. Here are three big evils to come into our lives, certainly health-wise. They are a mighty deterrent to all to avail of proper exercise, destroying what can lead to a healthy lifestyle.*

Lack of exercise is the biggest health problem we have in the world today, as it leads to ill health. This statement cannot be questioned or denied. The greater number of illnesses we have can be traced back to lack of exercise. This one trait in life is at the top of any recommendations to change one's lifestyle".

In front of me are bulging files, all marked 'Diabetes Mellitus'. They cover types one and two diabetes. Laid on top of each other they are almost one metre high. The upsurge of this ailment has appalled me because I have studied it comprehensively since I was told I had diabetes over 40 years ago. Explanation will be made later as to why I do not have the serious health problem. Just like so many who are told, sometimes bluntly by the doctor, *"You have diabetes",* it is doubtful if it was even there when diagnosed. Before then we heard little about diabetes compared to today. There are too many reasons why it has now become endemic. The medical profession and the synthetic drug industry have been, and continue to be, major contributors to the problem, by prescribing drugs. The ever-recurring theme of lifestyle is a major factor. If ever there was a need for abiding by my slogans *'YOU ARE WHAT YOU EAT, DRINK, SLEEP AND EXERCISE'* or *'CHANGE THE LIFESTYLE',* in relation to prevention and care of diabetes, it is now.

There is no known chemical medicine, which will eliminate the ailment. There are natural remedies, which will, and chief amongst them is proper diet of food and drink, all to be natural. Apart from not using my slogans and keeping to them, I repeat, "**One of** *the chief causes of diabetes is the over consumption of sugar, confectionery, sweets, chocolate and other sweetened additives which are offered as 'rubbish' foods or drinks."*

Fizzy, energy, many artificially sweetened and other sugary drinks also the thousands of other non-nutrients in the stuff offered as 'food' are enemies of diabetes. Fast or processed foods, almost all of which contain sugar and undesirable additives, as well as the many over hyped sugarised breakfast cereals must be avoided. In three words *'SUGAR IS DANGEROUS'.* Some bod wrote recently that it is a myth that people with diabetes shouldn't eat sugar. He is a liar or to put it nicely he does not know what he is talking about. One can only presume that he has a monetary interest in the sugar industry.

Sir Frederick Grant Banting, who in 1929 did so much for the future lives of diabetics when he discovered insulin, warned that *"Diabetes has increased proportionately with the per capita consumption of sugar".* He described refined sugar as *"A dangerous foodstuff".* What would he say if he were alive today? Recently a well-known professor described sugar as *'PURE WHITE AND DEADLY'*. Almost daily I refer to it as being dangerous and to be avoided.

Obesity, or being over-weight, even slightly, comes from an inferior lifestyle. It can lead to diabetes and to further complications which can arise. Being over-weight, like so many of our present day complaints, comes about through the type of inferior lifestyle the writer keeps labouring on and repeating.

Every pound of weight lost reduces the risk of diabetes. Dr. Susan Jebb, of MRC of Human Nutrition Research, Cambridge, told a conference that one study, which found overweight people who lost nine pounds on a diet and exercise programme, reduced the risk of the disease by 58% per cent. I repeat, see *Healthy Body Weight* caption.

The doctors, consultants and much of the medical profession, as already stated, are acting in a disgraceful or shameful manner. Drugs for diabetes are being prescribed far too soon. I have had many people visit me in desperation, saying how they were told by their doctors that they had diabetes. They had been put on medication but were able to turn away from this after change of way of eating, drinking and sleeping also taking exercise. Some of this is set out under *Doctors and Medical Profession* caption. Many patients are been advised incorrectly by the doctors. They have and are being slyly or deviously put on a lifetime of chemical drugs, the majority of them being healthy beforehand.

I cannot but restate, that drugs for diabetes are being prescribed far too soon. They should only be used as a last resort and all should be aware of this.

Some time ago trials and a survey carried out by doctors showed that 7 out of 10 patients diagnosed as having diabetes would need no medication, if they were advised and followed a recommendation, to just change their lifestyle or way of living. In simple language, their eating, drinking, sleeping and exercise habits needed much thought, with steps to be taken to make changes where necessary. Correcting wrong kind of lifestyle and requesting the patient to return in six to eight weeks would show up a very much different result, with much less need for prescribing of drugs, yes, perhaps over two thirds less. Just imagine the expense, drudgery and hassle, all of which can be avoided? Diabetes is not endemic, despite the hype within the Sickness Industry. This is just another money orientated scam, sad to relate.

A somewhat similar situation has arisen where prostate screening may be doing more harm than good. Where the medics screen for prostate cancer by measuring for levels of the prostate specific antigen (P.S.A.), which is a sign of or pointer to prostate inflammation, they are not recognising that there may be other conditions which can or may be the cause of the inflammation. It is a fact that the P.S.A. test is terribly unreliable, the result being that the 'cure' may be worse than the disease. I have had many seek information about prostate treatment, and who now live normal lives by the use of natural remedies.

Can anyone imagine the G.Ps. sitting patients down, giving them an amount of their time to advise change of lifestyle and way of living. In simple language many are being sent down a road of hell, being on drugs for life, not curing, probably worsening the diabetes, all because of the thoughtless, one can say callous ways, as the doctors prescribe drugs all too soon for the disease.

Many years ago my brother-in-law, a doctor, a wonderful man, who understood about the need for proper lifestyle, including diet, examined me. His words were, *"You have diabetes, but if not you are certainly a border-line case"*. He knew that at the time I drank, smoked and lived a terrible lifestyle. He referred to the food eaten, amongst other things. With his help and advice I changed my way of living in a big way. One of the results was that I did not have and still do not have diabetes. This is when my slogan *'WE ARE AS WE EAT, SLEEP, DRINK AND EXERCISE'* was coined and first used.

How many Doctors will act and advise today as he did? I well remember his attending to his dispensary duties, now called surgeries. There would be no more than five or six patients or callers on any morning. No need for any appointment, just roll-up. All this before the commercialisation, only in recent years, of the lucrative and money making Sickness Industry we have now.

Having dwelt on the fact, and one might say, accusing the medical bods, also the pharma drug-manufacturing companies, of accelerating the rise of diabetes to epidemic proportions, much of what I write here sets this out to a very large degree. There is very much further evidence that what I state is correct.

Enter here the Diabetes Federation of Ireland or its cross channel equivalent, Diabetes U.K. Both are charitable organisations, regarded as benevolent. No doubt both do some good. They have had different titles in the past. Both groups came from humble beginnings, before the drug industry and the medical profession took a huge and rewarding interest in these and others, which are regarded as

charitable health aid groups. Both organisations can also be bracketed with the chemical drug multi-nationals in the harm they cause, as well as their tunnel vision as far as treatment of diabetes is concerned. No doubt this will raise some hackles or ruffle some feathers. Let me proceed further and then what I write may cause them much food for thought, as they realise they are wrong in their approach to disease or illness, especially diabetes.

The diabetic organisations, as we know them, were first started by some three or four concerned people coming together in private houses. They were concerned because either one or other or a relative had diabetes. They wished to seek each other's advice and if possible find further information about the disease, which they too regarded as serious.

Today, we are plagued by experts. I don't remember any in those far off days. Then all thought sugar, like smoking, was the in-thing.

Yes, The Diabetes Federation of Ireland, Diabetes U.K., The Heart Foundations, Cystic Fibrosis Association, The Asthma Society and many of our charitable organisations started out in a very small way, as described. As a charity worker I have met with people who helped get more than one of them off the ground in the 1940's and 50's. Only very recently I spoke with a lady now over 80, who was a charity organisation volunteer, who told me some of the stories of which there are many, about their early pioneering work to help those who were ill. Almost all of these charitable organisations, societies or whatever name they are known by now, have been hijacked. The person referred to confirmed this.

They have been taken over, with intrusion by the medics, ably assisted by the pharmaceutical and chemical drug-processing conglomerates. There are lay people involved, most of them paid employees but all being dictated to by the Sickness Industry. The older, more sensible and demure persons, who have worked so hard for these organisations in the past, all voluntary, have been ousted, relegated.

What have we now? The chemical drug and medicine industry, also the medical profession, have infiltrated the charities, the important ones, and indeed some they deem not so important, but where they wish to be seen to be doing something. The G.Ps. are lining their pockets by prescribing chemical drugs, at the same time helping enormously to improve the finances of the mighty drug manufacturers. The Diabetes Organisations are examples of what I write about. Again I repeat, I am well aware of the much help these organisations or clubs give regionally and nationwide. I am also too aware of the power of the drug-manufacturing companies and the medical profession, the many with monetary interests and the control they hold over the charitable organisations. Where health organisations are deemed charitable there must be a question mark placed against them. Certain of them are indirectly part of what is big business, the Sickness Industry. Where does the charity begin or end?

Look at the list of multi-nationals and large drug companies who are seen to exhibit, support, sponsor or lend their name to the Diabetes, Heart, Asthma, Depression and other health awareness functions laid on. They cannot legally be looked on as charitable societies when infiltrated by industries which supposedly support them. This means they have vested monetary interests in more ways than one. Yes, regarding some of these health organisations or societies as charitable is questionable.

I made a point of visiting the Diabetes Federation of Ireland and Diabetes U.K. annual general meetings held in Dublin and London respectively. Diabetes Federation of Ireland promotion was titled, with extra publicity, Diabetes Health Awareness Exhibition. It was certainly an exhibition, medical presentation and drug show. I was not in the least surprised to see the road show, the merry-go-round, the carousel, as presented by another segment of the Sickness Industry.

The Irish A.G.M. was held in one of the largest hotels in Dublin. The exhibition and trade show did not come cheap. There were many trade stands.   Names appearing over them included: Pfizer, Roche, Servier, Bayer, Novo Nordisk, Eli Lilly, Merck Sharpe & Dohme, Glaxo Smith Kline, Abbot and others. They were all there for a reason and the main one was not anybody's better health, '*IT WAS MONEY*', as they advertised and promoted their so called sickness aids. Splenda, the producers of the controversial and questionable artificial sweetener of that name had their logo emblazoned in many places at the Dublin exhibition. Splenda were the sponsors.

When I asked an official of the Diabetes Federation why they had accepted Splenda, the makers of the sucralose-based sweetener which may be harmful and is being criticised worldwide, as sponsors, the reply was, *"We find it almost impossible to find a sponsor, so we have to accept them"*. I see this as irresponsible.

It is obvious that there is nobody to promote a health show like this unless they can make money out of what they do. I suppose it was a little bit better from the point of view of having one of the major drug-manufacturing companies as sponsors. I took many photographs and talked with people, spending some considerable time asking questions. The several instances I let my feelings be known it could be said *'I was not popular with some of the personnel'*.

Danone offered one of their pretentious 'foods' which is additive-containing, all free of course, and when something is handed out for nothing, with a highlighted brand name like Danone, the elbows were needed to get to the bar. I asked why the ingredients were not printed on the container. I got a shrug of the shoulders. I knew from experience that they were listed on the exterior wrapper, so I proceeded to retrieve some from the waste bin. I then read out some of the contents to the users. Aspartame was prominent amongst other things not natural.

When I put it to personnel on the Diabetes Federation stand about diet and the need to avoid so much that is harmful for diabetics I was just fobbed off. Eventually I was referred to a woman who was completely gormless about natural foods or food additives or anything pertaining to natural way of living or good health. I felt afterwards that this was done on purpose in order to get rid of an interfering nobody like myself. I was like a thorn in the sides of many as I continued to castigate their methods of selling more and more sickness. See *Pretentious Foods* Caption.

I really enjoyed myself at the diabetes bazaar because that is what it appeared like to me.

The need for the nine words I use regularly were not of any interest as far as most of them were concerned. These nine words are **'WE ARE AS WE EAT, DRINK, SLEEP AND EXERCISE'.** One can also include the other slogan: **'CHANGE THE LIFESTYLE'.** Nowhere is this more applicable than if with diabetes, but even more importantly to prevent the disease.

Not one stand or area was set aside to advise people about diet, lifestyle or their mode of living. Nowhere was there a line about the 'dangers' of sugar. Nobody mentioned anything about fast and processed 'foods', the harmful additive-filled nosh being offered as sustenance today. As I have said, my nine words were irrelevant.

The only stand with anything natural being exhibited was Flahavans, the porridge oat producers

A large stand with a big sign reading **'Think Pharmacists First'** was surrounded by many people. The prominent sign on it also read **'Free**

Consultations'. Another sign said **'Thinking Cold or Flu – Medicines, Vitamins'**. There could or should have been added, "All Synthetic, far removed from the Natural, which the Health Food Shop provides." An extremely big sign said **'Your Local Health and Medicine Expert'**. As one who seldom has reason to visit the purveyors of synthetic chemicals, who are major outlets for the legalised drugs producing companies, I decided to look in, or shall I say look on. Here was further proof that sadly today all too many are ingrained with a line of thought that there are 'pills for all ills.'

I restate my thoughts that **"It is crystal clear that prescriptions are being issued unnecessarily, one could say whether the patient likes it or not".**

Studies show links between diabetes drugs, bone fractures, heart attacks, with other complications and side effects. The drug companies concerned deny there is a problem, quietly withdrawing a chemical when a big furore arises and then only when put under severe pressure. Nobody is ever prosecuted, even when deaths occur, because of what has been administered.

Nowhere at the diabetes trade show or A.G.Ms. did I see a stand, which could have had a sign **'Do You Know What You Are Eating'**? or **'Do You Give Thought To Diet or Lifestyle? Come In and Talk'**. Advice about prevention of diabetes was not available. The people behind the drugs and medical goods being promoted are not interested. I repeat, **"It pays them to keep people ill".**

I read through the annual report of the Diabetes Federation of Ireland, apparently the first ever for such a large society. There were a few lines which read as follows; *'In Ireland, and in most developed countries, the instance of Type 2 diabetes is increasing due to reduced physical activity levels of all age groups and the ingestion of more frequent meals/snacks especially convenience foods, which tend to have a higher content of saturated fat and refined sugar. Diabetes and its complications are responsible for a tremendous personal and public health burden of suffering at the present time'.* This was just news, with not a warning given to avoid these harmful and unhealthy foods or the grossly over sweetened drinks we are offered.

The Federation should have given precedence to having a large room, which could accommodate many. There, nutritionists, naturopaths and some who fully understand natural, pure foods and drinks, also food and drinks additives, could advise about either their uses or avoidance, also of the need for exercise and proper sleep. There are many nutritional experts who understand the natural fully, but are seldom heard of, who are apparently no friends of the Sickness Industry because of their natural leanings. This was all ignored as drugs and medicines were highlighted and promoted.

A section of the report told us of sessions of a countrywide Interactive Workshop run by the Diabetes Federation of Ireland. The reader was informed that '**The key focus of these sessions was highlighting the importance of making healthy food choices for all in the family, not just the person with diabetes**'. The sessions allowed parents to explore the particular challenges facing children with diabetes, in particular understanding the significance of carbohydrates for energy and in managing blood sugars. They encouraged parents to look at portion sizes and the impact this can have on blood sugar control. The role of exercise on managing the diabetes was also addressed and the necessary food or insulin adjustments required. <u>The sessions referred to were held at six venues throughout Ireland, with less than 100 people attending in all, despite being well-publicised. Here is a glaring example of the mind set of many within our community, especially when the sessions referred to were free.</u>

Those with diabetes, and especially parents, should remember that their health and that of their children is their own responsibility, nobody else's. All need education about health and prevention of ill-health, not medication. Here was a wonderful chance to learn about this, but sadly only availed of by a very small number. This proves that many take no responsibility for their own or their family's health, thinking that they can turn to the doctors when problems arise.

At the Diabetes U.K. A.G.M. the only difference was the bigger stands and huge attendance. An over-powering feeling hit me as I watched the all powerful drug conglomerates talking down to the general public. It is plain that many people have become obsessed with the use of medicines and drugs, as was all too evident there.

When I was a boy few attended doctors. I certainly did not when cold, flu, tonsillitis, mumps, measles or whatever a few days or a week in bed would cure. This is mentioned because on view at the shows were insulin pumps and other sophisticated apparatus. All this alarmed me. Much literature was available. Here again, nowhere could I find a word about lifestyle or how to live properly to attain better health.

You may ask, *"Why do you visit these conventions of the Diabetes Federation of Ireland and Diabetes U.K?"* I wish to be convinced that my 80 odd years old friend and myself, a younger but sprightly octogenarian, are right, also to make certain we have our facts correct. It was highly apparent that the synopsis of the Diabetes organisations of Ireland and the U.K. has been hijacked and is now an integral part of the Sickness Industry.

All of this has been astutely built up by the medics and the drug-manufacturing companies. An extract from the annual general report of the Diabetes Federation confirms this. Here are just two paragraphs, which justify my allegations or charge. *'In terms of turnover, the Federation has never had it so good and funds are being used effectively to support the ever increasing Diabetes community. The value of the many initiatives can be measured in terms of the number of people with diabetes who are supported by the Federation, the number of people detected early and the increased awareness of Diabetes among the wider community'.* Note the words *'detected early'*.

Just think that over three quarters of these people could be free from diabetes if the medics were not so hasty in detecting. The following paragraph is a typical case of how the Sickness Industry is promoted and enlarged. It is as follows; *'Therefore, it is now more important than ever, that pharmaceutical companies continue to support the Federation and that the Health Service Executive continue to provide grant-aid to ensure that our many services can be maintained'.* Here is a prime example of *selling sickness*.

Do the pharmaceutical companies who had stands taken, who are the legalised drug barons of our land, do anything for nothing? They are huge money making businesses, not benevolent funds. Whatever health problems people have, they are brought on invariably by themselves. **I reiterate that all must learn that prevention is all-important, vital.**

Diabetes can be prevented, reversed, and even cured. One does not hear this from the doctor. This is all the more reason why people look after themselves and learn that the doctors are there only if it is absolutely necessary to pay a visit. The only time I find them helpful is on my yearly visit for what can be called an N.C.T. in Ireland or an M.O.T. in the UK, the annual check-up I advise all to have.

IN ORDER TO EDUCATE AND CORRECT THE ATTITUDE OF THE MEDICAL PROFESSION, OUR GOVERNMENT, THROUGH THE HEALTH SERVICE EXECUTIVE, WHICH IS THE HUB OF THE SICKNESS INDUSTRY, NEEDS TO TAKE THE LIFE AND DEATH, CRUCIAL, AND VERY WORRYING MATTER OF DIABETES VERY SERIOUSLY. TO BEGIN WITH THEY CAN TELL PEOPLE THE TRUTH ABOUT THE MANY USELESS DRUGS BEING USED AND THE NEED FOR PROPER LIFESTYLE.

SOME OF THIS IS SET OUT IN *'THE NATIONAL OBESITY TASK FORCE REPORT'* ALSO *'THE NATIONAL NUTRITION POLICY DOCUMENT'*, BOTH OF WHICH ARE APPARENTLY SHELVED, BEING GIVEN NO PUBLICITY. THIS IS SIMPLY BECAUSE, IF FOLLOWED STEADFASTLY, THERE WOULD BE LITTLE NEED FOR CHEMICAL DRUGS OR THEIR PRODUCTION AND PRESCRIBING. THE SICKNESS INDUSTRY AS WE KNOW IT NOW, WOULD BE DEFUNCT, EXTINCT.

Prevention, and above all, the treatment being prescribed so inaccurately, all too loosely, by the doctors, needs to be dealt with **now. NOW means immediately.**

The doctors and drug companies are running amok amongst the all too trusting patients, as the medics present the prescription pad as if they were holy people on a bible crusade. The difference is that the medicos and chemical drug purveyors are there for serious money. The scandal of diabetes diagnosis is that the majority do not have diabetes when diagnosed. As I have said, *"Many, many healthy people are unnecessarily being put on drugs for life"*. The detection, recognition and prescribing methods for diabetes are totally flawed. **IT IS A DISGRACE, A NATIONAL SCANDAL.**

It appears that the doctors do not want to know about the legitimacy of the outcome of the survey carried out by their fellow professionals. The main reason would of course be the danger of customer/patient loss or the consequences of the non-use of the prescription pad, their cash till. Diabetes is a lucrative money-spinner. It is beyond belief that simple words of advice, as set out by the survey team as already referred to, would reduce the instances of diabetes by some 70%. Here is further proof, if proof is needed, that the Sickness Industry is going down the wrong road in the erroneous and over-prescribing of pills, potions and medicines. Just imagine that 700 out of every 1,000 people diagnosed as having diabetes or being merely borderline, if that, are put on drugs for life. The epidemic of diabetes we hear about is sheer deception by the G.Ps.

I have helped many be free from the health problem, especially in recent years. A list of names of those identified as being diabetic, now made well, has been compiled. These, all too trusting patients, were wrongly advised or diagnosed by doctors who told them they had diabetes. **With a change of lifestyle and better way of living being advised, all are well, free from diabetes.**

To prevent the disease, a wonderful aid to better health is that of the use of Vitamin D3. One 1000 iu. capsule, from the health food store, taken daily, is a wonderful assurance for future better health, including prevention of diabetes. It must be taken with a diet of pure non-processed, additive free, unadulterated foods or drinks. Exercise and sleep patterns frequently need monitoring.

Adults and children who have a diet lacking in Vitamin D3 very often go on to develop diabetes, with symptoms of rickets now being diagnosed. Here again your health food store can help. See **Vitamin D3** caption.

RHODIOLA

This is a wonderful root extract, which can be purchased from your health food store in tablet or capsule form. Up to some years ago I was very dubious about Rhodiola, having had no experience of and with only some reports of its goodness. As a cynic, also being a questioner, I need convincing about the goodness of anything which is taken into the body. Rhodiola is an adaptogenic herb which helps boost performance of body and mind. It contains Flavonoids, which include Salidroside and Rosavin. It is excellent for fighting fatigue, improving mood and alleviating depression, but I must keep stressing that no medicine, natural or synthetic, will work on its own to help one to better health. The base is pure, non-processed, additive free food or drinks. Pure food is essential for better health, being a must in order to help be free from depression or other illness. Rhodiola will then prove to be an excellent aid. I have had much feedback about this herbal supplement, all of it very favourable. Because of this I have taken Rhodiola myself over the past few years and can highly recommend it for its aid to better outlook on life.

LEARNING

Anyone who stops learning is old, whether 20 or 80.
Anyone who stays learning stays young.
The greatest thing in life is to keep the mind young.
- Henry Ford

CHOLESTROL

HOW HIGH IS LOW CHOLESTROL? THE RIP OFF AND DECEPTION WHICH IS STATINS – CHOLESTEROL – STATINS

A few years ago I visited the doctor for annual check up, which in my talks, lectures and writings I advise all to have yearly. The first words uttered by the G.P. were, *"I'll check your Cholesterol"*. I stood up and rightly in my opinion looked down on the medic as he sat in front of a computer. I told him in no uncertain manner what I believe to be true, as do many who understand the cholesterol and statins related con and fallacy. *"This cholesterol lark"*, I said, *"Is an almighty scam and it is utter deception. Cholesterol is not a disease. It may perhaps be a symptom of heart disease or blocked arteries. This too is highly debatable"*. While his *'I'll check your cholesterol'* words had I am sure raised my blood pressure I continued, *"Until the Mercks, Warner Lamberts and later the Pfizers of the chemical drug-manufacturing and producing world latched onto a Japanese idea for another invented disease, now called cholesterol, it was unknown"*.

The word cholesterol, which up to recent years was not in our vocabulary or dictionary, except for a few lines, which were totally different from today's interpretation, has only come into being commercially in recent years. It originates from the old medical term, again difficult to find, Hypercholesterolaemia. Cholesterol is now an invented sickness of the drug companies, which the medics and drug giants have almost brain washed people into believing is a serious disorder.

Only later did I appreciate the fact that the doctor, whom I had talked down to, making no apology for this fact, had sat calmly through my reprimanding of him, without uttering a word. It struck me that perhaps he knew about the scam, which like the majority of the medical profession, he is part of. He made no answer. I had my annual check up, getting the all clear. If one is disciplined enough to follow the maxim *'WE ARE AS EAT, DRINK, SLEEP AND EXERCISE'*, following this through diligently, then the cholesterol and blood pressure levels should be normal.

I repeat, if all followed this advice also putting into practice the three words *'CHANGE YOUR LIFESTYLE'*, our hospitals would be less than one quarter full. I honestly believe this all comes from experience gained over the past 45 years, that if one monitors the blood pressure regularly, every four or five days, then keeping it right, one is well over 80% per cent of the way to better health. A good and easily read blood pressure monitor is a reminder to keep well. It is an invaluable investment.

There are of course those with what are called genetic problems. For instance there are those with extremely high readings of cholesterol, where medication will not lower it. Nobody dies from high cholesterol. I know a woman with a reading of 11. It cannot be lowered. This lady monitors her blood pressure almost daily and is in excellent good health. **Using my advice about healthy body weight she has lost 22 pounds (10 kilo) in 16 months.** I have had many others visit me who have cholesterol readings of eight and nine. All too many die from heart disease also stroke, as a result of high blood pressure. If people paid more attention to the heart and none to the cholesterol levels they would enjoy much better health. I repeat again and again, **pay attention to lifestyle**. See **Lifestyle** caption.

Most people who visit doctors are browbeaten, propagandised, and duped into the idiocy of the words which raise my blood pressure, *"I'll check your cholesterol".* It is nothing more than just a money-spinner operated by the medics and the drug companies. The relationship between them is all too cosy and intimate. This has been referred to on numerous occasions by those responsible in their own professional, supposedly regulatory, bodies. Despite glib talk also plausible admonition about correcting this incompatible, almost cartel like system, who does anything? Like much in the Sickness Industry, which is our Health Service Executive, the answer is '**NOBODY**'.

I cannot help emphasising throughout this book that people are being frightened into accepting the hype about cholesterol. For example, we are almost brow beaten into the belief that most of the margarine type spreads also butter substitutes will lower cholesterol. We already have warnings about cholesterol being too low and the dangers which can arise from this. When people buy these supposedly cholesterol lowering spreads this is working even further to lower the cholesterol figure. In simple words **'there is no proper control over how low one can go'**. This can be highly dangerous healthwise.

At my talks throughout the country, also in the shops where this oily processed margarine or butter look-alike stuff is sold, or elsewhere, frequently I question people about the various branded or so-called cholesterol lowering aids. With the very odd exception none realise what is in the carton or container. They don't read the labels. I asked, *"Why do you buy it?"* The answer is, *"I hear about it, or I see it advertised"*. The majority believe the advertising hype.

It should be added that people who understand about the ingredients, or are health conscious, leave those which contain additives on the shelf. They too, like myself, are fully aware that if a balanced diet of pure, unadulterated and natural food and drink is taken into the bodily system, plus some daily exercise, such as walking, and with proper sleep pattern, there is no need for these kind of processed, oily, overly hyped concoctions. The ordinary citizen is being duped into believing the jargon, not realising what is necessary by way of nourishment. The giant multi-nationals who promote this type of stuff have the lucre, the riches, to advertise persistently. See *Margarine* caption

We hear of the Food Safety Authority questioning the claims of the manufacturers, especially those who promote and advertise the spreads. If they are not satisfied then how can these products become part of the gigantic Sickness Industry. Some of these 'foods' contain what are called plant sterols, substances similar to cholesterol. Where humans need cholesterol, plants use the sterols for their nutrition. The human body does not retain these sterols and it is doubtful if anybody knows exactly how plant sterols work when they enter the digestive system. No matter what we are told, it is not just normal to absorb these 'foods' from the necessary amounts of plant sterols required daily for better health. Another factor is of their being mixed with 'food' and 'drinks' additives, which makes the whole process unnatural, no matter what ingredients are there. Turn to *Probiotic and Functional Foods* caption

If and when somebody shows me and gives me the evidence that all who consume the greasy products have benefited from their use, then I might retract some of my way of thinking. When taken with a diet of fast, processed, sugary, unnatural food and drinks, then it would be impossible to find evidence that they are beneficial. This logic, that they work in conjunction with or if taken with a balanced diet is meaningless, because a balanced diet of good food on its own is the answer to attaining better health. Sadly the majority do not understand what a balanced diet is.

Many I know, including myself, eat a balanced diet of pure food because we have learned fully to understand its meaning. We don't use margarine, butter substitutes or so called probiotics.

When healthy people are prescribed statins for what is described as high cholesterol they are on them for life. It is like the medic making a sale, which is a recurring one. I have not mentioned the pharmacists, who also benefit enormously. Not health-wise I add, but money-wise. What about the side effects of chemical drugs such as statins or indeed any drug? People give little thought to the chemicals being put into the body. Indeed little thought is given to anything partaken of. Fast, additive-filled and processed foods are an example of the 'garbage' or junk put into the most highly intricate system in the universe.

The supposedly cholesterol lowering statins or drugs curb, repress or stop the enzyme required to make cholesterol in the liver. They block the manufacturing of required nutrients such as Coenzyme Q10, which is known to benefit the health of the heart, and is indeed vital for many facets of better health. A huge side effect is that the statin drugs very often result in weakening also exhausting pain, in muscles and joints, with resulting tiredness and fatigue.

It is coincidence that a gentleman telephoned as I put these words on paper. He told me how his wife had been put on statins some months ago and had terrible symptoms such as described in this caption. **He said "Siobhan was in agony until deciding to throw the statins on the coal fire". These are his words.** Daily I get telephone calls asking for advice or how I can help the various health problems so many have. In some cases, just like this query, it is as a result of side effects of chemical drugs. I don't tell anybody what to do. I just tell them what I do or what I would do. They can then form their own conclusions after I have spoken with them. I repeat *"I certainly would not take statins or other drugs. I would not use margarine, butter substitutes, probiotics or anything processed or with additives. Almost all are unnatural, with little, if any, nutritive value."* They can be referred to as dead products.

Over the years I have told many that if lifestyle is changed the results can be dramatic. Cholesterol, blood pressure, depression, stress and hundreds of ailments can be a thing of the past. I repeat, **"The responsibility for people's health is in their own hands."** The pills for all ills mind-set, which is all too evident, is totally wrong. I reiterate that side effects from the use of statins include liver problems, bone and muscle pain, headaches, stomach pains, skin rash, nausea and much more. As I have stated, many people have told me of the effects of taking prescribed or indeed over the counter drugs. These include statins

A woman taking statins related that after three weeks she had some of the symptoms I have set out. More frightening was that she thought she was having a stroke. Like so many who have told me of their side effects problems, she gave them up and like all the others who did so, felt so much better. She stringently practices my advice about blood pressure, which is now normal. Like the many who have changed their lifestyles to help get the blood pressure normal this lady told me of how she feels so well now, having much energy.

When healthy people can be put on statins for a non-existent disease it is an almighty disgrace, bordering on the criminal. I repeat myself intentionally when I say many healthy people are being prescribed chemical drugs they probably don't need. Before 1980, cholesterol was almost an unknown word, except to certain chemical drug manufacturers, who were working furiously on the development of statins. It was not until the year 2000 that the word statin appeared in the Oxford Concise Medical Dictionary. Now the sales of the drug run into billions of euro or dollars annually. Here is non-existent ailment invention and **selling of sickness** on a colossal scale.

From 1985 to 2006, prescriptions issued for statins in the U.K. increased by almost 15,000%. There have been huge increases in the prescribing of Statins from 2006 to date for which no figures are available. Perhaps one reason for this is that the almost obscene over use of the prescription pad, the doctors cash till, might be discovered. I use the word obscene because it is disgusting, a bloody disgrace, that hundreds of thousands of people who are quite healthy should be made to accept advice which condemns them to a life time of taking chemical pills such as statins, which there is no need for whatsoever. In simple language these people prescribing them, whom I have previously referred to as 'pickpockets', are making billions for the drug companies, themselves and the pharmacies, by prescribing for invented illness.

The indoctrinated (no pun here) public are worried by the hype of what is supposed to be a serious ailment. Almost daily people speak with me about their supposedly high cholesterol. I repeat, a symptom it may be, but this is highly questionable. It is certainly not a sickness. It is nothing to worry about. I repeat again and again **"Keep the blood pressure levels corrected naturally, living a proper lifestyle, then all should be well".** Turn to *Blood Pressure* caption.

The Government of the day, and that includes the Health Service Executive which is the Sickness Industry, will not utter a word of condemnation. All are in it for the scandalous money being extorted from the supposedly ill. The Government will not act, knowing that the employment given, plus P.A.Y.E. and many other taxes paid into their coffers by the Sickness Industry associates will repay them many times over in the long term.

Regularly we learn that the country is now bankrupt. It would be crippled, impoverished, if the drug companies were liquidated. Maybe asking GOD to solve the Sickness Industry problems might help.

Ask anybody within the medical profession what the levels of cholesterol should be. Different people I speak with give me varying answers, none of them similar. When put on statins the patient given the prescription very often does not know what his or her reading is. Very many don't even ask. Ask the person taking the reading, often to be cutely dismissed or brushed off. I know all this from experience and from that of the many I speak with. Having written to the major manufacturers of statins, asking what is the safe cholesterol figure aimed for and what can the cholesterol reading be, both high and low, before it is considered dangerous. I have not had the courtesy of one reply, despite registering some of the letters of enquiry.

Recently, when at the wedding of my granddaughter in the U.K., I was introduced to a doctor and his wife, who is a nurse. When I aired my views regarding statins and cholesterol the G.P. agreed with me fully. His thoughts and words were more forceful and vigorous than mine in his condemnation of the statins and cholesterol charade. He was vehement when he spoke. I quote his words which I have on my pocket memo, which I always carry with me. It is like my camera, a good friend. When I asked what the levels of cholesterol are he said, *"Nobody really knows. When statins were promoted and marketed first the sales were minimal. We were told that a reading of eight was the norm. Then it came down to seven, then six, and eventually five. Then we were told varying figures be it five and a half and even four. Only a few weeks ago, when at my doctor friend's clinic, he told me he had a patient call for a check-up, where cholesterol reading was 2.4. The person concerned had been on statins for two weeks and there and then gave them up. He handed the statin drugs to my friend, the doctor, telling him to destroy them. There must be many like this patient, now no longer one, who realise that they have been sold the con, which is cholesterol, and who now spurn the drugs. This figure was dangerously low. It seems that the figures are pulled out of space. Does this not point to this being a scam as you say? What many don't realise is that when a person is prescribed statins that the lowering constituents are working all the time, therefore the person consuming the drug is at serious risk of too low a reading".* The doctor continued, " *Very often those who are taking statins may be consuming some of the products touted as 'cholesterol lowering'. This is where dangers arise. You rightly mentioned the seriousness of the relationship between low cholesterol and Parkinson's Disease, also the various health problems that can arise. I am part of this money rip off myself. It is costing the state billions, all for nothing. Me, and my profession, just flow with the tide, keeping our criticism and condemnations quiet. Pfizer's have artfully and cunningly been in the vanguard of marketing statins. They are chief amongst those who set the targets."* Remember this comes from a seemingly honest doctor. There are not many of them left.

Apart from the extremely serious and disturbing aspect of statins interfering with the necessary Coenzyme Q10 is the fact that too low cholesterol is highly dangerous to one's health. Let's revert to the vitally important Coenzyme Q10. This is said to enhance stamina, benefit heart and circulation, good to help reduce high blood pressure and to aid irregular heartbeat. It is good for gums and teeth and may help to prevent Alzheimer's disease also being an anti-aging aid. Already referred to is the relationship between Coenzyme Q10 and Parkinson's Disease

The very fact that statins interfere with these all so necessary aids to the healthy working of the body system and especially the prevention of Parkinson's and Alzheimer's Disease, tells all that it is time to shout **'ENOUGH IS TOO MUCH'.** Why nobody steps in to cry halt does not surprise me. In the greed for money, with statins having captivated the G.Ps., **'NOBODY'** will interfere. *Selling sickness*, such as high cholesterol, is a crying shame.

A few years ago news headlines and also many reports told of how one major drug manufacturer had dropped what was referred to as a new cholesterol drug. We learned that it was another cholesterol chemical to replace their popular brand, which was highly prescribed. This was coming off patent in the near future so the failed chemical was to be lined up as another money-spinner. The headlines in the newspapers gave some background to the failure, even telling us of the resultant side effects upon people who can now be looked upon as guinea pigs. The media was much more concerned with the loss of jobs as a result of the shut down. Questions can be asked **"Is there co-relation between the stopping of this drug and the fact that the statin producers have come too far down the figure scale over the years in telling doctors what the levels of Cholesterol should be?"** They can't lower their figures anymore in this extremely profitable, remunerative, travesty or sham. **Have they decided enough is enough in their lowering of the figures over the years? Have they agreed that we are perhaps below the danger line, where the side effects are really coming to light as reported in the many surveys being carried out? Do they now realise that there is huge evidence that lack of Coenzyme Q10, due to statin use, may cause Parkinson's or lead to Alzheimer's disease, perhaps many other health problems for which this enzyme is so vital?**

Despite the outcome or seriousness of this report and evidence, we find so called experts like Profession Peter Weissberge of the British Heart Foundation telling us that nobody should stop taking statins on the basis of the report. He speaks for the medical bods. There are many others, like myself, who are far from being experts, but we know differently. Our line of thinking is that, **'Statins are an insult to the thinking of the general public'.**

Other 'eggheads' or 'know-alls' have said it is unlikely that statins cause Parkinson's disease. If so, then why was the report released? The vast majority of them know little about Coenzyme Q10 or that it is available in natural supplement form, from the health food store. Whether it be food additives, chemical drugs, pills and medicines, even alcohol, the lobbies and quangos, especially in the Sickness Industry, are so powerful and the money to be gained so enormous that the health and well being of all is given scant consideration. After use of some of the chemical drugs prescribed, people have to die before action is taken and even then there must be more than one fatality. Single figures mean nothing except to those who are left bereaved.

It is evident that Pfizer's, Merck and other statin processors are now going down another road, that of increasing and promoting the sales of statins being produced. Throughout the world, we hear of proposals for statins to be prescribed for millions, the majority probably in good health. This can mean all of us. If the medical profession, aided by the drug companies, have their way, all will be on this chemical.

We are told of proposals to prescribe statins to all young and old, even if healthy, for the prevention of heart attacks, even for use by those over the age of 80. It has even been touted as being a water additive. All this despite there being no evidence whatsoever that heart attacks are being prevented by their use.

The use of statins in the U.K. and on the N.H.S., which is free for those with medical cards in Ireland, is costing the users and taxpayers more and more daily. The figures are astronomical. The more I see, hear, read and talk about the statin and cholesterol relationship the more I realise that Dr. Malcolm Kendrick in his book *'The Great Cholesterol Con'* is right in his findings. For details see *Bibliography* section. Dr. Kendrick tells us much, in well-chosen words. In one paragraph he wrote, *"I am not alone in my beliefs. There are many hundreds of doctors and researchers who agree that the cholesterol hypothesis is bunk. Many keep their counsel, others have been silenced, but a few have had the guts to speak out. However, their voices, unlike those of the implacable medical 'statinators', are not supported by a multi billion-dollar pharmaceutical budget".* This sensible medical man tells us *"I am deadly serious in my belief that the misguided war against cholesterol, using statins, represents something close to a crime against humanity. So close, that you may not be able to spot the difference".*

Dr. John Briffa, in his enlightening and informative natural news articles on www.drbriffa.com tells us *"All rationality and common sense seems to fly out the window when certain doctors and scientists start talking about cholesterol. When it comes to the science, it's clear that many are ignorant of or choose to ignore the stacks of evidence that clearly contradict their stance".* Need one dwell more on this cholesterol deceit.

In this book, *Selling Sickness*!, I am delighted to be associated with so many people who realise that **STATINS, CHOLESTEROL, ALSO CHOLESTEROL LEVELS, ARE AN ALMIGHTY SCAM, LET'S CALL IT 'DAYLIGHT ROBBERY'. At the same time I am saddened that our legislators have not had the fore-thought to recognise that there is outlandish selling of sickness for ailments other than cholesterol, with no curb or restriction placed on the issuing of prescriptions.**

OMEGA OILS – DO WE NEED THEM?

Only in recent years have we heard of Omega oils. Omega has always been known as the 24th and last letter of the Greek alphabet. The word is now used to describe what to the body are essential fatty acids (E.F.As.), namely Omegas 3 & 6. The fatty acids we refer to were being investigated as far back as the 1930's but in a trivial manner. It was not until the 1980's that the man who pioneered, researched and did more technical work on Omega oils than anybody else, offered us what is the most natural, pure and to me, also those who use it, the very best, namely, '**Udo's Choice Ultimate Oil Blend**'. It is better known as '**Udo's Oil**'. This blend contains the ideal amounts of Omega 3 & 6 oils.

Dr. Udo Erasmus is an international authority on fats, oils, cholesterol and human health. In 1980 his life took a significant turn when he was poisoned by pesticides. When conventional medicine was unable to provide help, he concluded that his health was his own responsibility and turned his attention to nutrition. Several years of research culminated in his best selling book, '*Fats That Heal, Fats That Kill,*' which earned him a PhD in nutrition. See *Bibliography* caption

In 1983, he began to pioneer technology for pressing and packaging edible, fresh oils, made with better health in mind, under the exclusion of the three main factors which can transform nutritious oils into what may be toxic ones. This latter includes light, heat, and oxygen. Until that time, oils were very often highly processed with destructive results, sacrificing health benefits in order to attain long shelf life. Indeed, many still are. Most cooking oils are an example of this.

I hold no brief for Omega Oils, including '**Udo's Choice**', but when I see the hype and commercialisation blurb that is Omega Oil today I just think to myself, '*Here is another money-making effort*'. After Dr. Udo Erasmus's success, where he seems to have left no stone and many seed grains unturned in his analysis and study, this was the green light for all too many to jump on what appeared to be and now is the Omega 'gravy train'.

Many so-called 'foods', including certain margarines, probiotics, milk, bread, and many other things offered as nutrition, claim to contain these essential fatty acids. One sees Omega printed in absurd places. Most of this indoctrination or publicity should be taken cynically or viewed with much suspicion. Let's use an old fashioned saying, '*It should be taken with a pinch of salt*'

These oils are regarded as being essential because the body does not make them. Even when the various products supposedly have Omega 3 in them, the essential 6 can be missing. In the processing the polyunsaturates can be turned into *'Trans fatty acids'.* The goodness is destroyed by improper processing, as with fast foods.

Many of those who promote, manufacture and in many cases process Omega Oils, conveniently ignore the intense or high importance of the correct ratios of Omega 3 and Omega 6 oils. One or other on its own can be dangerous, leading to ill health. Read, view or listen to the propaganda, which is not too strong a word to use, as the need for Omega 3 is highlighted, much of it bunkum. This is where Dr. Udo's early pioneering work holds the trump card over all other Omega Oils. What he promotes is correctly balanced. I hold no brief for any oils, just giving facts.

Like much in the food industry, especially regarding Omegas 3 & 6, we can certainly ask, *"Who do we believe, who do we trust"?*

In my archives, I mean my attic and elsewhere in filing cabinets, there is much which has been collected on the subject. It is preposterous that medical journalists, who supposedly write on health topics, can get away with what appear to be their views. All too often they do not give concise facts. In front of me are twenty-two sheets of A4 paper, all writing about and promoting the good of Omega 3 oils. Very seldom are we told about Omega 6. It is all about the need for Omega 3. I do know that there is a need for proper balanced intake of Omegas 3 & 6. These hacks should either give true facts, where health is concerned, or cease giving versions which can be terribly misleading, even injurious to health.

To be sure of the natural, visit an independent health food store and speak with the staff about the oils. These have all been formulated, using natural ingredients. The three main factors, which can turn nutritious oils into toxic ones – light, heat and oxygen, have been carefully monitored. This is vital for a pure natural and correct blend of Omega Oils. The Oils I write about and suggest the use of, are formulated from Genetically Modified <u>Free</u> Seeds, whereas many other brands are not.

Being told that fish oils are the best source of Omega is highly debatable. Scientists and so-called experts tell us that fish oil is far superior to seed oils as Omega Oils. As with many who have vested interests, we were informed by them that fish oils break down and are ingested quicker and to a greater degree than plant or seed oils. At the time of writing this idea has been disproved, with the opposite being the case. It is not coincidence that it is only recently we hear this, when over the years '**Udo's Oil**' presented no problems in this respect. The fact that fish oil only produces Omega 3 makes the debate more contentious. It is much easier to control the producing of proper ratio of Omega 3 and Omega 6 when using pure vegetable seeds. This, as I have stated, is vitally important. Here again pure is pure.

Dr. Udo Erasmus has done his research and calculations extremely well. For this reason I have much faith in his product. I do not agree with his daily requirement instructions. Using, as instructed on the label, I feel that one third to a half of what he suggests is sufficient daily. Using it this way it is much less expensive to obtain the required Omega 3 & 6 oils.

We are frequently being warned that our fish stocks are dangerously low. Only recently we heard that if over fishing is allowed to continue, as it is now, our stocks of fish will be near to extinction by 2050.

Very often when the question of Omega Oils, and other supposedly Omega containing oily fats, spreads or so called foods are mentioned or read about, I say *"How did we manage?"* As mentioned already Omega oils have only been touted very recently.

Today many eat food on the 'run'. The family, or indeed any group, seldom sit down to three meals daily of pure, natural, unprocessed, nutritious foods, like the older generations have been used to. Because of the lifestyle our Sickness Industry is booming, especially in recent years. If one puts into practice and diligently follows the maxim *'WE ARE AS EAT, DRINK, SLEEP AND EXERCISE'* the outlay would be little, if any, for drugs or remedies and that includes Omega Oils. I have to admit I keep a bottle of '**Udo's Oil**' in my fridge, all too often finding that it has been used by another family member.

Dr. Udo Erasmus found that nature always provides us with the tools we need to Heal and Thrive: Pure Water, Clean Air, Sunlight and Wholesome Nutritious Foods and Drinks, which give us the energy to exercise. These basic elements of nature, when used as a primary health care, will build strong and healthy bodies. Grass roots solutions to modern health concerns lie within our diet. Essential, natural, and unprocessed fats, enzymes, greens, natural probiotics, such as Super 8 and fibre are healthy foods, provided by nature, that can create better health and longevity by providing:

Nutrition: foods that contain the nutrients required to support our bodies thousands of normal functions.

Detoxification: the removal of toxins from our bodies that interferes with our built in programmes for health. Pure food and drinks with a proper lifestyle is as detoxification. **Detoxification, as we see it advertised regularly, is nonsense. Let pure natural unadulterated food be the medicine required. This is detoxing at its best.**

Proper Digestion: The correct breakdown of foods to facilitate the absorption of nutrients. When these foods are eaten and chewed properly, with nature in them, they act as natural, healthy supplements, with the ability to nourish and cleanse and so are powerful tools for good or better health.

A simple and inexpensive way of taking Omega 3 is to obtain Flax Seeds (Linseed), in its pure state, from the health food store. Grind in a liquidiser by putting in small amounts at a time, just sufficient to reach the tips of the grinding knives, in order to bring it almost to a powder. Store in a closed container and take one dessertspoonful on porridge at breakfast time and a second helping in the evening. Chopping and making the seeds into powder gives maximum benefit from the linseed.

MARGARINE – THE 'UNHEALTHY SCANDAL'

I cannot imagine there are many with a hobby of collecting empty food, pharmaceutical drug and natural remedy containers or packaging. My collection includes cartons, tubs, boxes, bags, crisp bags, plastic, glass, aerosol propellant substitute cream containing canisters, and other bottles or containers. At one time some of them contained foods, drinks and other items sold as food, much of it 'foodless', with little if any nutrition. Some of it was undoubtedly harmful to the body, no aid to better or good health, having been processed and with much unnatural added. Additives such as hydrogenated oils, monosodium glutomate and aspartame are three that come to mind.

The medicine, pills and health food store packaging is kept separate from those which contained food or drinks. **This packaging has been collected to record the hundreds of ingredients, additives, and the 'E' numbers used, all to provide much of which is just 'rubbish' and pretentious food.**

In front of me are dozens of margarine containers from past years up to the present. I repeat myself many times in this guide book, *Selling Sickness!,* when I ask *"Do you read the ingredients labels?"* If not then you do not realise the amount of additives which are in much of the so-called food on offer, including almost all margarines and so called butter substitutes.

Over time, but more especially in recent years, the wording on the plastic margarine containers has been changed dramatically. The margarine does not appear to have changed in texture, colour or taste. Some of the ingredients supposedly have, if one can bring oneself to trust the processors. We hear about trans fats, low and high fats, saturated and polyunsaturated fats, omega 3, with little, if any emphasis on omega 6, lo and high cal, also many additives, some with unpronounceable names. The person who shops for food is almost bamboozled. A lot of what we are led to believe in the advertising of these is balderdash and nonsense. When you have finished reading this article or caption I think you will have to agree that many of those who continue to churn out margarine and butter substitute spreads are not to be trusted. Similarly with much else offered as 'food' and 'drink'.

Let me take you back to the early part of the last century. To the writer, at some 80 odd years of age, that is not so long ago. The grease, which is margarine, was not being well received then by the people or the bureaucrats of most countries. There was much resistance to its use, even by Governments   Over the years changes and more changes were made to the product. Throughout those early years boiled fats were being used as the chief ingredient. It was discovered that hydrogenated oil might be the answer to some of the problems of producing margarine. Later still they turned to vegetable oils to make it appear better.   The oils were still hydrogenated in the manufacturing process and perhaps still are. The fierce competition changed the approach to selling the margarines.

Highly promoted and advertised, sales of the butter look-alike substitutes took off astonishingly. This was no doubt due to the advertising promotion of what was supposedly a 'healthy' butter substitute. Much emphasis was placed on its low fat content also its 'health' giving virtues. Little did the people realise what they were being offered.

In the early 1990s there were rumblings about the margarine industry, that the processed spreads had serious 'designer faults', to use an engineering term. This was discovered by those who were interested in better health, including those who wished to expose the pap for what it was and perhaps still may be. **The world was told that hydrogenated oils are highly questionable and could be a forerunner of bad health. Yes, we were informed that the highly processed oils could help clog up the veins, arteries and capillaries of those who used the margarines, imitation butters, or other 'foods' containing the oils.**

The manufacturers and processors tried to play down the utter seriousness of this discovery. There were claims, counter - claims, even denial on their part. **They would, wouldn't they?** They had made billions by unloading the hydrogenated oil based margarines on the unwitting and trusting public. This was just not over a short period but for many years, for decades. **Who knows what the consequences HEALTHWISE have been?**

The bubble burst, so to speak, as the truth about the 'dangers' of hydrogenated oils and fats emerged and were made public. It is a disgrace, totally wrong, one could safely describe it as a crime, that for decades the gullible public may have had 'disease giving', unnatural and processed

155

spreads foisted on them.   Yes, for decades, margarines have had hydrogenated oils and fats in their make-up, being chief amongst their main ingredients. Maybe turned into harmful trans fats in the processing, these perhaps damaging or lethal products have been ingested into the bodies of the altogether unsuspecting partaker

When the 'guilty' party's filibuster was faced up to they had no alternative other than to change their highly questioned methods once again.   They then maintained that they had backed out of using hydrogenated oils or fats. All of this was kept extremely quiet.

My collection of margarine boxes amassed up to that time was now more valuable.   Yes, not money wise, but as to the evidence of the seriousness of what had been sold as 'healthy' spreads, but which contained the suspect hydrogenated oils.

Within a short time the ingredients labels of the margarine containers read differently. They were changed by the processors, the manufacturers.   Suddenly we read *'No hydrogenated fats'.*   Within one to two years these words too were removed.   I deliberately use the words *astutely* or *cunningly* to describe this.   Why?   Because replacing the now dreaded hydrogenated oil or fats words were vegetable oils.   Now all very stealthily we see no reference to hydrogenated fats or oils.   All this was quietly and conveniently forgotten about. **OR IS IT?**

We have been left to sit or stand and stare, as we ponder and speculate on the audacity of these hypocrites who perpetrutated what might be considered as bordering on a crime against humanity.   I use the word hypocrites purposely because they sold the butter like, 'but not like', substances, telling us of its health value, when it was allegedly 'not safe'. Then they just changed their methods and procedures. All this, apparently without interruption, as they continued their almost similar ways of processing.   After their carry on of the past, who would trust them, no matter what they say about the oils, the methods or the additives used, being changed?

The margarine refiners as a result of the bombshell findings, that hydrogenated fats were unacceptable, now had to find another method to produce the grease like substance.   They had extricated themselves in the past, so enter here two words. 1. Fractionation. 2. Interesterification.   Try pronouncing the latter word!   All very interesting!

The fats, additives, and other processed ingredients could not be left out.   They were cheap.   Economics played a huge part in what had to be retained.   One doubts that health was anywhere on the list when change was urgently needed.   Now instead of hydrocracking of fats, or the use of hydrogen or other source being added to the fats substances treatment, they are interesterified. Various types of oils are used in the processing and conversion.

Interesterification has been known about for years but it is clear that many scientists, nutritionists and even those in the higher echelons of the food industry knew little about it. They did not have to. Until the margarine manufactures were forced into using it as a processing method because of the hydrogenation 'scare' there was little interest in the subject. Indeed the bods knew little about hydrogenation and now even less is know about interesterification.

This whole area of fats, trans fats and a multitude of fats is like entering a maze. The minds of those who use them in manufacturing, change frequently. **Eating purely natural, non-processed, additive free foods such as pure butter, is the only way to avoid them.**

Interesterification, like hydrogenation, produces molecules that are not natural. It hardens fat, but supposedly without producing oils that contain trans fats. Already questions are being asked about its use. Many remain unanswered.

Vegetable oils, when used in margarine processing, have been altered through chemical treatment, being no longer natural. When this happens they can be 'harmful' to health. Interesterified fats are now in much processed foods where cooking oils were or are being used. These include: margarines, fried foods, butter substitute spreads, chips, crisps, pastries, salad dressings and mayonnaise, breakfast cereals, crackers and confectionary. Even very many of the cooking oils on display can contain these 'contentious' fats.

Virgin cold pressed oils are excellent. Safflower oil, cold pressed and organic, is the Queen or King of cooking oils. It is pure, natural, being available from the health food store. It must be added here that a dessertspoon of Safflower oil, taken night and morning, is a marvellous aid to better health. See *Healthy Body Weight* caption.

As with the hydrogenated oils and fats 'scandal', can we believe anybody in the food processing industry? Because interesterified oils and fats have been in use as a substitute for partially hydrogenated oils in recent years, the process is not classified as a new additive or method. In the circumstances it was just a matter of change of routine and procedure. All quite simple, with little thought as to whether the produce is safer than the removed hydrogenated oils. With questions already being asked about the relationship between interesterification and better health, let us hope it does not take as long to deliver the outcome of tests being carried out as it did to inform us of the seemingly 'harmful' hydrogenated oils. In the meantime, we have interestified oils offered to us, being told of their goodness in relation to health. All who are interested in better health, like myself, will wait and see. Those who know nothing about the margarine 'scare', because of the silence, will continue to use the stuff to their 'disservice'.

You may well ask *"How do I avoid dangerous fats in food?* The answer is, as already laboured on, *"Eat nothing processed or with additives and that includes margarine or processed spreads, including butter substitutes. All are unnatural. "*

John Lonergan retired after 42 years in the prison service. He was governor of Mountjoy prison in Dublin for 22 of these. He was a young prison officer in Limerick jail in 1969 when a new governor was appointed. John remembers one change the new administrator made. He removed margarine from the prisoner's daily diet and gave them butter. The new governor must have known something about natural health, not using greasy spreads, as he arranged for the margarine to be replaced by the natural food, which is butter.   See *The Governor* in Bibliography section.

All my life I have used butter. Now in my 80's the advice I give is, *"Use it sparingly. "* The ingredients are purely and simply butter. It is just that.   There is no need for any ingredients section on the butter wrapper.

Put margarine outside or somewhere it will not be interfered with for some considerable time, perhaps years. It will not go mouldy or be touched by flies or insects. It will not be eaten by animals, even by rats or mice. During the winter freeze up it was put on the bird table with other fats when feeding the birds. They cleared everything, leaving the margarine.

The question must be asked again *'Do we have to wait for decades, as with the little known and conveniently covered up hydrogenated oils withdrawal, which nobody has been made accountable for, before we hear whether the highly questionable interesterified margarines are safe or otherwise?'*

The reader may well ask *'Why did we hear nothing about this alarming and worrying matter?'*   Yes, many questions could be and should be asked about this. Like the Thalidomide and other dangerous withdrawn drugs which can kill or maim, all too much is swept under the carpet in the name of big business. How many have given thought to the 'harm' done by hydrogenated oil? I have dwelt on it many times over the past 40 years. The alleged clogged up arteries, the questions about heart attacks or cardiovascular problems, perhaps serious illness or even deaths, will never be answered or known. The compo culture in this instance is without a shred of evidence.

The hydrogenated oil withdrawal exposé got a few lines in some newspapers. '*The Guardian*' was certainly the most informative.

There is a huge reason why people are not told about the dangers of many food additives or other food problems. This includes the hydrogenated oil disclosure. It is that the media receives so much money for advertising from the supermarkets and food purveyors that it is not in their interests to elaborate on matters like this. They will not rock the boat. As with all too much in life *"Money talks"*. The publication, M.A.P.S., which is the official directory of the Association of Advertisers, gives the going rate for a full-page colour advertisement in the *'Irish Independent'* as being almost €36,000 for a single insertion. *The various advertising outlets, which include newspapers, will only tell the all too gullible public what suits them, not us.* See *Advertising* caption.

I have mentioned about the processed oils used in the manufacturing of margarine. See **Cooking Oils chart** caption to realise that many of the oils used are over heated, steamed, pressed, distilled, refined, neutralised, bleached, deodorised, and with chemicals such as caustic soda used in the processing. They are highly unnatural. The same chart includes a diagram setting out how pure, non-processed, simply cold pressed oils, are produced. The latter mentioned pure and natural oils, too costly for margarine manufacture, have not been processed or interfered with.

Recently it has come to our attention that even the plastic containers in which margarine and butter substitutes are packed, in various types of receptacles and food containers, may contain the dangerous chemical, Bisphenol A. This is used to make plastic semi-rigid and flexible. *Is this the tip of the iceberg, another 'scandal'?* There are many questions being asked now about the dangers to health from the use of Bisphenol A in plastic. It is also regarded as one of the causes of obesity. See **Bisphenol A** caption.

I have studied and watched the use of margarine and butter substitutes for many years and this includes the people who eat them. My conclusions are that there is all too much theory, much of it on paper, also as printed on the plastic containers containing the stuff, but with little evidence that they are of any use to better health. With the odd exception, most people like a spread on bread. I repeat there is nothing better than butter used sparingly. It got a bad name because of the hype of the margarine manufacturers, including the low fat claims which are now turning out to be nonsense. Butter is pure and natural. It is food. Margarine is not.

What is amazing is that The Food Safety Authority took no action or accepted any responsibility for the use of the 'unsafe' hydrogenated oils or fats. They allowed the stuff to be sold for all too long after the first findings. Nobody was prosecuted for promoting or selling the highly questionable product, which for many, many years we were led to believe was extremely 'healthy'. All was kept quiet. In my dealings with this Authority also the Advertising Standards Authority of Ireland, I find they always have a politically jargoned answer, as they state the lax laws which exist in relation to 'food' manufacture or advertising, by way of defence. It often strikes me that they are a party to much which is 'unhealthy'. They too will avoid upsetting the manufacturers and processors. Sometimes one feels they are in cahoots with them.

Further evidence that nobody has or is prepared to look closely into the whole situation regarding margarine and butter look-alike spreads is the fact that when the story regarding the withdrawing of hydrogenated oils surfaced, nobody within Government, health or food circles, raised their voices or asked questions about their alleged 'harm to health'.

All concerned will not interfere where money and big business is concerned. The media, occupied with the thoughts of future advertising business, as described under *Advertising* caption, kept quiet, as did so many others responsible for our welfare. The margarine industry kept very quiet. They took steps to protect themselves by supposedly removing the hydrogenated oils and fats also the wording on the plastic containers. They did not inform the general public as to why they removed the 'unhealthy' ingredients or changed the ingredients blurb on the packaging. They will never explain why they changed the wording on the plastic containers. Let them truthfully answer the question **"Why did they remove or replace the greasy hydrogenated oils from the processed margarine?"**

There is one thing now very obvious. Margarine and butter look-alike spreads are being decried, as very many, including those who promoted these processed and converted greasy spreads in the past, are advising people that BUTTER is best. Turn to *Butter* caption.

COOKING OILS— HOW THEY ARE PROCESSED

The accompanying chart sets out how the many Oils we see on supermarket and food store shelves, or where used as boiled oils for cooking, such as in chip shops and other fast food outlets, are processed and produced. The highly transformed, converted and refined vegetable and seed oils, the end products, once natural, now very far from being so, are the chief ingredients in most margarines and substitute butter spreads. They are used for frying and cooking, whether commercially or in the home. Once heated and especially when brought to boiling point, the 'dangerous' trans fats rear their ugly heads. Despite all the hype, nobody understands how 'bad' or otherwise they can be in the blocking or clogging of the arteries or veins. Here the advice given must surely be, **'When in doubt, leave out, do without'**.

Study the production methods in the chart to note the processing, bleaching, deodorizing, injection methods, de-gumming, pressing, heating, crushing, chemical use and much else that goes into making up cooking oils, which as finished cheapened products are anything but natural. The lard and dripping used in bygone days for cooking purposes, and which many have decried, was natural. The processing, heating and additions, made to the seeds and contents, are an outstanding example of how grossly over refined, factory made, so called foods, are made cheap. This of course results in bigger profits for the manufacturers and their shareholders, with no thought given to the health of the user.

Note the small amount of work necessary to produce pure cold-pressed oils, as shown in the section on the right. Just as it is with anything PURE, the purchasing price is higher. Cold pressed cooking oils, when obtained from a reputable producer, as sold in health food stores, are purely natural, unprocessed. (Turn to chart on next page)

HOW COOKING OILS ARE PRODUCED

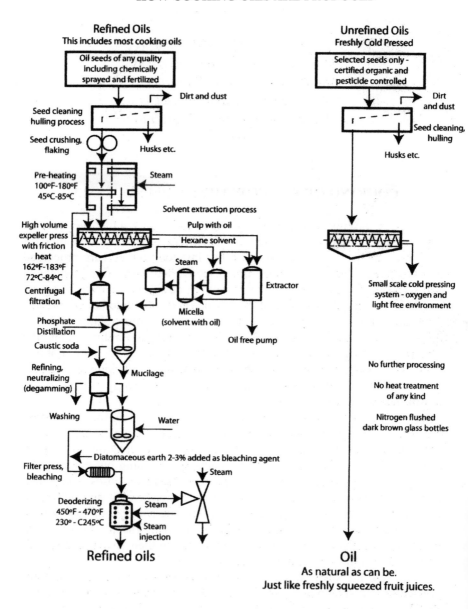

Refined Oils
This includes most cooking oils

Oil seeds of any quality including chemically sprayed and fertilized

Dirt and dust

Seed cleaning hulling process

Seed crushing, flaking

Husks etc.

Pre-heating 100°F-180°F 45°C-85°C

Steam

Solvent extraction process

Pulp with oil

High volume expeller press with friction heat 162°F-183°F 72°C-84°C

Hexane solvent

Steam

Extractor

Centrifugal filtration

Micella (solvent with oil)

Oil free pump

Phosphate Distillation

Caustic soda

Refining, neutralizing (degamming)

Mucilage

Washing

Water

Diatomaceous earth 2-3% added as bleaching agent

Filter press, bleaching

Steam

Deoderizing 450°F - 470°F 230° - C245°C

Steam

Steam injection

Refined oils

Unrefined Oils
Freshly Cold Pressed

Selected seeds only - certified organic and pesticide controlled

Dirt and dust

Seed cleaning, hulling

Husks etc.

Small scale cold pressing system - oxygen and light free environment

No further processing

No heat treatment of any kind

Nitrogen flushed dark brown glass bottles

Oil
As natural as can be.
Just like freshly squeezed fruit juices.

Taken from 'Health Is Wealth' Encyclopaedia

PRETENTIOUS 'FOODS'

Never eat anything that pretends to be something else. Yes, we have much offered as food, which is not. Buy only the natural – the good, additive free, unprocessed. Avoid 'food' or 'drinks' products with health claims. Have you every seen them on carrots, potatoes, vegetables, or other greens? Have you seen the goodness of fruit highlighted on any fruit? Foods that have reason to advertise claims for better well-being should be left on the shelf. Breakfast cereals, margarine, many probiotic and functional 'foods, butter substitutes or anything with vitamins or minerals or other additives are a prime example of this. I make an exception of porridge oats, which is pure food, but which has to be advertised because of the competition. Organic or pesticide free oats can be bought from the health food store. Any porridge oats, if promoted as fast food in plastic containers for use in the microwave, or if not offered as GM free, should be rejected if the plastic has bisphenol A in its make up See ***Bisphenol A*** also ***Probiotics and Functional Foods*** captions

Handed to me recently by one of the audience at a talk I was giving, with the words ***"I know you'll love this"*** was an aerosol tin of 'Elmlea' whipped cream substitute, or to me it is anyway. On the tin are the words ***"Tastes so good, so much fun"***. This can be found on the food stores shelves adjacent to or amongst the cream or whipped cream cartons. Cunningly omitted are the words 'Cream', which most people believe it is.

'Elmlea' is an excellent example of a specious, pretentious, adulterated 'food' product, far removed from the natural cream it imitates. The trusting innocent customer, desiring to purchase cream, reads the blurb. The ingredients labels are ignored. They have such small print that they are barely legible. The list of its make up reads: Water, Whey (27%), Hydrogenated Vegetable Oil (24%), Sugar, Milk Proteins, Emulsifiers: E472b, E475, E435, E471, E433, Stabilisers: E460, E466, E339, E407, Salt, Colour: E160a, Flavouring, Propellant: Nitrous Oxide. To decipher all this I used both reading glasses and a magnifying glass. What hope has the pitiable customer of understanding this at point of sale? There are dozens of so-called 'foods' and 'drinks', such as these concoctions, on the shelves of the food stores or supermarkets.

Months, perhaps 12 months after writing the above, I relate the following. It is rather strange, perhaps coincidence, that my good wife, who was expecting visitors, purchased two cartons of 'cream'. Having made a trifle the idea was to top it off with whipped cream. The first problem was with the 'cream', which had the word **whipping** printed in large letters on the plastic carton. Despite five minutes or more of using an electric whisk the white liquid remained as it had been when poured from the carton. It was at this point I arrived in the kitchen when the remark to me was, **"I can't understand why this cream will not thicken"**. It was then I discovered that the so called cream had been taken from a plastic container which had the 'Elmlea' brand printed on. This product has a different formula to the additive laden, cream like material, in the aerosol tin as already referred to. This **WHIPPING** stuff showed 70% buttermilk and only six Es, amongst other things.

Here is certain proof that unsuspecting people can be 'conned' into buying pretentious foods. Because we make a point of not purchasing any foods or drinks which contain additives, the lady of the house was really annoyed. As she said, *"Who would look at a carton of cream to read the additives, cream is pure, there is no need for an additive section on its container?"* When returned to the store and a complaint was made all of the jargon on the tub was carefully scanned. The store assistant had to put on her glasses to read it. She eventually found three words in very small print, which read, 'alternative to cream'. It is entirely wrong that big businesses are allowed to produce this kind of additive-laden stuff or permit it being placed alongside or amongst containers filled with pure cream. I repeat, **"The trusting or unwary customers place the additive made up white cream look-alike thing in the baskets or shopping trolleys, thinking they are purchasing pure cream"**. This processed mixture, had it not been bought for whipping, could have been used as cream in our home. The very thought of this is terrible! In order to be certain that my line of thought was not a form of perverseness I have since stood at the point of sale of cream in the supermarket, where Elmlea was on sale. **Spoken with were 28 customers. All, without exception, thought the product was pure cream.**

One has only to read the ingredients labels to see what is being put into the human system. Here is further proof as to why many are sick and under nourished. **THERE ARE MANY OTHER PRETENTIOUS 'FOODS' ON THE SHELVES IN THE FOOD STORES, ALMOST ALL CONTAINING ADDITIVES, WHICH WHEN PARTAKEN OF MAY LEAD TO ILL-HEALTH.**

A PERFECT PRAYER

Lord GOD
Please give me work to do
Please give me better health
Please GOD give me joy in simple things
Give me an eye for beauty
A tongue for truth
A heart that loves
A mind that reasons
A sympathy that understands
Please GOD that I will have neither malice or envy
but a true kindness and a noble common sense
At the close of each day
Please GOD give me a book or good reading
And a friend or friends with whom I can either be silent or speak with.
Amen
Benjamin Franklin (1706-1790)

DEPRESSION

THE RIDICULOUS WAY IT IS BEING TREATED

In my encyclopaedia '**HEALTH IS WEALTH, an A to Z of over the Counter, Proprietary Branded Natural Remedies and Good Food'**, there are two pages devoted to the subject depression. I cannot better the advice or remarks in that book. Nonetheless, I had to add a little, also to make remarks and offer some further advice. The main reason for this is because regularly I talk with, treat and help depressed men, but more especially women.

It is a subject, complaint or disorder I have had much success with, in treating and curing. I get annoyed when I see the ridiculous way that people with this problem are given treatment, much of it very unnatural. They are not sick when they are taken to or attend the doctor. There is never a question asked by the medic about lifestyle, diet, exercise, and mode of living or social life. No. What happens? Invariably these good people, now healthy, are turned into sick patients. They are treated by the use of antidepressant drugs, psychotherapy, counselling, with various other nonsensical or

165

pretentious ideas being suggested or used. *Selling Sickness*, making healthy people ill, is big, very big business.

Many have come to me who are nearly demented, feeling low, worn out. The majority of these have been attending the doctor, which has only worsened matters. They seek another therapy because they can see no way out of the miserable life they are locked into. Here is one ailment for which I get much thanks for my aid, as I help put depressive people on a better path. A lot of the thanks comes from relatives or others who had to put up with and try to help or take care of the person with depression, stress, nerves, or a combination.

Depression is not an illness. Nevertheless the medical profession tell us it is, treating it as one. They would, wouldn't they? There is money in it for them.

Certain members of the medical profession have stated openly, **"For much depression, lifestyle changes and psychological therapies can be as effective as medication".** This is near confirmation of what I have harped on continuously for many, many years. This again backs up my reasoning, **"Why use medication, all of it ineffective, for depression?"** Without doubt, **Change Of Lifestyle works Wonders,** none more so than for depression or mental problems.

Around me as I write are numerous files, some bulging with papers, records, case histories, all to do with depression. On my book shelves are many books and publications regarding health. I say this because apart from the natural health books, and many records sent to me or obtained from people like myself, who think and act by using what is natural, drug free, there is little if anything worth reading in the pile.

At hand are five or six useless books picked out at random, all to do with depression? Why do I buy them? Why do I pick a recently published one up from the library? Simply because I wish to or hope to learn something new from the author. Almost all are of drug or chemical way of thinking, researching and prescribing. I have learned little, if anything, from them.

Often I wish I could give some of the authors a good shaking. I do know that I could teach them much in relation to the treatment of depression, whether it be bipolar or other lesser form.

A 330 page book, titled *'Depression, The Way Out'*, which I have in front of me now, goes into detail about the use of antidepressants, counselling, counsellors and other therapy. This large book devotes 15 to 20 lines to diet and exercise. It would have been as well to leave them out, because what has been outlined is of very little value to assist one to better health. The other books give little or no information on the so vital subjects of eating, drinking, sleeping and exercise. What is written in them is mostly irrelevant. Pages should have been devoted to getting the message across about the need for change of lifestyle, change of eating and drinking habits, sleeping and exercise patterns.

Many who visited me in the past, who had depression, were well within a short time. With others it took longer. There were some who from childhood had various stigmas, with what were to them worrying social or esteem lowering problems. With them, the treatment is ongoing but not hopeless. For some of them it means continuous but simple and natural treatment and way of living. I have seen those who were treated the natural way, who felt so much better, perhaps cured, and have cried with joy as far as some of them were concerned. Perhaps this was because relatives who accompanied them at the outset could not see an answer to the problem.

A masterly example of how the drug industry and the medical profession have elbowed and shoved their way into the running of the various so-called health charities, is of their attachment to the AWARE Organisation which strives to help where there is depression. This has happened in Cystic Fibrosis, Cancer, Asthma, Diabetes and other charitable groups or societies, with the drug companies being supporters and sponsors. The doctors aid and abet, while prescribing their chemical drugs, none of which cure.

Some time ago I attended a meeting promoted by AWARE. **It was advertised as a lecture**, the subject being depression. The doctor who spoke is also a politician. He read from a paperback booklet which I had already studied more than once.

This highlighted the use of Drugs, Counselling, Psycho Therapy, Anti-Depressant Medicines, Mood Stabilisers, Electro-Convulsive Therapy and other methods of treatment. Mentioned were a dozen brand named anti-Depressants, including Prozac, Seroxat, Zispin, Tryptizol and Anafranil. Name one of these side effect giving chemicals that cures? **Conveniently perhaps, we were not informed about the top of the list of prescribed drugs, which is statins, or their extremely serious relationship to depression. By lowering cholesterol these drugs interfere with Serotonin concentrations, so vital to the functioning of the brain and mood. This can lead to suicide, Alzheimers, dementia and other mood related serious health problems. I have had people tell me that they were never informed about the highly serious danger of taking anti-depressants and statins at the same time.** As one who treats people the natural way I would look at some of the forgoing as mal-treatment, bordering on criminal. To me the advice in that booklet was irrelevant because the main aid to stop depression was not even given a word.

At the end of his reading, the G.P. held the publication up at arms length, having the brass neck to inform the audience that *"Everything they wish to know about depression is in these pages"*. I nearly lost my cool. My anger was rising.

Later,when the meeting was thrown open to discussion, I pointed out that the G.P. had not lectured as advertised, merely reading from an existing manual. I set out that he was far from being correct when he informed us that the information taken from the book was complete or entire. I pointed out that as a medical graduate surely he must know that **Hippocrates,** the father of medicine, had as his aim or slogan *"Let food be your medicine and let medicine be your food".* **Hippocrates** did not have to add the words natural, unadulterated, additive free and non-processed foods, because everything put into the body when he was alive was natural.

When speaking, I dwelt on and placed emphasis on the fact that the doctor had not mentioned one word about natures great aid, often a cure on its own for depression, that of exercise. Walking, which is an extremely suitable exercise, according to age and ability, to be at the top of the list. There too should be placed the need for diet of pure natural foods and drinks for any who suffer from depression, with need for proper sleep and sleep pattern. **If with a serious health problem seek advice before embarking on a strenuous exercise programme.**

I have mentioned about the goodness of meditation, but palming of the eyes is equally so, being much easier to do. See *Palming* caption.

Change of lifestyle must be included in the treatment of any ailment. On its own it is often the cure. An example of this is when a person is informed by the G.P., "You have diabetes. I am putting you on medication". Very often one can forget about the medication. Change of lifestyle or mode of living can very often put this serious health diagnosis right in a matter of weeks. **Taking the wonderful herb Rhodiola, which is available in capsule form, also a Vitamin D3 capsule, both obtainable from the health food store, is strongly recommended for depression, but diet of pure natural unadulterated food is number one.**

There are many who have depression, including Seasonal Affective Disorder, who do not realise or know they have a problem.The certain aid, dare I say cure, is almost always the change of lifestyle I keep referring to. It works wonders to help one to better or good health. I told the doctor who had read from the booklet that I thought it disgraceful that at the meeting, just as like many other conferences concerning sickness and ailment, a diet of pure food, additive free, unadulterated, was not and is not being mentioned and promoted. The 'pills for all ills' syndrome or idea is all that is promulgated or sold to those who are or have family or friends ill and unwell, whether in mind or body. I got a great ovation when I finished. My still small voice got the message about food and drink being as medicine over to the small audience. What about the hundreds of thousands in the outside world who are left unaware of the facts I spoke about? **Hippocrates** idea, which is as relevant today, some hundreds of years after his death, should be promoted throughout the nation. If taken up and followed by the majority it would save our exchequer billions. It should be remembered that *'When diet is wrong, medicine is of no use, when diet and liquid intake is of pure natural food and drink, medicine is seldom needed'.*

Those with depression, their families and the many others who help care for depressed people, need to promote the nine words *'WE ARE AS WE EAT, DRINK, SLEEP AND EXERCISE'.* It is the greatest antidote or remedy known. The medicos will certainly not dwell on the matter.

Almost always when depressed, with daily blues or even with maniac or bipolar disorder, the person concerned is suffering from malnutrition, being under-nourished. Very often many, but especially the elderly, are not eating and drinking sufficient natural and nutritional fare. Some as they get older think they don't need food, often existing on tea and toast How wrong they are. Often the immune system is weak and suppressed. The white blood cells are unable to conquer infection. One of the vital questions a doctor should ask when dealing with mood problems is *"Have you been ill or feeling sick recently?"* Part, if not all, of the problems can be solved if the answer is in the affirmative. Like with many ailments, the three words, *'Change your lifestyle'* if acted upon, can be the answer to *'Why Depression?'* Depression with many is only minor. Beware the doctor who can turn it into an illness. They seldom if ever ask about lifestyle, what is being ate and drank. The word exercise is taboo to the majority of them. If they were doing their job properly the person with or thought to be with depression, would be put sitting down in a comfortable chair, then spoken to and questioned for up to 30 minutes or longer to fathom out why there is a problem. This is how the doctors in days long past treated their patients.

If ever there was an example of treating a person naturally, the treatment of depression gives the answers simply. Living with somebody who suffers from prolonged anxiety and depression, even when mild, can make those who care for the depressed more susceptible to illness.

I have seen change of lifestyle with proper diet, sleep and exercise work, as if miraculously, for those who were with depression. **Drugs of any kind are a last resort in the treatment of depression, anxiety, stress or mind related problems**. Turn to caption *Undernourished and Sick Nation.*

AGEING

"If I realised I was going to live to be as old as I am,
I would not have grown as old as I did"
Chinese Philosopher.

ADVERTISING,

THE SERIOUS POWER IT CAN HAVE ON PEOPLE
- OFTEN   OVERPOWERING

Very much thought can be given to what all too often leads to stress, depression and feeling unwell. Yes, reading into the advertising blurb we are faced with can lead to illness. Many who view, remember and follow the advertising in the media, especially on the goggle box, the television, are addicted to them, particularly our younger generation. Regularly I question people, especially in the shops or at my talks, asking why they purchase such and such an article? They are mostly 'food' and 'drink', almost always processed, unnatural, full of additives and sugarised. The usual answer is, *"I saw it on the telly"* or *"I saw it on an ad".*

I quote from '*The Word For Today'*, which is a wonderful booklet with daily readings. It is published by United Christian Broadcasters and is available for a reasonable donation to help promote Christian thinking and doing. For full details of how they can be contacted see *Bibliography* section.

The quote is as follows: *'The average person is bombarded with about 300 advertisements a day, promising everything from whiter teeth to faster cars. It's a mega – billion – pound or euro industry designed to make us want what they're selling. But there is a subtle message being conveyed. In a word, it's discontent, and it eats away at us by creating a desire for bigger, better, more.   The Bible says, "WE BROUGHT NOTHING INTO THE WORLD, SO WE CANNOT TAKE ANYTHING OUT, IF WE HAVE FOOD AND COVERING, BEING CONTENT". It sounds simple enough: food to eat, clothes to wear, a place to sleep. But how we live doesn't bear it out. When Rockefeller was asked, "How much does it take to satisfy a man?", with rare insight he replied, "A little more than he has now. So does contentment mean not setting goals or aiming higher? Does it not mean enjoying nice things? No, it just means not letting all those nice things 'own' you. Learning to be satisfied is a process'.*

If all were to follow and be guided by the advice – *"Buy not what you want, buy only what you have need of",* imagine the savings and peace of mind which would follow.

Much of the advertising regarding 'foods' or 'drinks', when viewed or listened to, should be acted upon with extreme care, just as much of what we are given to understand is pure, but is not, can be related to advertising. Much is just hype. Those who ignore it enjoy better health, with peace of mind. Just as I believe that the off button is a central part of the T.V., the fast decrease of sound when the advertisements appear brings a smile and a chance to relax.

Many food adverts, with breakfast cereals, coke or energy drinks as an example, lead people to believe that 'unhealthy' food or drink is extremely good. Advertisements for the over sweetened breakfast cereals are an example of what I mean. Subtle is a good description. The highlighting of the snack nutri grain bar, which contains over 30 ingredients, some of which I would not regard as health-giving food, is a further example of the hype used for promotion. At the showing of the Athens Olympics on television, we had what to me as a natural food addict, were the annoying words 'Fuelling our Olympic athletes', flashing across the screen regularly. This plug was for nutri grain. We won nothing. Many like myself were not surprised. No wonder so many, especially our young people, get the message about diet all wrong, as some think of a balanced diet being an additive-filled, sugarised snack bar in one hand and a bottle of lucozade, coke or fizzy drink in the other. Diet coke, which is another example of what advertising can do to promote this additive collection in water, shows a list of ingredients which many, like myself, would not regard as being either dietary or healthy.

The advertising laws are so vague that they are often ridiculous where the health of all is to be taken seriously. Many are being manipulated and over influenced by the big 'food' brands. As with the Food Safety Authority, the Advertising Standards Authority is ambiguous, a smoke screen for big business, allowing it to operate as it does.

I feel sorry for young children who are freely allowed to loll about in front of the goggle box, often more interested in the adverts than the programmes being beamed out.

In days past youngsters went to bed anytime from 6 o'clock onwards in the evening, according to their age. Now one sees them, often as young babies, viewing up to or perhaps after 10 o'clock. Here is a primary reason for illness in so many today. They get little or no exercise but of ultra vital importance as far as their future health is concerned, there is a lack of sleep. Sufficient and proper sleep at the right time is one of nature's medicines. It sets young people up for life, costing nothing. I saw a heading in the *'Daily Telegraph'* recently, which read, *"Children have no escape from aggressive advertisers".* How very true. Another heading tells us, *"Getting children hooked on certain products can guarantee loyalty for a lifetime to big brands, much being unhealthy."*

Recently, when in a hotel at breakfast time, I counted 28 people who were eating. All of the adults, except one, were on what is called '**The Full Breakfast'**, which included bacon, eggs, sausages, beans on toast, even chips. All this is totally non-nutritious. Almost all were cooked in hydrogenated or interesterificated oils. Some children had glasses of lucozade or coke with their first meal of the day, the most important one. Many of the adults were reading the national newspapers. It was Thursday, which is the popular day for the Tesco, Supervalu, Dunne's Stores, and other food store advertisements.

I often wonder how many people read these displays. I certainly do not. At a going rate of well over €30,000, yes, almost €36,000 for a full page in colour, as set out in *M.A.P.S.,* the Media and Services Directory of the Association of Advertisers, did any of them realise that indirectly they were paying for these adverts? This advertising brouhaha is not to be seen on the same scale in the U.K. Here is another reason why food is so much cheaper there.

Brass neck and being brash mean the same thing. When one sees the extremes that advertisers go to in setting out what can very often be untruths, it points to the trusting or naivety of the reader and those who take the plugs seriously. Here is an example of the people who are brow beat, let's add intimidated, into believing the advertising hype as set out.

The *Irish Farmer's Journal* sets an alternative example. This excellent paper is purchased every week, not alone for its farming content, but for much other informative articles, including health, cookery, home economics, horses, weather reports and a host of things which make enjoyable reading. One does not need to have an interest in farming to purchase and enjoy the news, information and advertising within its pages. We could certainly do with much more reading matter like this informative farming weekly paper.

Here's an example of sham or 'deceitful' advertising, where TESCO WERE CAUGHT DOCTORING TRACTOR NUMBER PLATES. The top brass in Tesco and their servants never cease to amaze me. An example of their sheer brass-neck can be found in the pages of *'Irish Country-Living'*, where a Co. Meath farmer explains how he saw pictures advertising Tesco, with his farm machinery being used in the campaign, with the number plate having been changed to

172

give the impression that the photograph was taken on a named County Wexford producer's farm. This was all done without his being asked, with no form of acknowledgement, so that Tesco might get the message across that they were selling Irish vegetables. All should be aware that every little helps Tesco! With this kind of carry on it would be difficult for anybody to trust them or believe anything they say.

'*Irish Country-Living*' is the magazine which accompanies '*The Irish Farmer's Journal*'. It is apparent that the whole set up was 'deceptive', but Tesco have no qualms of conscience in this respect. They were furthering their own ends as they got their illusory message to the all too trusting public. How low must a multinational like this stoop in order to promote its foods, all too many of them containing additives and perhaps 'foodless'? This is one of the many ploys big business uses, to enrich the shareholders.

In front of me is an advert., which tells us little. It is a picture of seeds. The wording informs us '*Heart Health Oils from 18,000 seeds crammed into every tub*'. This is for an 'original' margarine, which I presume is another processed, and additive-containing spread. I certainly would not believe that this is the original, the very first of the grease filled margarines. I have old, not ancient margarine boxes but the original 'original' must be way before my ageing lot, some of them shabby. All show changes made to the stuff over many years. Like much of the advertising hype, the number of seeds could be just hype too, if not counted. The healthy oils referred to are not cold pressed. The oils used in commercially produced margarines are processed, chemicalised and therefore not natural. See *Cooking Oils* chart and caption which describes how they are processed.

Over the years we have had health scares and other hair and mind raising stories about additives, foods, drugs and other associated things, which pertain to better health. Like much of what I write in this book, most of these stories seldom, if ever, get an airing or a line in the media. Writers, like myself and others with similar interests in what is pure and natural, have submitted articles, also writing to the letters pages. This is all for nothing, not even an acknowledgement. Why so, one can well ask? The answer is simple but a disgrace. The newspapers will keep quiet. They will not upset the lucrativeness of their take from the mighty 'food' and drinks advertisers.

As is usual the press will tell us what suits them. News, especially bad news, is selected. Some of the editors are single-minded. I did not use the word simple. They are often self-opinionated and with fixed views. Read the leading articles of certain of the national dailies to see what I mean. These should be written impartially, but where there are three sides to the stories, yours, theirs and mine, theirs is usually printed.

So much for advertising, often too forceful, sometimes sickening. If one does not feel unwell on reading some of it, the end product that is advertised may often lead to illness. By this, I mean the adulterated, additive laden, unnatural and processed foods and drinks which are promoted.

MEN'S HEALTH

In my book *'Health is Wealth'* I wrote about 12 lines under the caption Men's Health. At the time I felt **'What is the point of writing more or indeed anything regarding men and their health'.** Big strong man, it won't happen to me, is the idea of most men. I know, I was one of them. Now I speak with many who have realised, like myself in the past, that when the age of 40 is reached, the body, too often not properly serviced, begins to give trouble. One can't go out and buy spare parts for it or press the rewind button. I repeat again, *"We spend the first half of our lives living it up, destroying the body, and the second half trying to undo the harm".*

Proper maintenance, **with emphasis on prevention,** is vital for men of all ages, from their youth onwards. Those under 40 don't appear to bother. As I said, *"The attitude is, it won't happen to me".*

Most men avoid seeing their doctor, hoping illness or health problems will go away. They would rather remain silent, tolerating the symptoms, very often feeling uncomfortable, even with pain, not seeking advice. It is amazing how those, who to their friends, work companions and others, project a strong unabashed slant, then being brought to their senses by a woman when in full command. My writings, suggestions and advice would not be accepted by most men, without almost a falling out, whereas a female quickly gets the message across.

I admit I wrote little in my original book *'Health is Wealth'* about **Men's Health** but I have been amazed at the huge number of men who purchased the book and also by the many who made arrangements to visit me for advice, as they sought help. I have been proved partly wrong where men don't seem to care about their health. The vast numbers of male telephone calls, letters and personal callers, as well as the books sold to men, showed me that they just need prompting. Many don't have much wrong with them until they reach their 50's, but that is all the more reason for them to look after themselves when younger. **In their 30's and 40's prevention is easy. They don't have to suffer either mental or physical illness in silence.**

With a little thought and often a change of lifestyle, including a diet of pure natural foods and drinks, most ailments of the future can be avoided. How many men know that by taking daily just one tablet of calcium bone formula, osteoporosis and arthritis may be prevented. Where there is a woman in the home this is a vital medicine too. See *Calcium* caption. Prostate gland troubles can be alleviated, lived with, reversed also prevented, by taking Zinc, Saw Palmetto, Pumpkin Seeds, Pulsatilla and/or Lycopene, also Vitamin D3. Other men's health problems which occur or can be prevented which come to mind are sexual or colon problems, where the man is too shy to seek help. Blood pressure, being overweight, fear of heart disease if it is in the family, smoking and indeed one can safely include many of the over 1,000 ailments listed in my book, *'Health is Wealth'*, can all be easily taken into perspective and treated successfully.

For all listed here and in the book mentioned, there are natural, no side effect remedies, all of which I have seen work, whether for prevention or cure. They are all available from the health food store. It makes one realise that another of my slogans or mottos is highly applicable. It reads: *"Your health is your own responsibility".* Nobody will worry about it except the affected person and if one sets out as a youth or man to look after one's self there should be little problems.

I know, I've been through all of this before realising, when in my forties, that I had to do something. My doctor relative was responsible for frightening me into acting to change my lifestyle. I repeat again and again and especially to the reader, *'YOU ARE AS YOU EAT, DRINK, SLEEP AND EXERCISE'.*

Men are good at many things. Looking after their health is not one of them. It is a simple discipline to do so and be healthier.

We've been taught to rely on every new miracle remedy, depending on the yearly influenza shot and counting on guaranteed protection by the use of chemical drugs, which don't cure. More importantly, many have forgotten to live healthily. Everyday lifestyle is of huge importance when it comes to enjoying better health.

It involves a few basic principles:

* Eat simple nutritious natural food, additive, preservative and colour free.
* Eat at regular hours, making time to do so.
* Eat only what you need to maintain your ideal weight.
* Exercise. You may be surprised how enjoyable and refreshing regular outdoor activity can be, especially walking.
* Respect your body's need for rest. Sufficient sleep is not a luxury: it is a necessity.
* Use lots of water – inside and out!
* Avoid the health destroying habits of smoking and alcohol. Preserve the life you have, don't destroy it. Give very serious thought to the fact that the human body system is the most co-ordinated set up in the entire Universe. It is a marvel, being beyond comprehension.
* Enjoy life. Be positive. Put your trust in GOD. Most of modern day synthetic medicine, when taken, can lead to ill health. There are many alternative and natural remedies that offer you better health in an increasingly disease-ridden world. Visit your local Health Food Store to discover the good of natural remedies.

Acknowledgement is made with thanks for some of this information to
The General Conference of Seventh-Day Adventists as a community service.

EXERCISE

"The sovereign invigorator of the body is exercise,
and of all exercise, walking is best".
Thomas Jefferson (1743-1826)

WE ARE A SICK AND MALNUTRITIONED NATION

Our hospitals are full. There are waiting lists. There are insufficient beds for the sick. In some hospitals, patients on trolleys wait in the corridors. There is a shortage of doctors, even with the number of foreign medics increasing. To put this all in perspective, one short sentence sums it up. **'WE ARE A SICK NATION'.** The vast majority do not realise that they are part of a nation suffering from malnutrition. Many are undernourished, without sufficient energy. They do not realise it. It is a fact of life, accepted by all, because they are unaware of their state of health. Get up and go is not there, but they do not recognise it.

Last year there were big headings in the Irish national newspapers. They read: 'MALNUTRITION costs up to €1.5 billion per year. At the same time the U.K. newspapers reported that nearly 250 National Health Service patients were dying of malnutrition every year, also that the cost of treatment was estimated to be £14 billion sterling the previous year.

Professors of Nutrition, Marinos Elia in Southampton and Michael Gibney in Dublin told us that proper nutrition for older people can easily be provided with oral nutritional supplements, informing us further that they have consistently been found to provide huge cost benefits. To them they may appear cheap but telling us of giving them as proper nutrition is utter nonsense, pure idiocy. Note that these two learned people are Professors of Nutrition. Is it any wonder we are a sick and under-nourished nation, with individuals like this advising us. Just as many get the idea that they can take vitamins, minerals or supplements in order to make up for deficiencies in their diet, so too these nutritional, dare I use the word 'experts', have a similar way of thinking.

I repeat, and keep quoting my findings and those of many others, that if without pure natural additive free and nutritious food, a proper balanced diet, we will remain a sick and undernourished population. **No supplements, and I repeat the words NO, will take the place of any real food.** They will help one attain better health, but only if taken as a combination including pure good food and natural drinks. **Supplements taken otherwise can be dangerous and certainly do not lead to good or better health.**

I mention elsewhere in this book that old, elderly and sometimes even not so old are under the illusion that as they get older they need less food or nourishment. They are totally wrong. Those who care for them should also know and remember that as one gets older, more and better food is required for both body and mind, to help keep one feeling younger and healthy. I am partial to good foods or if not I would be run down, unhealthy, without energy. Many are existing on a diet which leads to illness or even slow death. They become ill and turn to the doctors' for healing. They will only offer pills and potions, none, and I repeat none, of which are cures. Many are probably harmful to the system. G.Ps are prescribing chemicals, which when mixed with the junk and fast food diet being eaten, are perhaps a cause for further illness, lethargy and unwell feeling. As **Mike Adams** in his wonderful advice notes on *www.naturalnews.com* tells us, *"Many are on a diet of death"*. He tells of how the use of junk, fast, dead, processed, additive-containing, GM and unhealthy so-called foods can be highly dangerous. These kinds of 'foods' contain little or no nutrition. They are best left on the store shelf.

Sugars and processed carbohydrates are being used to excess. Colours, additives, preservatives, also thousands of chemical and artificial ingredients are in the 'food' chain. Pat Thomas tells us in the excellent and hard hitting book *'Living Dangerously'; "Food is inexorably linked with health. It is the bedrock on which a healthy life is based. It is the body's buffer against the onslaughts of an increasingly toxic environment".*

"Yet today most people do not eat food in any reasonable sense of the word. Instead what is eaten is an approximation of food. We eat meat by-products enhanced with meat flavours to make them palatable. We eat processed, quick cook microwave and oven meals that contain more preservatives and other additives than they do nutrients. Even the cereals eaten at breakfast time are so highly processed and nutritionally poor that the manufacturers have to add vitamins to them so that they can be classified as foods".

"Each day we put this nutritionally poor, unbalanced stuff into our bodies and then wonder why our bodies don't function properly". See *Bibliography* section for details of the book *'Living Dangerously'*

Over cooked and boiled oils, probably hydrogenated or interesterificated, are used. Animal products, including offal, are in the processing of some so called foods. Because people are undernourished, due to the 'rubbish' food many partake of, here is one of the main reasons for the much illness, lethargy and under-nourishment so many have to contend with now. See *Margarine* caption regarding this subject.

Sugar and sugary products, which are mostly over-eaten, are hugely responsible for some forms of cancer. These are amongst the chief ingredients of fast and junk foods and drinks.

Dr. Chi Van Dang, who is a director at the John Hopkins School of Medicine reported that *"cancerous cells are such junkies that glucose and sugar deprivation contributes significantly to their demise".* I repeat what I have set out elsewhere in this guide to better health, "Sugar is evil, it should have health warnings on the packaging".

The vast majority very often unwittingly eat or drink what they are led to believe is good for them. The advertising hype or propaganda has many brain-washed into believing that bad food is good food.

Much of the stuff offered as 'food' or 'drink' contains ingredients which have little if any nutritional value?

Throughout this book the question is asked numerously, *"Do you read the ingredients labels?"* Sadly all too many do not. Worse still they do not understand them. There is nobody to whom they can turn to find out what all the E's and the funny named ingredients mean or what their make up is. All are kept in the dark. Because there is nobody to educate the gullible public about what they are purchasing, the consumer accepts the stuff without question.

What should be unsettling or worrying is that they are unaware of the consequences of putting the junk into the bodily system. Stand near the checkouts in any food store. View the trolleys and baskets. Those who think like the writer, who understand the harm of artificial and many other additives in either food or drink, realise that it is appalling and a scandal that the general public, the consumer, can be conned into buying so much which is adulterated, additive-containing, processed and often unhealthy. As the elderly lady, who is the subject of a story elsewhere in this book, said in the supermarket, "I never saw so much stuff we do not want, it is not food".

Restaurants, tearooms, and cafés are now joined by the recent arrival of the 'deli'. This is an abbreviation or truncation of the word delicatessen. It is taken from the French term, delicacy. The dictionary description is **'A store or department in a store, which sells table delicacies which are either ready to serve or require little preparation'.**

These 'deli' fast food stores, which are on a par with many of the fast food outlets which have sprung up in recent years, offer 'food' which is seldom a delicacy, but is always delicious to the taste buds. This is all part of the strategy, the ploy, of enticing the gullible public to purchase the fast, processed, junk, sold as food. The fast 'food' industry plays on the aspect of flavour, longing, desire and palate taste.

The restaurant, café or dining room will have seats. In the deli one stands, waits to be served and then usually eats on the run, when walking or perhaps driving. This certainly does not lead to better health, adding to the harm which may come from the junk food purchased. **Who has a lunch hour break now?**

Many times I have stood in the queue in the deli, fast food outlet, or the fish and chip shops, just to see what is being prepared, offered and purchased. Obesity and being overweight comes about because of what people don't eat. This means that natural food should be used. Much of what I describe here regarding what is being eaten or drank, as produced in the 'deli' and fast food shop, can only lead to obesity or ill-health.

We hear of how large portions of food are to be avoided at mealtimes. I know thousands like myself, who eat any size of portion we wish to, and never have to worry about our weight. Why? Because we eat pure natural food such as porridge, salads, various types of grains and pulses, eggs, wholemeal bread, whole wheat pastas, potatoes, fish and fresh meat, also vegetables, all properly cooked. In short, we only eat what is additive free and natural. Eating this type of nutritious food, whatever the portion sizes, will not add weight. We eat as much as we wish to. If you wish to read further about this subject turn to *Healthy Body Weight—How to be the Right Weight and Brimful of Energy* caption.

As one interested in better health, as an addict to good, pure, natural, additive-free and properly prepared food, I can honestly say that having viewed the fast and processed stuff, sold as sustenance, I have felt ill on occasions. To see the boiling oils in the chip shop fryer, so very unhealthy to the consumer, or the sausages, processed burgers, chicken nuggets, pies and other additive-containing fillers in the fast food outlets is a revelation to a natural food enthusiast.

In my travels as I give talks in various parts of Ireland and the U.K. I can't help but notice the full Irish or English breakfast, according to the country one is in. All look alike, with various oily cooked and 'unhealthy things' in the big fry up.

The subject of my talks is about the use of natural and pure food, also the use of natural remedies, where applicable. The slogans used, '*WE ARE AS WE EAT, DRINK, SLEEP AND EXERCISE*' or '*CHANGE YOUR LIFESTYLE*' have helped many to a changed and healthy lifestyle. The full breakfast is noted as I eat my porridge and then brown bread and honey. The big fry up can be a combination of beans, bacon, eggs, sausages, black or white pudding, liver, chops, toast, chips, onion rings, mushrooms or potato bread. The grease laden mixture can be a forerunner of clogged arteries, atherosclerosis, bad circulation, varicose veins, ulcers and dozens of other ailments, many of them serious. Fried food is an enemy of one's circulation. The partaker is either not aware of the consequences or does not care about their well-being. Eating this kind of food gives no nutrition or aid to future health. It can be described as 'killer food'. The best place for the pans or deep fry utensils, usually stainless steel, used to fry this kind of unhealthy food, is in a recycling centre.

We are indeed a sick and undernourished nation. Could this be the main reason why our hospitals are full to overflowing? It is not to be wondered at. I can hear the doubters, the sceptics say, *"This is nonsense".*

Again I pose these questions. **"Why are our hospitals full to overflowing? Why are the doctor's surgeries full, with waiting lists? Why do we have to make appointments? Why did we have none of this until recent years?"** 20 to 30 years ago, we had none of this carry on. We had no illness as of now. Neither had we fast, processed, additive-filled or factory made up 'foods', much of which is unnatural. Here again it is not coincidence too that the Sickness Industry has only grown and expanded during this time.

Many pharmaceutical chemical manufacturing drug companies have become huge multinational conglomerates as they take over one another. Aided by the medical profession, the Sickness Industry has expanded to be the largest commercial unit in both Ireland and the U.K. One can safely say that many within the medical profession are the servants of the almighty legalised drug pushers as they over-prescribe chemical drugs, none of which are cures.

It must be retold that it is not coincidence that up to 20 years ago, even less, we did not have the vast amount of fast and junk food as available now. **Only in this time have we seen the huge increase in the deli's and junk food manufacture, preparation, processing and sales.**

In the past, people ate mostly in the home, sitting at the table. Usually the family gathered together to enjoy their food – pure and simple – discussing the topics of the day, with much conversation. There was no rush, no urgency as of now. People lived then. Many just exist now.

In those days the vast majority were used to partaking of additive-free food, usually when having the most important meals of the day, breakfast and dinner. Dinner was at midday until this meal acquired the pseudo or pretentious title of lunch.

Again we can hear the sceptics, the doubters, saying, *"But people are living longer now".* Very little of this can be attributed to the use of prescribed drugs and certainly not to the eating of fast and processed so-called foods. Very much of the longevity of life has to be attributed to the easier living standards of today. People do not have the hardships, labour intensity or privation of former times. There is no hard work as done manually in the past, often working long hours in atrocious conditions. We now have the tin box on four wheels, the car, jeep or van. Electricity, wall-to-wall carpeting, central heating, and home insulation, as we now have, were unknown. There is now no need to milk the cow to obtain milk. The fire does not have to be stoked up to boil water or cook, often by the light of a paraffin lamp or perhaps a candle. Now at the flick of a switch we have heat and power. The fridge, the freezer, the many mod cons we have today, were unknown. Many of the 'mod cons' referred to have only appeared within the past 50 years. To the octogenarian writer this is not so long ago.

One can dwell further on this subject of long living and ask the question: *"Where people are old and in extreme ill health, very often bedridden or seriously incapacitated, is there any sense in prolonging their lives?"*

Regularly I visit nursing homes, institutions or places where there are old or infirm people. Sometimes I place myself in the position of those who need constant attention and care, those who are unable to do little or anything for themselves. If I am ever like that, with the next world beckoning, then the call could not come soon enough. Living long lives is not always right for some. Yes, many are living longer, but at what expense and I don't mean monetary wise. **Those I write about or refer to would perhaps be better off in the next world. Monetary wise the only beneficiaries are nursing home proprietors and their staff, the doctors who prescribe medicine to assist the prolongation of life, also the drug manufacturers. Here again there are no cures.**

We are undoubtedly a sick and unnourished nation, living in this modern age where **MONEY** is the *god*. The sceptic, the doubter, or indeed you the reader might rightly ask, *"What has money to do with sick, malnourished people?"* Big business today is all about money. The Sickness and Food Industries are a prime example. Mentioned in this book more than once is the influence the giants of the chemical drug industry have. This statement also concerns the medical profession, the pharmacists and those who believe there are pills for all ills. Many of them are not interested in cures. With the very odd exception they have produced none. Stoppers of pain perhaps, and little else as an aid to better health. The principle line is money, profits for themselves and where relevant the shareholders. Our good health is not their business.

The fast and junk food industry is no better equipped to aid our ills. As already stated, the ingredients all too often leave much to be desired. Hundreds, aye thousands, of artificial things go to make up the all-too-often foodless stuff sold as 'food'. We have drinks and food flown half way across the world, some then sold as fresh. To know what is right for a balanced diet is almost impossible. Even the nutritionists and dieticians can't be sure unless they are trained in naturopathy. This would be foreign thinking to almost all of them. **Diets filled with pure natural additive free foods and drinks are the requisites for good or better health.** I re-quote **Hippocrates** words, which are the answer to the ill-health and malnutrition which so many suffer from. They are, *'Let food be your medicine, let medicine be your food'.* The father of medicine was not referring to the junk which is offered as food today.

In the Bible we are told of how the wise and learned prophet Daniel asked for himself and his companions to be given vegetables and greens. Also he requested that only water be served. They did not want to eat food or drink the wine from the King's table. We are told how Daniel and his three friends looked better than any of the young men who ate the King's food.

In the modern kitchen you can find many things except natural or good food. We know a family who in the now deceased 'Celtic Tiger days' built a very nice five bedroom house. They have two children who are constantly ill, visiting the doctor almost weekly. This fact is mentioned for a reason. The nicely designed and laid out kitchen, with every facility and mod con, has a large breakfast bar in the central area. **The wife and mother can't cook.** She started school at the age of three, taking her second masters degree aged 29. She openly admits that she never learned to cook, with the microwave being the gadget she uses regularly. **It should be mandatory that cooking be classified as essential learning, whether at first, second or third level education. Sadly many don't know how to boil an egg now. All too many have got their priorities wrong.**

Mentioned are the regular visits of the children to the doctor, even if only with a sniffle. The parents too are frequently ill. This can be attributed to the diet, which is atrocious, the main reason for having many ailments. Like the majority in our country they are malnourished, not realising it. When we visit them, I would not raise what to me is the serious matter of nutrition. These nice people are not the kind who listen to advice. 'I keep biting my tongue.' The highly educated parents appear to know it all, but sadly don't.

In my travels around the country, which I love, I go out of my way to collect menus from various cafes, restaurants or hotels. Some of them are not very inviting types of eating-places. In front of me is a selection of these menus, which contain lists of various kinds of foods, much of it, foodless. Starters, where provided, are usually par for the course, similar in wording, similar in taste, mostly fast foods provided by the chief supplier in the country. In other words they originate from the same processing supplier, but perhaps put together in warehouses many miles apart. When these menus are read by those like myself, who enjoy and appreciate good food, they appear as sickening, making one cringe with contempt. Even four star or supposedly high-class hotels offer many fast and processed foods on the menus, all purchased from the manufacturing or processing outlet referred to. For dessert one can be offered Raspberry and Orange Charlotte Double, Chocolate Mousse Cake, Orange Jelly and Lime, Bavarois Slice, Caramelised Lemon Tart or various other over sweetened and therefore 'unhealthy' deserts. If all knew the make up, additives, the contents of these sugarised and over sweetened things, also realising the harm they may cause to the health of the partaker, they would not be eaten. With the odd exception I have yet to read the words *Fresh Fruit Salad* on a menu. Yet we are harped at and told regularly to eat our daily portions of fresh fruit.

Where once we had bacon, cabbage and potatoes, Irish stew, colcannon, roast lamb with pure mint sauce, Lancashire hotpot and many other Irish or English dishes, we have much which is foodless being offered. What happened to boiled potatoes in their jackets, which are the epitome of good food? Now we have chips and more chips. These are fried in boiled oils, very often hydrogenated, which can perhaps be lethal to the body. Walk into any restaurant, it does not have to be a fast food outlet, to see them pile up the fast, very often-terrible stuff, offered as food on the plates. Here is an example of good food, the potato, being destroyed. Feeding young children with this kind of fare is bordering on criminal.

Imagine eating *'Lunch Specials'* as shown on a menu I read from: Sausage, chips and can; bun burger, chips and can; batter sausages and can; chicken fillet baguette and can; chips baguette and can; hot dog, chips and can. The menu also shows 19 different kinds of burgers, all with chips, more chips and more cans.

I hold menus with Chinese, Japanese, Thai and French 'foods', all of them picked up in Irish eating places. One can have a lunch of curry sweet and sour, chop suey, szechuan and others with unpronounceable names of so-called food, many with rice or chips. The white rice is just a filler, with no nutritional value, like much of what it is served with. Brown rice, which is pure food, unhusked, is one of nature's gifts to all, being highly nutritious. Brown rice is slow to cook. Fast food is the norm, therefore white rice which is of no nutritional value, is much quicker to cook. It is not natural food, being just a filler, having been processed to remove the invaluable health-giving husk.

Visit France, Thailand, China, Japan, even the U.K. and look for Irish foods. I have yet to find any in these countries except in the odd case where I know Irish food is provided, with the chef or cook being Irish. When it comes to alcohol, here is one of the chief causes of ill-health, as is coffee.

Only in recent years have we learned that there are wines other than Vin De Pays, Asti, Black Tower, Blue Nun or other cheap brands. Now that we have attained cosmopolitan and widely travelled status, such as the week in the Costa del Sol, Lanzarote or other resort, much it appears has been learned about wines. Journalists turned wine buffs, now write pages about various kinds of wines. Almost all now know that there are two kinds, red and white. I usually read between the lines and regularly laugh at some of the idiocy written. Some of the wines sold at ridiculous prices cost little to produce. Many are French and can be bought there for small money.

To me the finest wine is pure organic red grape juice, being 100% natural, not from concentrate, being non-alcoholic, or a bottle of Chilean Merlot. These contain the resveratrol found in certain red wines. They are a marvellous health aid, belonging to the intricate synthesis which are polyphenols. These compounds are being linked to better health in many ways. They can help to prevent heart disease and cancer, two of our biggest killers. See **Resveratrol** caption.

Coffee and the drinking of the liquid is certainly no aid to better health. It is highly caffeinated and can become drug like. I quote from *'Health is Wealth'* as follows. *'The drinker becomes dependent on coffee without realising that it can be a health hazard, leading to headaches, constricting of blood vessels, reducing absorption of minerals, especially Iron, also causing imbalance of Calcium. It is a stimulant and to be avoided'.* Give me weak tea regularly or pure organic grape juice diluted half and half with pure water. A glass of cool clear water, provided one knows the source, is best of all. To be certain of pure and clear water it must be filtered. See **Water** caption.

Most of the pizzas which one sees stacked in the coolers in supermarkets are about as nutritious as a pig's ear. The latter would probably be better to eat. How many read the ingredients labels on the pizza packaging. I have one in front of me, purchased in Ireland, in a supposedly cheap German supermarket, where much of the food and drink is overly additive-filled. It has a list of additives, which is so diverse that it is extremely difficult to find the bits that might be food. The 'hotch botch', which is called pizza, is factory-made, best left on the shelf.

Home made pizza, which contains purely natural foods, and I mean nutritious food, is delicious. Very few know how to make them, just as the many who cannot cook or produce nutritious homemade fare.

We are indeed a sick and undernourished nation, not underfed, being overfed, just eating the wrong foods and eating too much of what is 'rubbish'. Only today I visited a home, after invitation, where there are five children. They are constantly ill. The diet of the family is scandalous. It is Saturday and the children, including teenagers, are not at school or college. The dinner was being eaten and the fare on the plate was, to me, disgusting. There were tinned beans, chips, sausages and lashings of tomato sauce. There was white bread and an amount of confectionary. The contents of the plastic margarine tub, with its *'proven to reduce cholesterol'* blurb, was highly obvious. The tiny print on the container stated *'if taken with a balanced or healthy diet',* or words to that effect. Who reads or searches for these almost undecipherable words? Here is an example of the use of foods, which are anything but healthy, as a diet. Sadly all too many are unaware of what constitutes a balanced diet, as was this mother.

On the table too were little cartons of yoghurt style liquid called Vitalinea. The tiny worded advertising spiel told us 0% sugar. I repeat 0%. Would someone please tell me how you can promote a product where 0% of a particular substance is or is not in something? The small print, which I needed a magnifying glass to read, showed this, also added sweeteners, Aspartame and Acesulfame K, which are unnatural, the former now under serious scrutiny. They are certainly highly questionable as additives. At least sugar is pure, they are not.

Compare this to Glenilen Farm Natural Probiotic yoghurt, with no added sugar or artificial sweeteners, as produced in Co. Cork. The ingredients label reads; fresh pasteurised whole milk, skimmed milk powder, live probiotic yoghurt cultures *and nothing else*. It specifically stated **AND NOTHING ELSE.** What a change to see one of the very few **natural** yoghurts on the shelf. The others, which I suggest, are Killowen, Glenisk, Yeo Valley, or there may be a small pure yoghurt maker in your area. I mention about natural yoghurts to make comparison with what the mother of the children was providing. **Almost all yoghurts are unnatural with additives of some kind.** One has to search for the good. There is available, 'rubbish' food in abundance.

Also on their table was Carie brand dairy cream substitute, which the unfortunate mother thought was real cream. This cream, if that is nice enough word to describe the stuff, contained additives and is certainly not real dairy cream as described on the aerosol tin. Real dairy cream is pure and natural, additive free. Skimmed milk, the largest ingredient in the Carie processed mixture, is what one obtains by separating the cream from milk. 'Carie' creamlike liquid was much removed from real dairy cream in its pureness whatever about its colour. Here is a typical example of what is pretentious 'food', as available on the shelves for an unwitting housewife, such as the mother referred to, a cook, a provider of food for the family. Here is another lady who does not read the ingredients labels and is therefore not aware of much that is being bought as food, but which is not. I did not discover until late in the conversation that both herself and the husband smoked. As I have told many, often in forceful language, **"They have their priorities totally wrong".** I felt like a beaten or failed man. It would be impossible to advise this family of how to be healthy if they did not forego the slow-killing cigarettes. I did impress on them the need to read the ingredients labels and to avoid the unnatural. See *Pretentious Foods* caption.

I genuinely felt sorry for this nice person as I spoke with her. She had no idea about cooking proper nutritious, health giving meals. Being completely ignorant of what was in the stuff she purchased as food made it more difficult. There are many families such as this where both parents may be out of work, where there is limited income or to put it bluntly, a shortage of money. Older people too are often unable to make ends meet.

The tendency with many is to resort to purchasing processed and additive-filled 'food', which appears to be cheap. Cheaper may be dearer in the long-term, as it very often leads to ill-health and malnutrition. There is much, which is natural and highly beneficial to better health, in supermarkets, butchers, fruit and vegetable shops, and especially in the health food store. It just means a little thought and searching for. Learning to cook and present simple meals can be likened to a major investment in good or better health. See *Eat Well On A Limited Budget* caption

I repeat, *"I am convinced that if the lifestyle of the people of our nation was changed, our hospitals would only be quarter full, if that"*. Our doctors would be working part-time. Many of the drug companies would be in liquidation and the Sickness Industry would shrink. The Government, the food industry or the money-orientated bods who manipulate the Health Service Executive purses, all provided for by the taxpayer, will ensure none of this can happen.

In one half of the world there are millions starving because they have no food. In the half we live in there are millions with seemingly plenty, much of which is processed, factory made, unnatural. The majority of the latter mentioned are plagued with ill health because of what they are eating, or rather what they are not eating.

Show me the doctor who advises better health with change to pure, nutritious foods, which are the greatest medicines known

WE ARE INDEED A SICK AND UNDER-NOURISHED NATION, with all too many suffering from malnutrition because of what people are taking into their bodies, believing it to be good food.

GET ON YOUR KNEES

Get on your knees and thank GOD you are on your feet

CANCER

Over many years I have collected much information about cancer and the terrible scourge which it is. My 'hide-out' from which I work, also my office and the attic, are the archives which I sometimes delve into when seeking information, knowledge or help.

Regrettably I have no answer to the dreaded disease, but I do have much advice and information which can help one prevent cancer, or to live with it. The disease is something I do not advise people about. It is beyond my remit. All too many being treated for cancer by the medical profession die. As a layman, if I treated some and they recovered there would be little about it, with perhaps the reasons for the cure being given as other than my help. If just one of those people I gave help to died I would be looked upon as being a pariah, a fool maybe. Sadly there are many within the medical circle who can do little. Almost daily we hear of some breakthrough which will bring relief or cure. None cure. Yes, there is often remission or respite. Name for me any drug that cures cancer or other disease? It will be very interesting to see the results, in the long term, of the use of the much hyped Gardasil, the unproven and controversial vaccine which is being prescribed to help prevent cervical cancer.

There are many, many myths about cancer. Among these stories or handed down beliefs are that:
• Breast cancer is not preventable.
• The only treatments are chemotherapy and radiation.
• Mammograms are best for cancer detection.

These three disclosures are untrue. I am convinced that the veins, arteries and the body's circulation system can be cleared or made to work better, as I have done, following two heart attacks some years ago. I know, as do many of my naturopathic friends and a vast number of people who have treated themselves naturally with success, that cancer can be prevented or aided the natural way.

As one who for the past 45 years has lived a life of using natural and additive free foods and drinks, always emphasising and dwelling on the need for prevention in relation to health, I now hold my hands up and ask, "Does it help"? Call me a sceptic if you wish and I will not be annoyed. Apart from the two heart attacks referred to, where I went down the road of successfully treating myself by the use of natural remedies, also following the advice of my slogan, **We are as we eat, drink, sleep and exercise,** I have never been ill except when with mumps, measles, chickenpox or colds when a youngster.

At 82 years young I was diagnosed with stone in the kidney. It proved to be much more serious than that curable problem. Within a very short period from then, the diagnosis was a malignant growth on my kidney.

I was referred to St. Vincent's University Hospital in Dublin. There I was cared for by a medical team which was supreme, excellent, and to me incomparable. There are many adjectives which could be used to describe the thoroughness and rectitude of the highly trained medical specialists, which included surgeons, doctors, nurses and allied health care specialists. All were highly trained in their various disciplines, working gently and assiduously as they resolutely went about their tasks. The caterers, cleaners and all concerned with the highly successful running of the hospital carried out their duties in a thoroughly proficient and painstaking manner. I cannot praise all sufficiently.

On my first visit to St. Vincent's University Hospital, which was for diagnosis and interview, I was told that were three options open to me. I could have drain out/wash out and chemotherapy, do nothing or have an operation. I decided on the latter although warned of the seriousness because of my age. There were several appointments kept over the next few weeks as I went for scans, x-rays, superscans, blood tests, E.C.G. and other tests.

My first day in hospital was a day of preparation by the medical staff. It was also a time of continuing prayers as I asked Almighty GOD to perform what to me has been a miracle. This too may have been and continues to be because of so many friends, neighbours and relatives entreating with GOD on my behalf. The parting words of a very good friend on the day before entering hospital were, "GOD be with you, we'll pray the rosary for you every night". Sadly not many families kneel to say the rosary, the trimmings or other prayers now. Several prayers are included in this book but the call to GOD which I said regularly was that given to me by another friend, with the words;

LORD GOD, please shield me from harm
Guide my medical team
Please give wisdom to their minds
And skill to their hands.   Amen

There are many who face up to the misfortune which is cancer and without doubt prayer is an almighty aid and help.

Very early next morning I was taken to the operating theatre and after other mild preparations I was told, "You are now being put to sleep". Some four to five hours later I woke up, after what I imagined was a few minutes. My first thoughts were, 'Oh they haven't even started yet'. My fears were unfounded as a voice said, "Good, you are awake now, all is done". I then discovered that I was snugly tucked in between the snow-white sheets of the bed I had been returned to. Having been wheeled back to the ward, I had at this time, various tubes connected to my body as well as an oxygen mask. One by one they were taken away over the next few days. My diseased kidney had been removed successfully.

The morning after the operation I was put sitting in a chair, later standing up and being helped to take some steps as I walked a little. Eight days later I went home, having been told that all was clear also that I must not lift or carry anything, not to overdo the exercise, being advised to use the stairs and not to drive for six weeks.

From time of diagnosis or probably from some weeks before then I lost 42 pounds, almost 20 kilos. I set this out to highlight how cancer just gnaws at the body from onset of the disease. Arrangements were being made for me to enter a nursing home for convalescence but the only home I wished to see was my own. I knew that my good and loving wife would provide all the restoration required.

Having been told by the surgeon, who was accompanied by some of his medical team doing the daily rounds, that 'I had been a magnificent patient', their words, they could not understand how or why I had healed so quickly. It was explained to these good people, all medical professionals, that I attributed my fighting and recuperative powers to my lifestyle, all of which is harped about and repeated constantly throughout these pages, also in my talks given throughout Ireland and the U.K. Good food, drink, exercise and proper sleep are better than any medicine.

The advice about prevention of cancer, as set out in this book, is the way to fight ill-health, including helping to stop the occurrence or re-occurrence of cancer. I have gone into an amount of detail here regarding my fight with cancer, hopefully now concluded. This has been done in an endeavour to assure any who find themselves in a similar situation, that a positive mind, not worrying about the outcome and perhaps using the power of prayer as I did, can be invaluable ways of fighting any disease, including cancer.

GOD'S GUIDANCE

**A nation without GOD'S guidance is a nation without order.
Happy is the person who keeps GOD'S law**

THE EXPERT WORLD CANCER RESEACH FUND REPORT

This eye-opening and amazing report gives colossal food for thought. This to me is one of the greatest blows ever struck in the endeavour to make people see sense and realise that synthetic or chemical drugs will do little, if anything, to give one better or enjoyable health. In simple words, as spoken by Hippocrates so many years ago, *"Let food be your medicine, let medicine be your food"*. In the defence of drugs against natural remedies, or more especially against good nutritious whole food, the old rigmarole is wheeled out that *'There is no scientific evidence'* that food or natural remedies are better. Read further to discover why 'The Expert Report' is not being publicised in any form by our bureaucrats, with the general public certainly being kept ignorant of its contents, being made fools of. We can rightly ask. *"What kind of people govern us"?*

Note that it was issued in 2007. Now, some years later, the all embracing and exhaustive work, which included half a million studies, is under wraps. These studies were done over a number of years and tell us much. They have not been given recognition by the medical profession or the medical bureaucrats who are supposedly responsible for the health of the nation. It is not in the interests of the Irish Medical Organisation or the British Medical Association, to inform the public of how to prevent illness naturally. They are in the sickness business and hope to keep it working and expanding. Cure or prevention are not their worry, or at the top of their lists.

Have you heard about the report? If not, why not? Like the withheld **National Policy Nutrition Report** compiled by an Oireacthas Sub-Committee, which since 2004 has been kept secret from the people, the **Expert World Cancer Research Fund Report** is locked away too, not to be highlighted. The **National Obesity Task Force Report of 2005** is another highly informative report about the health of all. This too gathers dust, as our legislators, especially the so called **HEALTH SERVICE EXECUTIVE,** appear to go out of their way to hide anything which can lead to prevention of illness. Here are **THREE REPORTS** which would lead all to be healthier and without most of the illness or disease we have now. As I have said, dispensing the 10 recommendations you will read about would bankrupt the drug companies and our Government. The latter is already very nearly bankrupt. Many within the pharmaceutical drug-manufacturing industry would be liquidated. Read on to realise, that if we wish to be healthy, including helping to avoid cancer, that prevention is the answer.

Here are their findings as issued by *The Expert World Cancer Research Fund Report (W.C.R.F.).* These are the vital parts of the report which gives the all-important 10 recommendations for cancer prevention. **It tells us that it is the most comprehensive report on cancer prevention ever produced**.

It took six years to produce and looked at all available research on cancer prevention. An initial 500,000 studies were screened down to 22,000, and then it was decided that 7,000 of these studies met the rigorous standards for inclusion in the report.

The literature review process was done by nine independent universities, which then presented the information to a panel of 21 world renowned experts who reviewed the comprehensive collection of evidence, drew conclusions and made recommendations. Because of the thoroughness of the report and the expertise of the panel, people can read the report's findings, confident that it is the most reliable and comprehensive information available on cancer prevention.

W.C.R.F. has developed 10 recommendations, based on the conclusions of the expert report panel, that certain foods and lifestyle choices affect the development of cancer. They state as follows:
Our recommendations are based on our findings, which contains the most comprehensive research available on cancer preventions. Outlined are the practical steps you can take to reduce your risk.

The 10 recommendations are as follows:

1. Be as lean as possible without becoming underweight. Convincing evidence shows that weight gain and obesity increases the risk of a number of cancers, including bowel and breast cancer.
Maintain a healthy weight through a balanced diet of natural food and regular physical activity to help keep your risk lower.

2. Be physically active for at least 30 minutes or more every day. There is very strong evidence that physical activity protects against cancers including bowel and breast cancer. Being physically active is also key to maintaining a healthy weight.
Any type of activity counts – the more you do the better! Try to build some into your everyday life.

3. Avoid sugary foods or energy-dense foods (particularly processed foods which are almost always high in added sugar, low in fibre, or high in fat). *Energy-dense foods and drinks are high in fats and/or sugars and can be low in nutrients. These foods increase the risk of obesity and therefore cancer. Sugary drinks, such as cokes and fruit squashes also contribute to weight gain. Fruit juices even without added sugar, are likely to have a similar effect. Try to eat lower energy-dense foods such as vegetables, fruits and whole grains instead. Opt for water or unsweetened tea in place of sugary drinks.*

4. Eat more of a variety of vegetables, fruits, whole grains and pulses such as beans and other greens. *Evidence shows that vegetables, fruits and other foods containing dietary fibre may protect against a range of cancers including mouth, stomach and bowel cancer. They also help to protect against weight gain and obesity. As well as eating your five a day, try to include whole grains (e.g. brown rice, wholemeal bread also brown pasta and/or pulses) with every meal.*

5. Limit consumption of red meats such as beef, pork and lamb and avoid all processed meats. *There is strong evidence that excessive consumption of red and processed meats are causes of bowel cancer and that there is no amount of processed meat that can be confidently shown not to increase risk. Aim to limit intake of fresh red meat to less than 18 oz (500grm approx), cooked weight (about 24 to 26 oz (700 – 750g raw weight) a week. Try to avoid processed meats such as bacon, ham, salami, corn-beef, also some sausages. All plastic covered and vacuum packed meats should be avoided.*

6. If consumed at all, limit alcoholic drinks to two for men and one for women a day. *Since the 1997 report, the evidence that alcoholic drinks can increase the risk of a number of cancers, including breast and colon cancer, is very much stronger. Any alcohol consumption can increase your risk of cancer, though there is some evidence to suggest that small amounts of alcohol can help protect against heart disease. Therefore, if you choose to drink, it is advisable to do so in strict moderation.*

7. Limit consumption of salty foods and foods processed with salt (sodium). *Evidence shows that salt and salt preserved foods probably cause stomach cancer. Try to use herbs and spices to flavour your food and remember that processed foods, including bread and breakfast cereals, can contain large amounts of salt.*

8. Don't use supplements to protect against cancer unless eating a varied and balanced diet of pure, unadulterated nutritious foods. *Research shows that high-dose nutrient supplements can affect our risk of cancer if the diet is not good, so it is best to opt for a balanced diet without supplements if eating pure and natural foods.*

Recommendations **9** and **10** don't apply to everyone, but if they are relevant to you, it's best to follow them.

9. It is best for mothers to breastfeed exclusively for up to 6 months and then add other liquids and foods. *Some evidence shows that breastfeeding protects mothers against breast cancer and babies from excess weight gain.*

10. After treatment, cancer survivors should follow the recommendations of cancer prevention. *The report found growing evidence that maintaining a healthy weight through diet and physical activity may help to reduce the risk of cancer recurrence. And always remember – do not smoke or chew tobacco. Smoking or using tobacco in any form increases the risk of cancer by a multiple factor also other serious diseases.*

In the report we thought we would hear something about a chemical pharma drug breakthrough, which would end all cancers. Instead those, like myself, who believe in the use of natural foods and drinks, exercise and proper sleep, lifestyle discipline and the simple respect for the wonderful, awesome bodily system, have had our views proclaimed and highlighted. **LET'S SAY, "WE HAVE BEEN VINDICATED MONUMENTALLY."**

This report, where it is apparent that nothing was left to chance, has not and seemingly will not be publicised. This points to sheer contempt by the Government, also The Health Service Executive/Sickness Industry and the various Cancer Charities, for the suffering cancer patients as well as for the many people who can help prevent the terrible disease. If the information and the 10 recommendations were publicised, not alone would we have cancer prevention aid in a huge way, but the health of all would also improve tremendously. As I have said already in this book, *"Our hospitals would be almost empty"*. Many blame the Government for the woes or points at issue, often undeservedly, but rightly so in this instance. With this vitally important information being withheld, the only people who can arrange for the publicising and advertising of the World Cancer Research Report are the legislators, those who govern or in this case

pretend to, as they do nothing, withholding the crucial and so necessary information.

The Health Service Executive, which as the Sickness Industry is the biggest limb of our bureaucracy, will do nothing to air the vital knowledge and data in the report. With all this weighing on my mind, just now I have spoken with a friend, a Teachta Dála, a member of our parliament, better known as a T.D., but on the opposition benches. When I put all this to him, we discussed the future, questioning if the recommendations were given headlines. We talked about setting them out in pages of our newspapers, especially the regional or local ones. **"Look,"** my friend said, **"It all comes down to politics and more so economics".** He continued, **"Consider that the foreign trade for the pharmaceutical drug and medical components industry is almost 40% of the total exports from our shores. Much of this goes to America, the biggest prescription drug junkies in the world. Neither in this country, the U.K. or America will the cosy cartel between private health insurance companies, Governments and the Sickness Industry, which includes the drug conglomerates, be subject to the slightest interference or intrusion. I must agree that if the ten recommendations, as set out by the W.C.R.F., were to be known on a countrywide basis the health of all would improve dramatically but the drug industry would be decimated. No Government will allow this to happen".** I repeat, **"The welfare and robustness of the economy is, in the opinion of our legislators, of much more importance than the health of those whom they supposedly govern".**

After reading this book, *Selling Sickness!*, all can rightly ask, **"Is this suppressing or hiding of the various reports acceptable to us?"** also **"What kind of democracy, what kind of a country do we live in?"** A dictatorship would be better than this kind of conduct or carry on, where the democratically elected parliament refuse to publicise, also withholding and suppressing reports which are vitally important for what is, in the opinion of the vast majority, if not all, the most important thing in life, namely, **GOOD OR BETTER HEALTH**. When put into two words this means **OUR HEALTH**.

With almost 50 years of experience with regard to natural health, I know that the 10 recommendations from this very, very important report are the answer to many of our health problems. Because of the pig-headedness of the Government, especially in their quest for money to keep the economy afloat, many are condemned to a life of ill health, being kept ignorant of the contents of the Expert Report of the World Cancer Research Fund. The full Report is available from the W.C.R.F. UK, 19, Harley

Street, London, W1G 9QJ – Tel: 00 44 207 343 4200, or **wcrf@wcrf.org**. What I have set out about the 10 recommendations gives the important and salient points as issued by the W.C.R.F. The Cancer Research Fund produced them and I have outlined them to you, the reader.

PAUSE

Many people worry about what others think of them.
They should pause to consider that the others referred to,
are too busy looking after themselves and their problems

DRUGS – CHEMICALS – WHAT DO THEY CURE?

With the exception of Penicillin, to which some are allergic, also Aspirin, there is not a drug that I know of, or have heard of, which cures. Most are unsafe, whether prescribed or bought over the counter.

Penicillin, which was derived from a mould, has been and is the one outstanding antibiotic I would accept as being a wonder drug. Aspirin is the other one, which if taken as prescribed, can give excellent results. Its use can lead to internal bleeding but only if mixed with other drugs or more especially if taken with fast, processed or additive-filled so-called foods. Who gives thought to this or the mixing of alcohol with Aspirin? Little thought is given to taking any chemical if drinking alcohol before or after the use of any drug. This can be extremely dangerous.

Many doctors do not give sufficient thought to the prescribing of drugs. There are extreme dangers if anti-inflammatory and anti-depressant drugs are combined. The doctors are not always to blame. Many are on prescribed anti-depressant medicines, often buying over the counter so-called 'remedies', taking them without consideration as to the health consequences. Michael Jackson and Heath Ledger died because of the abuse of prescription medication. We heard of the medics being implicated in these tragic affairs. Where the doctors are concerned this will probably be the last we hear of the sad affair.

Even as I pen these words a relative in his 40's has died, because of a mixture of drugs and alcohol. His close relatives did not know about the dangers. Apparently this young and extremely nice man did not realise or know of the harm of the mixture. We were told that death was accidental. Others have died similarly. Surely if taken as prescribed this would not be abuse, especially if warnings are given by the G.Ps. and pharmacists regarding the dangers of mixing alcohol with prescribed and other drugs.

The doctors who prescribe a mish-mash of the chemicals should not allow the system to be abused. Their responsibilities are huge and they should be made fully aware that their use of their prescription pads, to earn huge money, should be curtailed.

Researchers tell us that the flu jab has been found to be useless. Scientists tell us that Prozac and similar anti-depressants do not cure, saying that a placebo would be equal. Prozac is nothing short of being a myth, to be avoided. Many drugs are addictive and should be shunned.

Drugs, which are costing the nation millions, make no difference to depression. Exercise, proper diet and lifestyle, also therapy, should be prescribed instead. I must ask the doctor for a prescription for this cure and watch his reaction. Will they tell us we need a change of lifestyle? Certainly not. See *Depression* caption.

I have seen the uselessness of taking many of the prescribed and other drugs. All too many who have turned to me over the years, asking for help by the use of natural remedies, draw attention to the naked truth that the drug-manufacturing companies and those who prescribe, the medical profession, are going down the wrong road.

Chemical drugs, pills and medicines are not the answer to our health problems. Indeed many healthy people are put on them. The result is that they are sick people for the rest of their lives or until able to come off the often harmful medication, which sadly is all too often **NEVER**.

The sceptics, the medical and indeed lay people 'know-alls', also those with vested interests, will try to tell us of the ineffectiveness of anything natural. They use the hoary chestnut or cliché that there is no scientific evidence to support their use. I suggest that they gather together the many thousands of people like myself, also the alternative health practitioners we have. Arrange for us to ask those we have helped to better or good health to meet. Croke Park would be an ideal venue. There would be many unable to gain admission to the packed hallowed grounds if the day out was advertised and given publicity.

The sceptics would be silenced. Do these scoffers realise or are they numb-sculled to the fact that almost all, if not all, synthetic chemical pharma manufactured drugs do not cure?

Many drugs are just stoppers of pain. All too many are injurious to better health. Will people ever learn that a safe synthetic or chemical medicine is a useless one? Need we add more to convince the sceptic, the doubter? Public confidence in the drug industry, the medical profession and the Sickness Industry is at an all time low. Many who are unwell are afraid to seek information or help, having been through the torturous route of terrible side-effects.

I have not digressed on the serious matter of drugs not curing, the side effects or the harm, which they can cause. So many products, which are sold to us, with promises of improving our health, only improve the medical profession's and the drug company's bank balances. **It has been found that many, especially the elderly, do not take their tablets or pills because of the fear of feeling unwell as a result of the side effects, the result being that in many homes there is much medication which remains unused. This is costing the taxpayers millions. Nobody could put a figure on this waste simply because of the fear of many to speak out and other doubts which lead to this. Older people are certainly reluctant to speak about this problem. I learn much from young family members.**

The often terrifying and adverse side effects of synthetic medicines are kept quiet by the Sickness Industry. Often they are conveniently neglected or silenced. Some of these side effects are everlasting, causing serious problems in later life.

The advice or writings given with or on the pills and medicine bottles or plastic containers advise about their use, but are often unread. Frequently there are warnings about the need for care in their use, of side effects. There is often advice not to drive, to operate machinery or of the care needed. The majority do not bother to read the warnings or other information. **IT IS OF VITAL IMPORTANCE TO READ THE ADVICE OR WRITINGS GIVEN WITH, OR ON MEDICINE BOTTLES OR CHEMICAL DRUGS CONTAINERS, WHICH INFORM ABOUT THEIR USE.**

I keep harping and repeating about the need to avoid additives. Nowhere is this admonition more relevant than with chemical drugs or medicines. Many are full of synthetic and other dubious additives, which are not natural. Young children and babies are given medicines which contain dyes, preservatives, sweeteners and other things which are not allowed in natural food or drink for children under three. Most drugs used to treat babies have not been tested on the young. It all comes down to money. The drug companies are unwilling to use research and development facilities because trial costs are exorbitant. **The profits for the shareholders are the prime object**. The juvenile's health is not their problem.

Regularly we hear or read of drug trials, which we are told will lead to an antidote or cure for some prevailing illness. **'Research'** or **'New Research'** are words highlighted, as is the good side of the story. The other side of the information regarding side effects or other unacceptable health problems are conveniently omitted.

All this reminds me of the photographs and write-ups about new fashions, which are often seen in some newspapers or their weekend magazines. They are also in glossy periodicals. A family in the fashion business, the rag trade, told me how young people come to the store with cuttings from the papers or magazines, enquiring where the depicted wearing apparel can be purchased. We agreed that the fashions enquired about, are just like the 'researched' chemical drugs mentioned. Almost all of them are not seen or heard about again. Scientific studies on drugs are often pretentious, as all too often we have drug trial disasters, with human beings used as guinea pigs.

I keep saying that it is my reasoning that certain of the media are in league with the drug and medical industry. Some years ago a full page was devoted by a tabloid, advising how **'Wonder Drugs'** (their description) will make us mentally sharp, improve our performance at work, referring to them as 'Miracle Medicines' or 'Smart Drugs'. Scientists have referred to them as 'Cognition Enhancers'. One by one, little by little, silently, these terrible drugs are being prescribed. My mind is not improved, just numbed, when I see the names, because I understand the dire consequences of their use. I would not give Modafinil, Ritalin, Rimonabant, Propranolol and others mentioned, to my worst enemy. I would destroy the drugs. The terrible chemicals mentioned, and the many unmentioned, will certainly destroy the human system. They will do this to the human body in the long-term, or maybe not so long-term. It is beyond comprehension that any doctor would suggest or advise the use of these drugs.

When consideration is given to the wonderful and intricate workings of the body, it is unbelievable that the Sickness Industry does so much to destroy the magical workings of the human system. Using the many chemicals prescribed by them, especially the over prescribing and mixing together of them, is insensitive and should not be tolerated. When it comes to the treatment of what is put into the stomach, it is plainly visible that no consideration is given to the future health of people for whom these very often dangerous drugs are prescribed.

As mentioned elsewhere, the drug companies have perfected the art of sickness invention. Quiet often we hear of some ailment with a new name. They then proceed to make more lolly for their shareholders as they promote sales by advising doctors to prescribe what can be dangerous drugs. Here is just one of the reasons why the pharma drug-manufacturing industry is not to be trusted. The very bottom line is **'MONEY/PROFITS'** for the Sickness Industry. The top and most other lines, as far as the patients are concerned, is that **DRUGS DON'T CURE.**

KEEP YOUNG

We do not stop playing because we grow old,
we grow old because we stop playing

SUGAR AND SUGARS

In my book **'Health is Wealth'** I have decried and railed against the use and blatant over-use of the 'unhealthy' substance, which is sugar. It has control of the taste buds, having no nutritional value, with enormous evidence of its harm to humans. It is not a food. We hear, read and see the advertisements giving all the watered down information about the dangers of fats. The big majority do not understand about this, the main reason being that there is frequent change of direction in the fat line of thought, with claim and counter claim. Unequivocal evidence shows that sugar, which is a fat, is the enemy of good or reasonably good health. It is being taken into the body excessively, with the oversupply sugar being converted into fats called triglycerides, which are deposited into the fat cells It is in most made up, processed or manufactured 'foods' or 'drinks'. Sometimes the blurb, usually on a plastic container, tells us **'No Added Sugar'**. Read further to discover that the ingredients label tells us it contains artificial sweeteners such as Saccharin, Acesulfame K, Splenda and perhaps others. All can be equally 'dangerous' to better health.

The consumption of sugar and I don't mean over-use, leads to all kinds of serious health problems including: obesity and being overweight, diabetes, high blood pressure, heart and circulation problems. There is no need for the householder or caterer to use sugar.

Study the history of the stuff. There are many books written about it. In their writings those with no vested interests in the product tell sad, inhuman stories of sugar production. The general public are oblivious to its dangers to the system. There should be a health warning on sugar packaging. One can easily reply and with good reason, saying **"The warnings that smoking can kill are ignored by almost all smokers"**. Sugar is equally as dangerous but in a different manner.

Repeated here is an extract from the report by the renowned and distinguished John Hopkins School of Medicine, which has and continues to do so much to fight cancer. Dr. Chi Van Dang, from the school, tells us **"Cancer cells are such sugar junkies that glucose deprivation contributes significantly to their demise"**.

Read the ingredients labels of much, which is sold as 'food', to discover its flagrant overuse. Take sugar into the system at your peril. This is not scare-mongering. How often do we see the advice, **'Cut down on sugar'**. My advice is **"Cut out sugar to enjoy better health"**. It can be another silent 'killer'. Artificial sweeteners too are not natural, to be avoided. The sugars referred to are all refined, processed, unnatural and certainly to be abstained from. I repeat the words which a well known and respected Professor used, as already mentioned, **"SUGAR IS SNOW WHITE AND DEADLY"**

SELF – CENTRED

**People who live in their own little world
never get to enjoy the world of others**

WATER

THE FLUORIDATED AND DISINFECTED WATER WE ARE EXPECTED TO DRINK

Water is now a chemically laden liquid, which we are forced to drink because of the pigheadedness of our uncaring bureaucrats. I ask two simple questions. *"If we live in a so-called democratic country, why is it that despite the majority being against fluoridation, Fluorosilicic Acid and Chlorine are offloaded into our water"?* Furthermore *"Why is Ireland the only country in Europe where fluoridation of water is mandatory?* Fluorosilicic Acid is a chemical, a waste by-product of the fertilizer industry. We are now officially told that it may be a cancer risk. This is in well-documented Epidemiological Literature associating hip and other bone fractures with drinking water which has been fluoridated.

The number of cases has increased dramatically over the past 20 years and is rising alarmingly. This chemical is an enemy of good bones and can lead to osteoporosis.

It has so much bad publicity and danger warnings that it is very obvious our Government doesn't govern. Most members of the Irish Expert Body on Fluoride and Health need their heads examined as they promote the chemical waste product. The population who have to drink the water which contains fluoride, more especially babies and young children, are being set up to be long-term clients of the Sickness Industry. The majority of those who promote the use of the unwanted, unlicensed, untested, so-called medicine, which is Fluorosilicic Acid, are medics, or in some way connected to the Sickness Industry. Here again it is obvious that it pays them to keep people ill.

Have they looked into the fact that it may be part of the obesity problem we have? To control the amount of the acid used is impossible because we have an overdose of the chemical. It is in many prescribed and some over the counter medicines and toothpastes. Fluoride is in most of the reconstituted fruit juices, fizzy, energy and juice drinks also many other foods or liquids where water is in the make up or processing. Many are taking well above the safe amount into their bodies, especially as already stated, our young people. Here again is one of the reasons why we are a sick nation. It is fair to assume that anything mixed with water contains an amount of fluoride, unless filtered before use. There is no way to control the amount being ingested into the body.

In May 2010, the Scientific Committee on Environmental Health Risks (SCHER) stated in its Pre-consultation Opinion: *'Water fluoridation is a rather poor and crude measure of systemic fluoride treatment, without a detectable threshold for dental and bone damage".* *"Systemic exposure to fluoride in drinking water is associated with an increased risk of dental and bone fluorosis in a dose-response manner, without a detectable threshold'.*

This last sentence means that any level of artificial fluoridation causes health damage to many people who are forced to consume the unwanted fluoride, which is the unlicensed chemical medicine Fluorisilicic Acid.

Barry Groves, author of the eye opening book *'Fluoride, Drinking Ourselves To Death'?* gives the reader and the drinker of fluoridated water much food for thought in the words set out here and taken from his book. *"No safety tests have ever been done on Silicofluorides. There are no proper studies on the effectiveness of Hexafluorosilicic acid in reducing dental cavities or caries either. Many of the components of the 'product' that is used for water fluoridation are known to be extremely harmful, yet no safety testing data is available for it anywhere in the world. Any claim that fluoridation is 'safe' is at best wishful thinking and at worst a lie."* AS THIS BOOK, *Selling Sickness*!, GOES TO THE PRINTERS, NEWS HAS COME THROUGH THAT OVER 20 STUDIES NOW SHOW THAT FLUORIDATED WATER CAUSES BRAIN DAMAGE IN CHILDREN. Surely no other evidence is needed. **Adding the untested chemical and unlicensed medicine, fluorosilicic acid, to our water must stop.**

THE JOY OF WORKING

When it comes to the work we do daily, it would be nice and certainly food for thought if we could be like **Thomas A. Edison** (1847-1931), who said *"I never did a day's work in my life, it was all fun."* As I went through life I can honestly say the same. All work, including the help to those who were and are unwell, has been joyful.

COSMETICS, TOILETRIES AND SKIN CARE PRODUCTS CAN VERY OFTEN LEAD TO ILL HEALTH

When one realises that over 60% of what is put on the skin is absorbed into the body, this should give much cause for concern. That is of course if we care about our skin. Who doesn't?

The worrying fact is the rate of absorption, or indeed the assimilation of chemicals into the body, some of them perhaps toxic.

The deodorant maker **Biosen** did a study, which confirms what I write about. This found that the average British or Irish woman, 'hosts' 515 chemicals on her body every day. It tells us that moisturisers could contain more than 330 chemicals and perfumes up to 400. **Biosen** also said most of the pollutants are self inflicted by women who sprayed deodorants, slapped on moisturiser or other creams, also applied lipsticks, giving little thought to the harm they may be doing to the skin and of course indirectly to themselves.

How many seek information about what is in body lotions, shower gels, shampoos, conditioners, make-up, creams and other skin products? Do so and be surprised at the chemical ingredients of much. Learn to read the ingredients labels. Many skin allergies and much skin discomfort is caused by synthetic and chemical additives, including preservatives. Recent tests have shown that most lipsticks contain excess lead in their composition.

In their book **'Cosmetics Unmasked'** by **Dr. Stephen & Gina Antczak'** we are told that one quarter of the chemicals used in the toiletries industry are harmful. It surprises me that the figure is so low. Recently I was handed a plastic container of one of the biggest selling shampoos, at the same time being told *"Read the ingredients label of this. Please read through to the very last synthetic chemical or ingredient"*. To find anything natural is difficult. The list reads **'Aqua, Sodium Laureth Sulfate, Sodium Lauryl Sulfate, Cocamide MEA, Zinc Carbonate, Glycol Distearate, Sodium Chloride, Zinc Pyrithione, Dimethicone, Cetyl Alcohol, Parfum, Sodium Xylenesulfonate, Polyquaternium-10,**

Magnesium Sulfate, Sodium Benzoate, Butylphenylm Methylpropional, Ammonium Laureth Sulfate, Hexyl Cinnamal, Sodium Diethylenetriamine Pentamethylene Phosphonate, Linalool, Magnesium Carbonate Hydroxide, Benzyl Alcohol, Alpha-Isomethyl Ionone, Geraniol, Etidronic Acid, Citronellol, Limonene, Sodium Polynapthalenesulfonate, Methylchlorisothiazolinone, Aloe Barbadensis, DMDM Hydantoin, Methylisothiazolinone, Disodium EDTA, Tetrasodium EDTA, Anthemis Nobilis, Tocopheryl Acetate. Just imagine putting this mixture on one's head. It is not to be wondered at that we see so many people with little or no hair. I have used, as shampoo, pure natural olive oil based soap for many years and have a good head of hair. The big problem is that it is grey!

The instructions on the container of the additive mixture as set out, many of them chemicals, tells the user to avoid contact with eyes. Tell me how one can do this. The fact that it may be harmful to the eyes is sufficient reason, if any is needed after reading this, to refuse to buy the chemical filled liquid. This is just one skin, hair, nail product picked at random by a friend. This is a shampoo which is highly propagandised and advertised. Many of these concoctions are a nice way of calling soft soap or washing liquid a shampoo.

There are all too many, call them 'beauty products', like this, with questionable additives. Just as with the food additives, many are used to cheapen the product, not to the purchaser, but so that the manufacturers can make their, often extreme, profits for the shareholders. I worked in this business many years ago. The mark up was often ludicrous. It was part of my education in life regarding the use of chemicals. **Environmental exposure to hair sprays, lipstick and the skin care or cosmetics referred to, can trigger many ailments including arthritis and other autoimmune diseases.**

Skin is made good by what is put into the body, not on it. Pure natural foods and drinks, regular meals, proper sleep pattern and exercise, with a good natural food supplement or two are the ingredients needed. I know, I see it every day.

'Perfectil' is an example of what I mean as an aid to better skin, hair and nail health. Sold under the Vitabiotics brand it is a natural progression from vitamin enriched external beauty products. These advanced nutrient capsules have been developed by doctors, with input from nutritionists, at the University of Reading Department of Nutrition, to provide deep nourishment for skin, scalp, and nail tissues. Each capsule contains 25 nutrients to help maintain optimal cell maintenance and cell renewal, along with antioxidants to help protect delicate tissues from the aging effects of the sun. For radiant beauty, 'Perfectil' also provides natural plant extracts with a proven role in maintaining a healthy complexion, also vitamins and minerals *essential* to blood circulation and strong tissue formation. This product is free from artificial colours, preservatives, gluten, fat, starch and yeast, and is produced under fully licensed pharmaceutical manufacture, with strict quality control. It has been developed without testing on animals.

There are other supplements claiming to be good. I have recommended 'Perfectil' for years because it is a wonderful combination of all that is health giving, I have taken them in the past in conjunction with a diet of natural foods and drinks. **Natural, pure food, combines with 'Perfectil' or similar type natural supplement, as recommended by health store adviser, as a recipe for excellent skin, hair and nail health.** I hold no brief or monetary interest in any of the things suggested throughout the pages of this book. Anything suggested for use as an aid to better well-being is because I have witnessed or been told of the good results of their use, before recommending them.

Unblemished skin, shiny, lustrous hair and good nails are all indicators of good health. This can all be had by simply following the words of my slogan **'We are as we Eat, Drink, Sleep and Exercise'**. A supplement to good diet of pure foods and drinks, such as 'Perfectil', can work wonders. Use the natural to be naturally well.

I get hot under the collar when I see claims by shampoo makers that they are anti-dandruff. The removal may be for a day or two, if that. Dandruff or scurf can only be cured, banished, by internal treatment. New Era Combination D Tissue Salts, obtainable from the Health Store, take only a few days to allow one be free from dandruff, with the removal of scurf taking a little longer. Cure from the inside is the only answer to the problem, as with much else where lotions, creams, ointments, and external applications are used. With a little thought and discipline, including the aids mentioned, one can have healthy skin, hair and nails. See *Tissue Salts* caption to read more about these wonderful natural salts of the earth.

There is much which is natural in the Health Food Store, including pure and natural cosmetics also skin, hair and nail products. Pay a visit and don't be afraid to ask questions. One can learn much there, where everything sold over the counter is natural. **Many cosmetics, toiletries and skin care products should not be used, because as I have already stated, they can often lead to ill-health in the future.**

In my book 'Health is Wealth' there is an article setting out the nonsense of where children under the age of two, because of an E.U. directive, must not be allowed use toothpaste when brushing their teeth. **How many parents or those responsible for young children know this?** This came about because of the use or rather ill-use of the toxic fluoride in our water and most toothpastes. Fluoride is being put into our water supply against the wills and better judgement of many, including myself, probably doing much harm to the body, especially the teeth. See *Water and The Chemicals In It* caption

As I put these words on paper the following report has been handed to me. **'A survey by the British Dental Health Foundation found that half of under fives suffer from tooth decay and a quarter of parents do not even think children need to brush their teeth twice a day. The survey found two-thirds of parents thought that brushing one minute was sufficient, when two minutes is recommended, and that a fifth of children under five are left to brush their teeth unsupervised'.**

My advice to all who visit, also at my countrywide talks, whether in U. K. or Ireland, is to **"Use a natural fluoride free toothpaste, obtainable from the Health Food Store".** Follow the advice above and remember that children, including those under the age of two, need to brush at least twice daily, if possible after each meal. They should be supervised and taught how to brush the teeth correctly.

Emphasis is placed on the advice to use natural toothpaste, such as Aloe Dent, which is available from the Health Store. Made by Optima Health and Nutrition, it is excellent, being pure and natural, chemical free. Compare this with chemical, additive-containing toothpastes as sold by supermarkets, pharmacists, stores and many other outlets. Reading the ingredients labels should be enough reason to put one off using the latter, especially if they have fluoride in their make-up. They should be avoided. Toothpaste chemicals, many of which enter the body, may lead to illness in later life. The teeth will certainly not be kept healthy by using unnatural, chemical and fluoride made up, additive-containing toothpastes.

TRUE FRIENDS ARE ANGELS
Angels exist that do not have wings.
These we call true friends.

John Hayes

HEARTBURN OR INDIGESTION

One frequently sees gaviscon, rennie and many other chemical made remedies highlighted for relief of heartburn and indigestion. They are given huge publicity through advertising, because the mighty drug-manufacturing companies who produce them have the wherewithal, the big money, to do so.

A simple but purely natural remedy, with no chemicals whatever included, is to use Charcoal tablets or capsules. Yes, the same charcoal as is used for the barbecue. It is powdered, purified, refined and made up under strict laboratory technique, as are all natural remedies, as sold by the Health Food Stores. I have recommended it to thousands, using it myself when necessary. It takes only a few minutes to bring relief. Doctors will not advise its use. It will not be found in the pharmacy, food store or the filling station. Again it is too natural, cannot be patented, therefore with no money to be made from the pure and simple ingredient.

There can be burning or big discomfort in the chest with heartburn or indigestion. The sufferer should be asked crucial questions. **Do you regularly suffer from indigestion or heartburn?** These two ailments, if prolonged, can lead to stomach and big digestion problems in later life. **Does anybody ever consider that the problems are almost always caused by what is eaten, or by the lifestyle?**

Corrections in the in take of food or drink are almost always the answer to the problem. There should be no need for treatment long-term. Charcoal is an excellent remedy, but it is far better to take steps to prevent Indigestion or Heartburn, usually by change of lifestyle, with much thought given to what is eaten or drank.

A PRAYER TO BE SAID ON AWAKENING

Almighty GOD, I welcome this new day
It is your gift to me – the first day of the rest of my life
I thank you for the gift of life this morning
I thank you for the sleep that has refreshed me
I thank you for the chance to begin life all over again
LORD, this day is full of promise and opportunity
Help me to waste none of it
LORD, this day is full of mystery and of the unknown
Help me to face it without anxiety
During this day, please GOD may I become a more thoughtful person
a more prayerful person
a more generous and kindly person
and a more healthy person
LORD, bless this day for all of us **Amen**

PALMING. SOMETHING ALL SHOULD DO

Many years ago I learned of one of the simplest methods to aid relaxation and to eliminate stress. This easy to carry out exercise requires no output of energy. It is not a physical exercise. Palming, like a natural tranquilliser, leaves one feeling at ease. People with stress, depression, tiredness, feeling out-of-sorts, and other low moods have told me of how it has helped them. It is a huge aid to better and clearer eyesight.

We know that meditation is extremely good for relief, even cure of depression. See **Depression** caption. Those who understand or learn about how to live naturally, practicing the nine words: **'We are as we Eat, Drink, Sleep and Exerci**se' know that meditation has proved to be an excellent aid or even cure for many kinds of illness. Meditation must be learned. It needs much discipline.

It is not just something to start doing without help or aid of a teacher. Up to now, like much else simple and natural which can be used to aid better health, the medical profession do not wish to know about meditation. They will certainly not prescribe meditation, because there is no money for them in this natural aid. They will certainly not tell one about palming. Palming is to me as good or perhaps better than meditation. It is much easier to use than meditating. It is simple and easy to do, if and when one wishes.

Pull a chair up to the table. Sit comfortably, with perhaps a soft cushion beneath. Place the elbows on the table. Put both hands together with the palms open. With the tips of the fingers resting on the upper part of the forehead, place the palms over the eyes, shutting out the light as far as possible. It will be impossible to do this completely but don't worry, just do your best. Close the eyes, feel restful and sense the relaxation of the mind and body. Remember that the eyes and the brain work in very close cohesion. Palming helps both in a huge way. One can palm the eyes for as long as it is comfortable and relaxing to do so. Some can do it for hours, others for shorter or even short periods. A small minority have told me they cannot do it.

As an impetuous person with a very active mind and brain, I would have thought I would be impatient or not persistent or persevering. This has not been so as I palm my eyes regularly. I believe that palming of the eyes is a marvellous way to ease tension, stress, depression, tiredness and much else. It can be done at one's leisure or discretion and wherever one wishes. It is certainly a good aid to better eyesight.

Palming and much invaluable information about attaining better eyesight by eye exercises is available in the best selling book, **'Better Eyesight Without Glasses'** by W. H. Bates M.D. See *Bibliography* section for details. I have met those who by following Dr. Bate's instructions have been able to put their glasses away. One must be fairly disciplined to do so. I mention this because I gave up after a short time, but now continue with palming frequently. At the same time my belief in palming is undiminished.

NUTRITIOUS, DELICIOUS FOOD,
TO WHICH I AM VERY PREDISPOSED

This is not a **recipe** book but I just have to include a few **recipes** of what I like best. These are economical, easy to prepare and cook, as well as being natural and health giving. Here is thought of food as well as food for thought.

SIMPLE BROWN BREAD
INGREDIENTS
I mug of wholemeal flour
I mug of strong white flour
Half mug of wheat germ
Half mug of pinhead oatmeal
Teaspoon of bicarbonate of soda
I pint of milk (Buttermilk optional)

Method. Put all dry ingredients into a bowl and mix. Add milk and mix further. Mixture will be quite wet. Pour into two greased or oiled bread tins. Bake in a pre-heated oven – gas mark 6 or 200F electric fan oven, for approximately one hour. When cooked remove from tins. Place on a wire tray. The bread can be frozen, if desired. This recipe has been given to thousands of people. Many of those who use it tell of its goodness. When working and living away from Ireland, I was often asked, **"What do you miss most?"** My reply has never varied. It was **"The brown bread, the hurling and the quality of life"**.

ONE-MINUTE PORRIDGE

Many people don't know how to make porridge. It is simple. An excellent rule of thumb or guide is to add one-and-a-quarter mugs of water to a half mug of porridge oats. If so desired use half milk/half water. Place the liquid in a saucepan. Stir in the oats and bring to the boil. Simmer for one minute, stirring frequently.

The porridge will become thick and creamy. Serve with honey and milk if desired. It is delicious, nutritious, being a simple and wonderful start to the day. The goodness of oats is mostly unknown. Suggestions are to add linseed, ground pumpkin seeds, especially if with prostate problems, also bran, wheat germ, lecithin, and/or any fruits available.

Any person who skips breakfast is foolish. It is the main meal of the day. Forget the sugarised, additive-containing, cardboard-boxed cereals one sees displayed. There is probably more nutrition in the cardboard than the contents. Porridge is just oats, pure and simple. It is free from additives. The only other breakfast cereal without additives which I have found on the shelves is Shredded Wheat.

BREAD AND BUTTER PUDDING

Usually when bread and butter pudding is served it is overly filled with butter and eggs. In a well-known hotel we visit, which serves good Irish food, this is their recipe for delicious afters. It is healthy and with all natural ingredients, being easy to prepare and cook. It is the nicest bread and butter pudding I have eaten.

INGREDIENTS

6 slices of brown-bread cut from a loaf, with crusts cut off
115grms (4oz.) polyunsaturated, fat free margarine (obtained from the Health Food Store)
60grms (2oz.) brown sugar
115grms (4oz.) sultanas
1 heaped teaspoon mixed spice
285ml (half pint) full cream milk
2 large eggs

Method. Grease a Pyrex dish or cake tin. Spread the margarine on one side of each slice of bread. Sprinkle some of the brown sugar on the bottom of the dish, also the spice. Cover with approximately one third of the bread with the margarine side down. Sprinkle on half of the sultanas. Add another layer of the bread with the margarine up. Add the remainder of the sultanas. Top off with the remainder of the bread, with the margarine side up. Break the egg into the milk mixture and whisk. Pour the liquid over the pudding. Leave to stand for 45 minutes so that the bread absorbs the liquid. If desired, sprinkle some spice and more sultanas on top. Bake in a pre-heated oven at Gas mark 5 (190°C) or 375°F for electric oven for about 40 minutes, when it should be golden brown. Serve on hot plates. I find this is more than a bread pudding. It can be eaten cold at breakfast, lunch or whenever. This is one of the very few times I would use pure, natural, fat-free margarine, instead of butter.

LIVER CASSEROLE – SERVES 4
INGREDIENTS

4 to 6 slices of liver – see over
1 medium size onion
Approx. 75 mls of cold pressed olive oil or safflower oil
(obtained from the Health Food Store)
I Oxo cube,
I dessert spoon of Worcester Sauce,
1 dessert spoon of Tomato Puree
Small amount of flour.

Method. Pigs or lambs liver can be used. Pig's liver contains much health giving goodness. To remove the bitter taste from the pig's liver, soak in milk for half an hour, and be surprised how delicious it can be later. Pat the liver dry on kitchen roll paper. Toss in flour. Fry lightly on both sides to seal the juices.

Peel and slice onion and fry lightly. Drain on kitchen paper. Make gravy with the little fat left in the pan, adding flour, one Oxo cube, and one dessertspoon each of Worcester sauce and Tomato puree. Place in oven proof dish (Pyrex) and cook in a moderate oven for 40 to 50 minutes. It is delicious and nutritious.

Many tourists and visitors have told of their disappointment at the 'food' being provided now in Ireland. Much of it is not native to our country. They say that if they wish to eat Thai, Chinese, Indian, French or other foreign type foods they can go elsewhere. Many visit us to sample the Irish food as provided in the past. Little of it is available anymore. Things like Irish Stew, Colcannon, Irish Beef and Guinness Casserole, Wild Salmon, Braised Leg of Wicklow Lamb, Baked Virginia Ham, Steamed Puddings, Apple Dumpling, Homemade Mayonnaise, Saddle of Irish Lamb, homemade mint sauce, and many other Irish dishes of the past have disappeared.

All too often on the menus provided in most cafes, restaurants and indeed many hotels, there are foreign dishes, panninis, quiches, pizzas or numerous other international named foods, often 'foodless'. Many of them are fast, additive-filled, factory made and have appeared only recently on Irish menus. If it were not for the many additives used, much would certainly not be attractive to the taste buds, the palate of the eater. This is to be expected because much of what we are offered as 'food' is made tasty and highly palatable before and during processing.

Many eat these kinds of meals with no thought as to whether they are healthy food or not. Many visitors to our land tell of their disappointment and of not being able to enjoy Irish food as produced in the past. Sadly, many tell us they will not return.

CHEWING FOOD PROPERLY

Most people do not give thought to the need to take time to chew food properly. Not doing so can lead to various health problems. All too many just gobble down what is eaten, often doing so on the run. It would be wise and prudent to give serious consideration to this, at the same time remembering that there are no teeth in the stomach!

ELDERLY PEOPLE

HOW THEY ARE BEING 'MALTREATED' AND MISDIAGNOSED

This subject is something I have repeatedly harped about over the years. Many elderly people in nursing homes, hospitals or even their own homes are being 'overly treated', one can add aggressively. A recent U.K. Government review has discovered that many are being prescribed medicines and drugs, merely to keep the patient quiet, often for the convenience of the nursing staff. This is just another of the disturbing and all too many pharma chemical drug scandals which we hear or read about regularly. University College Cork, in a report, also referred to the abuse. It was found that General Practitioners failed to prescribe the ideal medicine for more than 22% of elderly patients. I have been given evidence of this by relatives of senior citizens, also by psychiatric nurses with whom we are friendly.

Research carried out, examining 6,680 prescriptions handed out by G.Ps., showed there were large variations in the prescribing, which included patients who were being prescribed as much as 19 different medicines or drugs. The average per patient was five different prescriptions. It is a very thorough report and with many disturbing facts.

There are many cases of the misuse or mis-prescribing of drugs to the elderly. One of the biggest reported was by the B.B.C. recently. It could affect you, an elderly relative, or friends being cared for in nursing homes, institutions, hospitals or even if being treated in the home. **Many are being prescribed dementia drugs – often referred to as the chemical 'cosh'**. An official U.K. government evaluation has found that they are being prescribed to keep the patient quiet, very often unnecessarily. In simple language, the drugs are used to help keep the patient more compliant. Of extreme concern is the fact that in these findings the drugs are being prescribed wrongly in up to 60% of cases.

What the medical bods do not wish to know about is that Dementia can be reversed by use of natural treatment, even cured. Yes, people with this problem can get back to living normal lives. Over the years I have helped many do so. Here again is *Selling of Sickness.*

My book '**Health is Wealth**' tells the story. Proper diet of natural unadulterated foods, plus change of lifestyle, is almost always the answer. To this can be added light exercise, proper sleep pattern and perhaps taking certain food supplements.

Elderly patients are over treated in a huge way for high blood pressure, also the myth which is Cholesterol. **My views on the con which** is *Cholesterol* are set out under that caption.

Almost daily I see people who have been badly affected by taking the statins prescribed for Cholesterol. The side effects are many, while all of the time there is no need to take the drug, the biggest selling, so-called medication in the world.

Blood pressure control is almost always kept right by choice of lifestyle including proper diet. See *Blood Pressure* caption.

I have received many reports of elderly patients being 'maltreated', a little of which is set out here.

Many times I have witnessed friends and others placed in a nursing home, or other institution. They were usually reasonably healthy and mobile, but very often a huge burden on a family trying to look after them properly. All too often, when placed in an institution or perhaps a nursing home, these people are turned into sick patients, deteriorating in a very short time. Some ended up like zombies.

The inappropriate prescribing has led to healthy elderly patients suffering significant adverse drug reactions, often requiring hospitalisation. These wrongly prescribed drugs are regularly killing patients. As with the over prescribing of antibiotics, the side effects and harm of many chemical drugs, also many other things which are reported almost daily as being wrong in the Sickness Industry, the question must be asked, **"Who does anything to correct all this mismanagement and 'maltreatment?"**

SALMON

THE UNNATURAL BATTERY REARED CAGED SALMON WE ARE OFFERED AS 'FOOD'

Enter a restaurant, even a cheap café, pick up the menu, note the words now frequently used to describe a portion of salmon. Seldom is it referred to as a fillet or steak of the fish. The usual descriptive word is darne of salmon.

When I see this word darne, another French word which has recently come into the menu descriptions, I feel really annoyed. The word means steak. Why don't the people who use this word realise that there are many in Ireland who do not understand the many French words used in the food descriptions printed on menus. The word darne is not even in the French dictionary in front of me. It is in a gastronomical edition. Few look at the latter, except those with cookery interests. Why can't we use the language people are used to and describe it as steak? Recently, when in one of Ireland's leading restaurants, just for my own satisfaction, when reading the menu, I asked the waiter what darne meant. He did not know. Perhaps the hostelry owners have an air of loftiness or pretentiousness. There is no excuse for his lack of knowledge in this respect, which goes to prove the point I make.

Having travelled extensively in France I have yet to see a gaelic word used in their food details. With a love of good food, I have enjoyed myself there, but nowhere have I found food better than good plain Irish dishes, many of them simple, especially in my home or other peoples homes. Nowhere in Ireland or France have I found Stéag a bhrádáin or Stéag Salmon. What is wrong with using our native language, which sadly many Irish don't understand, instead of being snobbish to the point of using the French? We have strayed from the recipes, preparation and cooking of the nutritious Irish food served in the past.

There are many worrying aspects concerning the consumption of the farmed, battery-caged and reared, artificially-fed and chemically-treated salmon. Salmon is now offered amongst the bottom range of fish prices. On being offered salmon on the menu in the past it was regarded as an elegant treat because it was wild fish, being pure and natural.

The artificially produced fish are sprayed continuously in order to try to eliminate the lice which they are almost always covered with. Battery reared caged salmon is now totally unnatural, being fed additive-filled rations, much of which is factory produced and processed. Nobody would eat commercially farmed salmon, with its stark grey flesh, except that the farmed salmon industry scientists came up with the idea of an unnatural colouring, which when fed to the fish turns the tissue pink. To make the battery caged and unnaturally reared salmon marketable, a 'dangerous' chemical is used to artificially colour the flesh.

The colouring additive residue, which is in the flesh of the battery-reared fish, is liable to and may be affecting the eyesight of the consumers. Some years ago the E.U. issued a Directive to the effect that the chemical used was to be reduced considerably, telling us of the dangers. How can this be policed? Will officials be sent out in the boat every time fish are being fed? The battery-caged salmon producers will use what they consider is necessary to colour the horrible looking grey flesh. They are not interested in people's eyesight.

To the majority, salmon is just another fish dish. They don't realise the conditions under which the fish are reared or fed, often with chemicals and other unnatural food ingredients, as stated. The processed, factory produced so-called feed is very often highly unnatural. This is also especially true of the flesh colouring additives, which are unacceptable. To all too many, salmon on the menu is accepted without thought as to how the fish are produced, also as to how it arrived on the table. The fact is that it is reared as chickens are, battery caged, certainly not as wild salmon are.

It is not realised that the fish being produced in a mercenary manner are disinfected, being treated with chemicals and insecticides to kill the pervasive lice which are lethal to wild salmon offspring, the grilse. The farmed salmon is not natural. The chemicals in and on the salmon flesh are probably entering the body. Who knows the consequences? Where salmon is on the menu, very many, including myself, practice the slogan 'WHEN IN DOUBT, LEAVE OUT, DO WITHOUT'. This means almost all salmon, unless it is wild, including that which is tinned. Because natural salmon is now a delicacy it is almost unobtainable.

Some years ago there was a big scare following a study by scientists from the State University of New York. This claimed that Scottish farmed salmon was contaminated with high levels of cancer causing particles.

Natural wild salmon, with its natural pink flesh, which we delighted in eating in the past, is now almost wiped out. We are reliably informed that over the next four or five years the deadly sea lice, which are coming from the farmed salmon, could completely wipe out wild salmon. This can and is happening, year in and year out, where the migratory grilse fish continue to use areas which join up with the many salmon 'farms' which are around our coasts.

In order to try to conserve the little wild salmon stocks left, now being decimated, thousands of net fishermen have been deprived of their livelihood. Net fishing has been banned. In the past there was sufficient wild salmon to allow them net fish as they did. Then the cry went up that they were the cause of the shortage. This all started several years ago. The momentum for the ban grew and they have been the innocent victims.

Now there is conclusive and unarguable evidence that the farmed salmon industry is responsible for the demise of wild salmon stocks. This of course was not taken into consideration when the Net Fishermen were accused and let's say 'Found Guilty'. In all too many cases this kind of skulduggery has happened over the centuries. The landed gentry were often all too anxious to interfere in the past. It seems times have not changed in this respect. It is not the landlords who are now the inciters. It is our Government, who bow to the whims of the fish farm industry.

It is not coincidence that it is only in the past 20 odd years, since the commercial battery caged fish farming commenced, that the terrible

217

incidence of fish killed by the sea lice has escalated, with an extremely lower amount of wild salmon in our rivers and weirs.

The salmon farm industry had denied that their businesses are the cause of the demise of wild salmon. They would, wouldn't they? Their rejoinder has been, 'Prove it'. It has taken time but now they have been proved to be the guilty parties. This said, the question remains **"What is being done about it?"** Again the answer is *'NOTHING'*. Those who govern will not interfere with **'Big Business'**, which the fish farming industry is now. Here again **money** talks.

Many salmon farms go out of business only to spring up or be resurrected bigger than ever. Our Government remains unmoved. The Minister responsible is unmoved too, as if paralysed. **Unless something drastic is done in the near future wild salmon will soon be another species which will disappear**.

We are now told that The National Organics Standards Board has decided to allow farmed fish carry an organic label. What an idiotic idea. **Various natural things have been tried to turn the horrible looking grey flesh 'pink'. None have worked**. It is extremely doubtful that there is anything natural which can be used for the purpose. The producers revert to and use 'dangerous' chemicals to enable them produce pink fleshed salmon which might be acceptable to all who eat the unnatural fish, at the same time using chemical insecticides which kill an amount of the sea lice.

Those responsible for issuing organic licenses, can be classed as being 'foolish'. Here is something, which with the present set up, should not be accepted as being organic. How reckless can things get? Those who promote farmed salmon as food are doing the country a disservice, all of which leads to a serious question; **Should farmed salmon which is offered as food have a health warning attached?**

MARRIAGE

The working on it or of it. In the modern era, which is a continuation, carry on, (no pun intended) of the permissive age which broke out in the 1960's, we hear much about sex, cohabiting, the single parent, also the relaxed or liberal approach to all of this. Sadly, there is all too little heard about marriage or the joy of it today. Very often we hear of the break-ups between couples, of divorce and separation, litigation and the break up of homes. In many cases there is all too little love, trust or sincerity. Love used to be love, just that. Now all too many regard love as sex, with little or no discern or contrast. The children's thoughts, imaginations, or their future, is often given little thought, frequently resulting in a 'tug of war' situation. This is all very sad.

Mixed marriages were often the cause of family rifts in days of not so long ago. Who cares about this nonsense, if one is a believer. Those who were and are bigoted enough to help cause religious divisions had little reason to think so. Lets call it ignorance or misguided thinking.

Despite the fact that we are supposedly more educated now and shall we say "Should know better", there is all too much disharmony in marriage. I can't speak for cohabiting couples. One has the feeling that not 'tying the knot' gives either one the liberty to walk away from what would normally be a married, GOD fearing and therefore serious relationship. Anyway children need parents.

There are numerous incidences where the bickering, in-fighting, unpleasantness and animosity between couples could easily be put aside. If there is any sense of love and devotion between the two concerned this makes it easier. What many couples forget is the need to work on marriage or living together. There must be give and take, also dialogue. To the ordinary person, this latter word means sitting down and talking, having respect for what the other says. Shouting at one another or a slagging match gets people nowhere, only making things worse. **There must be give and take in a big way.** Ever notice how easily we accept friends as they are, yet sometimes have trouble doing that with the person we are married to? **Doesn't a partner in life deserve at least the same respect, loyalty, patience, gratitude and appreciation given others?**

I put these words together about 'Marriage', the working on it, or of it, for a good reason. It is my belief that if those who have problems, minor or major, just sat down together quietly and spoke rationally, the majority could settle their differences and 'bury them'.

Let me tell you a story. There was this couple who appeared to have irreconcilable differences. Demeanour, tone of voice, body language, and attitudes were terrible amongst each of them. Things deteriorated over quite a period of time, with short and often very long spells of silence, not speaking to each other. In between something might happen where both would come together, often for months. This something might be to solve a problem, maybe family, perhaps financially. The couple had no financial problems. Their home was paid for and well-kept by the house-proud lady, an excellent cook and mother. They had little reason to bicker, but did so. Things got more and more difficult until eventually the wife could take no more. She packed her bags, taking chattels, goods and necessities required to live simply, and left the family home.

There was some little communication between man and wife, with the threat of divorce and separation being raised, after about 12 months. The man concerned was convinced that the woman had Seasonal Affective Disorder, commonly known as S.A.D.S., and that she was to blame for the constant bickering and in fighting that went on. He was heart-broken, although on the exterior he appeared positive and resolute. He was always self-opinionated anyway! He did visit his wife on just one occasion and felt he got a very cool reception, even though the lady was quite friendly.

Some 14 months after they separated he took up the telephone and with some trepidation, call it butterflies, he dialled the number. After usual salutation he said, **"I would dearly like to come and talk with you."** The reply from the good and nice lady was **"I would like to talk with you too"**.

A date was made and kept where both sat down to talk. It transpired that one would not contact the other, being afraid of a frosty or cool reception, which would of course, mean further hurt. Pigheadedness and stupidity kept this couple apart. Later they told each other that while waiting for the date to be kept they felt like as if they were going on their first ever coming together.

I've told how both met. The flame of love, which was always there, was rekindled. They sat down to talk and now many moons later they are still talking enthusiastically. Their differences were put aside. They work together to make things work. Oft times the tongue is bitten by both, to use a cliché. Both realise that it takes two to cause friction. They now spend happy times together.

This story is told because there must be thousands out there in this modern day and age, who have, or are going down the road or path set out here. It takes little, other than common sense and the fact that it has to be remembered that there are two people, neither of whom is perfect, or indeed right. There are three sides to every story or happenings like this, the man's, the woman's and the other side.

I tell this very true story in the hope that it will help others. You the reader may not have a problem like this but may know someone who has. If so pass it on. It could mean mending a broken marriage or relationship. This story is told because I was one of the two people concerned. I am now convinced that it was not my wife who had S.A.D.S., it was myself. I realise that I was far more wrong than right. My devoted wife has consented to, and helped me write this caption. **We both hope that it will carry the message, that all is not lost if one has courage. At the same time we must realise that,** *'TO DEAL WITH A HURT ONE NEEDS THE GREATEST GRACE AVAILABLE; THE GRACE TO FORGIVE'.*

SUPPLEMENTS

Do we need them? It is often stated that as long as we eat a 'well-balanced diet' we will get all the nutrients we need. However, not everyone knows what a well balanced diet is. Survey after survey shows that even those who do believe that they eat a well balanced diet fail to get anything like the ideal intake of vitamins, minerals, and other essentials. Nutritional deficiencies continue to be problematical, even in populations of modern well-developed countries, particularly amongst the elderly.

Central to the concept of optimal nutrition is that long-term nutrient deficit can lead not only to deficiency states, but also to mild symptoms of ill-health, such as fatigue, frequent infections, dry skin, mouth ulcers, and much more annoying simple health problems, as well as increasing the risk of chronic disease. These risks may be greater in certain vulnerable sub-groups, such as the elderly, the very young, or the ill and infirm.

Vitamins and minerals reduce the risk of death from heart disease, stroke and many other forms of sickness, serious or otherwise. The best advice with Multivitamins is to ask the staff in your local Health Food Store to guide you through their pure and natural range. The majority are friendly and helpful. Confide in them and tell them if you have a health problem or what you hope to achieve. **Always support your locally owned health store.**

Buying a Multivitamin and mineral product should be the corner stone of your nutritional supplement programme. Go for the most comprehensive you can afford. Some Multivitamins seem expensive until you actually compare the number of nutrients included and their strengths. Food supplements are best taken with food, ideally with breakfast or midday meal.

Unless the diet is well balanced, with food which is pure and natural, additive free, the taking of supplements, including vitamins and minerals, will be of little benefit. Some are of the impression that a bad, or fast food and low nutrition diet, can be overcome by taking food supplements. They would benefit little, if anything, perhaps doing harm. It will be nothing in comparison to combining a balanced, pure, natural additive free food diet, with the natural supplements. Remember, natural supplements are safe if simply and safely used!

DISCIPLINE AND DILIGENCE

Diligence calls for being self-disciplined, motivated, alert and most importantly following through earnestly. Ill-health is a result of being undisciplined. The word discipline is used frequently in this book, as all are advised to avoid the many additive filled, sugary, unhealthy foods and drinks, much of which is foodless, which are available. **Often it is not will power, which is required, but more importantly won't power.**

'SMOKED' FOOD AND 'THE DANGERS'

In my condemnation and criticism of food additives over the years, the finger has often been pointed at 'smoked' food flavouring. In 1989 we were warned of its dangers. That was the first time I realised there was a question mark about its use. There have been various scares about its 'dangers' to health, especially concerns that it may increase the risk of cancer.

In the past we had fish, bacon and many nutritious foods smoked, using oak and beech timber as the base for natural smoking to produce the flavour. The fast food scientists then produced artificial smoked flavoured liquids. Now foods are dipped in a processed solution or have the flavoured liquid painted or sprayed on. On the 'food' store shelves we see artificially smoked ham, fish, barbecue sauces, burgers, crisps and other fast and snack 'foods'. These are highly unnatural and may be dangerous to health.

The E.U. is considering a ban on artificially smoked flavouring amid concerns that it may increase the risk of developing cancer. There is evidence that there is an increased risk of certain cancers where there is a high consumption of smoked foods where chemical or unnatural smoke flavouring is used.

As is usual, when an outcry like this arises, we have the politicians, know-alls, or their ilk telling us, *"This is daft, over the top, a ban is disproportionate to the possible risks".* One fool tells us, *"People have been eating smoked food for generations without any health problems being noted".* Why do I use the word fool? The politician who has the temerity to make this foolish statement needs enlightenment about how food additives, including artificial smoked flavour, may be the real causes of the illness and health problems, and perhaps some of the cancers, we now have. **He certainly does not understand or realise that artificial smoke flavourings have only been used commercially in recent years**. Before this, foods were given their smoked aroma or taste by use of timber smoke. To put it simply, they were smoked naturally. The politician's use of the word **'for generations'** is, therefore, stupid and foolish.

Take 'smoked' fish for example. It is dipped in the synthetic flavouring or has the liquid brushed or sprayed on the product being given the smoky taste. It has colour added, if not already in the stuff being painted on. This gives the fish the lovely taste and hue one associates with timber-smoked products. Various foods are done in different unnatural ways where artificial smoke and flavours are being used.

In Ireland there are only a small number of natural curing and smoking treatment businesses left now. One is William Carr and Sons Limited, Curraglass, Co. Cork. Tel: 058 56216. Another is Burren Smokehouse, Kincora Road, Lisdoonvarna, Co. Clare, Tel: 065 7074432. Their naturally cured fish is available in many supermarkets and food stores or direct from the producer by mail order. Seek out the natural brands if timber smoked fish and food are required.

We are now told that members of the European Parliament have a fear that any new measures to curb the battery caged fish production will impact unreasonably on the domestic industry. One presumes this also means the 'food' industry. **Which is of more importance, the health of all or letting big businesses do what they like to provide the 'food'?**, in this instance unnatural, chemically and artificially flavoured battery caged and reared fish.

The whole scenario regarding the sale of so-called foods is bordering on the ridiculous. Who knows the difference between *"Irish Smoked Salmon"* and *"Smoked Irish Salmon"?*

See **Food Labelling** caption if you wish to read about the comical way this has been devised or wangled. Here is another case of *'When in Doubt, Leave out, Do without'.* As with so much of our additive-filled 'foods', it is advisable to arrange for artificially smoke flavoured so-called foods including salmon or other 'smoked' fish to be left on the shelf and not to be eaten. Turn to *Salmon* caption.

PREVENTION

Disease prevention is much easier than trying to cure.
Why not follow this advice.

BLOOD PRESSURE HIGH – ALSO KNOWN AS
HYPERTENSION

It is alarming, a terrible indictment of our Sickness Industry, who have guided it to the pinnacle it is now at, that so many are on medication for **HIGH BLOOD PRESSURE.** Daily I meet those who tell me they are on blood pressure treatment. This, like all so much we hear about, such as diabetes, depression, dementia and many other ailments, can be controlled by use of pure natural foods, drinks, exercise and proper sleep pattern. This is what is called, '**Looking after yourself'**. All this, plus a few supplements from the health food store can actually cure people, including the majority who have blood pressure problems.

A blood pressure monitor is essential to help keep one informed on a daily or regular basis of the pressure readings. I've seen many restore their blood pressure to normal, including myself, by using natural methods. Of utmost importance is the Diet, which must be of pure natural foods. Avoid alcohol, smoking, including passive, also salt and sugar or so-called foods which contain either. We obtain far too much of them, as they are almost impossible to avoid. All supplements or remedies mentioned in *Selling Sickness!* are natural, being available from independent health food shops. They may be taken with anything prescribed by the doctor, unless otherwise informed. Always tell them what you are taking or what you intend to take. They will know little or nothing about them, unless familiar with natural remedies or additive free food, which is highly unlikely. What one does is their own prerogative.

Combined with the kind of diet suggested in this book, one can take hawthorn capsules, rutin, also kelp tablets, a good multivitamin tablet or capsule, with extra vitamin D3, lecithin granules and Hofel's brand garlic capsules. The latter gives all the goodness of this invaluable root, but without the sometimes unacceptable odour of the bulb.

If overweight, steps should be taken to lose the excess. This is most important. See *Healthy Body Weight* caption. If the advice in that article is accepted fully, adhered to, and carried out, a four-fold purpose is being combined. Weight will be lost, blood pressure will be lowered, general health will be much better, leaving one with an abundance of energy.

Exercise is vital. If with health problems or on medication be advised by your doctor before serious exertion. The exercise suggested is walking, which can be to one's own pace, depending on how energetic the feeling is. Avoid foods with colour, additives, preservatives or anything unnatural. This includes margarine, butter substitutes or so-called low-fat spreads. Like most yoghurts, also the over-hyped probiotics or functional 'foods' promoted, they contain additives and more. Only eat pure natural unprocessed foods.

Have fish, fruit and vegetables as often as possible. Use low-fat milk. Sugar or anything with sugar, also cooking oils and fried foods are enemies of High Blood Pressure. Learn to read the ingredients labels. I repeat, eat only what is pure and natural. Visit your Health Food Store, telling them what you intend to do and be guided by their advice as well as what is mentioned here. I've seen many who've brought their blood pressure back to normal by taking exercise, such as walking, regularly. Combining this with the suggestions made has helped many control their blood pressure naturally. *I reiterate that I don't tell anybody what to do, only setting out what can be done, what I have seen many do successfully, also what I do myself.*

ALCOHOL

Alcohol is evil. It has been the cause of illness, accidents, home and family heartbreak. Nothing good can be written or said about it.

WHY NOT SAY 'NO' TO PRESCRIPTION DRUGS?

Read the above words again, because all prescription drugs, and I mean all, have side effects. When mixed with other drugs or perhaps with the unnatural ingredients in the 'foods' we are offered, they can do long term damage to health. Many, far too many, who complain of being tired, lethargic, depressed or with a worn out feeling, are on prescription or perhaps over the counter, so-called remedies. Many who complain, often looking haggard, being in need of good nutrition or perhaps a tonic, can blame much of their problems on the use of prescribed or other chemical drugs. Many of our present-day ailments, some major, have been caused by the prescribing and over prescribing of synthetic drugs and so called medicines. Change of lifestyle is the chief remedy. It could not be more natural. **PRESCRIPTION DRUGS ARE NOT NATURAL AND TO BE AVOIDED IF AT ALL POSSIBLE.**

SIMPLE LIVING
We should simplify our lifestyle to allow ourselves,
also others, to simply live

TWENTY MILLION POUNDS IN PRIZES FOR IDEAS THAT IMPROVE THE HEALTH SERVICE

Some time ago we were informed by the National Health Service in the U.K. that cash prizes totalling £20 million sterling were being offered by the Department of Health to come up with ways of cutting costs or discovering breakthroughs.

The Innovation Challenge Prize, launched by Lord Dalzi at London's Science Museum, asked for suggestions on how to make the Health Service more efficient, or perhaps come up with ways to tackle the many issues, such as childhood obesity.

The Department of Health said it expected ideas to come from University departments or teams of doctors who will plough the money back into research, but the scheme was open to individuals. Note how the money would be ploughed back into research, more jobs for the medics and scientists. Not a single mention of prevention of illness. I submitted a reasonably short, but concise, thoroughly informative application, setting out my views of how to empty many of their hospitals. Included were recommendations as to how to tackle the overweight, diabetes, heart, cancer and hundreds of other health problems reported daily. **Prevention** of illness by natural methods was the keynote, the main and all-important thing, just like I have promoted daily for over 45 years. The theme, as prepared, was based on my slogans *'We are as we Eat, Drink, Sleep and Exercise'* also *'Change of Lifestyle Works Wonders'* with ideas of how this could be incorporated into the running of the N.H.S. Now some considerable time later I await even the courtesy of a reply. Maybe I will receive a sterling cheque, as I wait in hope!

My remedy is too natural, too simple. The medical bods who are responsible for running the Sickness Industry system, in this case the National Health Service of the U.K., like their counterparts in Ireland, are deaf when it comes to mentioning the use of anything natural or simple. They certainly will not listen to any suggestions about **prevention**, this being a word which appears to be anathema to them. My assertion that there is no money in it for them is highly obvious by their reluctance to even acknowledge my entry. They don't wish to hear about natural food and drink, exercise or the need for proper sleep and sleep pattern. **This, the greatest medicine known, is ignored by the medical profession.**

The resultant well-being of the majority would help wreck the already sick and depleted economy of the U.K. The Sickness Industry as we now know it, would collapse. As is usual, the economy and politics come first. The health of the nation is way down the list, if it is there, as the Sickness Industry continues to thrive. **Hopefully the Sterling cheque will arrive ......sometime!**

ENTHUSIASM

Enthusiasm is the baking powder of life.
Without it one would be flat, with it one rises.
Better health leads to enthusiasm.

VARICOSE ULCERS ELIMINATED AND CURED

My sympathy and understanding are with any person suffering from or trying to banish Varicose Ulcers. They can be eliminated and cured. All that is needed is a little time, patience and an amount of discipline.

Many have used my formula to fully cure the skin breaks and soreness, returning to walking normally, without difficulty or hindrance. My experience of this terrible treatment is an example of how to recover. Many who suffered similarly, now cured, have praised the methods, thanking me.

My bad luck was to put my foot and leg into an uncovered gully opening, where building works were being carried out. This happened on a dark night. In so doing the skin was damaged and torn on one side of my leg. Usually cuts or scrapes received would heal quickly. Not so in this case. The result was that I attended the doctor, somebody I avoid if at all possible. The leg was dressed, being dressed and redressed twice weekly for some months. Eventually I was referred to the hospital because there was no improvement. There I was examined by a Vascular Consultant who gave me about two minutes of his time. He directed the nurse to dress it again but to be frank it was the same only different. This time I had an elasticated stocking put on over the dressing. At the same time I was given a letter for my G. P. The direction then was to continue visiting the nurse for more dressings.

Only then did I realise that this carry on could go on forever. There was no way that the skin would heal by putting on fresh dressings, twice weekly. The foolishness of dressing and redressing, with no sign of cure in sight, should be stopped.

It was then I went down the road of treating myself. I started using Manuka Honey - plus 10 strength, but after 3 or 4 months there was no improvement. **I was then set on the road to recovery by my good friend who runs a health food store called *Carmel's,* in Ennis, well known in Co. Clare and surrounding counties.** This extremely knowledgeable person, who is a wonderful ambassador for natural health, told me, *"You are using the wrong type of honey, you must apply Manuka Honey - plus 25 strength. It is much stronger and highly efficient as a treatment".* Handing me a jar, the lady said, *"Use it".*

I must stress that no medicine will help if the patient is under nourished, run down or in need of good natural food. Proper and regular meals of natural food, aided by taking a natural Multivitamin also extra Vitamin D3 by use of a capsule, are amongst the secrets of better health. To help banish the Varicose Ulcer I smeared the Manuka Honey - plus 25, over the open wound for five or six days, each morning.

I left the leg uncovered except at night-time when it was protected from the bed sheet. Sometimes I slept with my effected leg outside the bed covering. During this time I found it best to keep the leg up by day, only walking when absolutely necessary. As it became drier I put some Tubi Grip covering over part of the foot and the leg to protect the scab which was forming. Sometimes when I had a sock on over this, it would break in a small area. If not careful the scab could be pulled off if it stuck to the Tubi Grip material, as happened to me on more than one occasion. Where it was necessary I used a thoroughly wet face cloth to fully moisten the covering, allowing for easy removal. It is most important to be careful in this respect, because a new break in the skin can trigger off more problems, meaning further treating of the area. After five or six weeks the honey had formed a thick scab, which I was able to remove as the leg healed. It was like peeling off old wallpaper.

The need for care cannot be over emphasised. Some months later I damaged the skin on the other side of the leg, when I slipped off a ladder when cleaning the windows of my home. So began the rigmarole of treating again. This was tedious but I had learned so much first time around that it made things very much easier. Within weeks both sides of my leg were completely cured and I returned to one of my favourite hobbies, which is walking.

There are thousands of people who have vascular problems, such as written about. They are attending the doctor, more often the nurse, having treatment by way of regular dressings described. It is like a never-ending course of action or procedure. This ridiculous method of hoping to clear ulceration of the leg should be done away with. Here again is proof that the natural way works.

The patient may be in bad health, very often in need of proper nutrition, pure food and maybe a food supplement or two, especially the wonder vitamin, which is D3. They may lack vitamins and minerals or the immune system can be weak. Never will either the doctor or consultant question the patient about this. I harp on this because I meet with and advise people daily, seeing many who are malnourished and unhealthy. Reasonable good health is over half the battle to recovery, including healing and cure of Varicose Ulcers. The Manuka Honey - plus 25 strength, is a marvellous aid, an excellent benefit.

It is obvious that the consultants and doctors ideas are to keep people coming back. Few are cured, therefore the Sickness Industry thrives. Simple natural remedies, such as mentioned, are unacceptable, being taboo to these professionals, as here again they proceed down the wrong road in pursuit of lucrative and bountiful monetary gains.

FOOD IS BETTER THAN MEDICINE

When diet is wrong, medicines are of no use.
When diet is correct, medicine is of no need.

THE CHEMICAL DRUGS-MANUFACTURING INDUSTRY:
THEIR ROLE IN SELLING SICKNESS

Do you remember the time when the mythical Celtic Tiger was alive? There was this insatiable greed for money by bankers, developers, builders and others who were there for easily-obtained money. Then came the crash. Many of the businesses, including some banks, went to the wall or had to be bailed out. Many were private or shareholder enterprises, self-supporting, provided they made money, which some of them didn't in the end. Compare all this to the pharmaceutical chemical drug industries. There was little effect to them on the demise of the so-called Tiger. The greed for money by many within this set up is continuous.

We do know that there was a call for the saving of approximately €700 million within the H.S.E. section of the Sickness Industry also the letting go of temporary staff, including sub-contractors who also employed many. Many were asked to take reductions in salaries.

The only other people to suffer will be the general public, the patients, including the extremely patient taxpayer. Some staff were offered redundancy, there being a disappointing uptake. There was some small amount of shutting down of parts of the sickness industry also withdrawal of beds. A recruitment embargo was agreed. Maybe this was no harm. We heard and read much about proposed drastic cuts. We have seen little which can be called drastic or radical. There were certain salary cuts, most of them minimal when one considers how the private sector has fared and all of that without much complaining or whimpering.

The comparison is that the private sector had all the problems and much more so because it was self-financing, whereas the **sick** Sickness Industry is kept out of a big hole by the Government. The taxpayer pays directly and indirectly to keep the money guzzling carousel afloat.

What of the chemical pharmaceutical drug-manufacturing and Distribution sector on its own, remembering that it is part of the Sickness Enterprise. Here again little, if any, serious redundancies, wage and salary cuts or closing downs were reported. The Government has made no demands on them. It is not in the interests

of those who profess to govern to say anything to, or about, the mighty chemical drug producing establishments. They are as a protected species. With the many thousands of jobs at stake taken into account, the politicians will nurture the legalised drug processing giants. They will be looked upon and treated kindly to prevent them from upping sticks and departing for cheaper shores and labour. Low corporation tax and various other tax incentives mean that the coffers of the nation see smaller returns. Eyes are closed to much which could be changed to help stabilise the national finances. Alright, we gather much from P.A.Y.E. also V.A.T. and in other ways because of the huge employment given, with Ireland being the capital of the European drug-manufacturing industry.

But and there is a big BUT, the huge source of revenue to our finances, which is Corporation Tax, is relying mostly on payments from a small number of the pharmaceutical companies as well as some I.T. companies. The near bankrupt financial side of big business, also other smaller struggling businesses, have been badly hit by the down-turn in the country. They too must pay Corporation Tax, where applicable.

Regularly we are told of the transfer of millions by the pharmaceutical drug-manufacturing industry to the parent companies or head offices in some far off land. American companies are allowed to cash in on a tax amnesty, planned to allow businesses to return profits earned in Ireland so that they may be invested in creating jobs in the United States or elsewhere. The results are that millions of euro are transferred out of the country. The up side of all this is the employment given. Recent figures show a workforce of over 24,000 in the medical device and chemical drug-manufacturing industry, with exports which are approx 40% of our total foreign trade.

We learn of the industry being in a healthy state and of the decision to move into the pharmachem chemical drug sector bringing immense benefits to Ireland. The same cannot be said about the majority of those exposed to the use of the chemical drugs or medicines which they produce. We saw pictures of official openings, also the many words of welcome to the chemical drug firms as they enlarged or opened new facilities and recruited. Headlined too was *'Why it is a boom time in Pharmachem City'*, meaning Cork'.

In an article headlined **'A NATIONAL TREASURE'**, the then Minister for Enterprise, Trade & Employment spoke of the contribution the pharmaceutical drugs processing sector makes to the Irish economy and the importance of continued investment in Research and Development. Elsewhere we are informed that the self claimed drug combines spend very much more on advertising and promotion than they do on research and development. When our leading politicians adopt this attitude, entirely monetary, what hope is there for the future health of our nation as people are plied and treated with drugs and more drugs, many being harmful or with serious side-effects, the very odd one *perhaps* being a cure.

Some years ago an Oireachtas Health Sub-Committee issued key recommendations into adverse side affects of pharmaceutical drugs, also other worrying aspects of the whole chemical drug-pushing scenario. Let's call it *selling sickness*. Among the other contentious issues of which there are many, was *'The influence of the Pharmaceutical Industry and the persuasiveness of its promotion of drugs, which was referred to as 'unhealthy'.* It mentions *'Generally excessive' reliance on Drug Therapies and the high incidence of prescribing errors"*

There is on record **the question of compiling a register of 'Significant Benefits', which doctors receive from pharmaceutical companies.** This was supposed to address the risk of potential conflicts of interest. The report or recommendations questions the part of the Irish Medicines Board (I.M.B). This body is apparently funded through fees to services for drug companies. We are learning of the carry on within the Sickness Industry regularly. There are many other recommendations but space does not permit their insertion. Seldom, if ever, are they acted upon. It appears '**NOBODY**' is responsible as more and more lip-service is forthcoming.

Somebody said recently *"**DOCTORS, OF ALL PEOPLE, SHOULD KNOW THAT THE MILDEST PHARMACEUTICAL PERK CAN HAVE DANGEROUS SIDE-EFFECTS'.***

Like much within the Sickness Industry *'The over worked Irish Medical Board'* has not got around to solving the recommendations put forward by the Oireachtas Health Sub-Committee despite its having being issued several years ago. Procrastination or inaction on acting upon the proposals put forward is a good way of keeping, what to them are contentious issues, at bay. Time allows for convenient forgetfulness. It has been called sweeping under the carpet, which is something the medical profession organisations or umbrellas are very experienced at, as was Lord Widgery who issued the lying report about Bloody Sunday in Derry. I state this to emphasise that sweeping under the carpet is now referred to as being '**Widgeried**'. It is noted that high up on the Oireachtas Health Sub-Committee concerns was that of the issues of adverse side effects of chemical drugs. **In 10 years time the question may be asked, *"What was done?* I bet handsomely that the answer will be 'NOTHING'. I repeat Ms. Nobody sits on the backside and does nothing.**

In a large media spread headed *'**Big Pharma search for acquisitions tells of take overs and the gobbling up or coming together of*** *huge drug multiplies, with money seemingly no object'.* Many billions are mentioned and change hands. Within a 12 month period there were at least six big takeovers or mergers. Chief amongst these were Pfizer's take over of Wyeth for $41 billion and Merck's acquiring Schering Plough for $68 billion.

Alongside these kind of mind boggling deals, the drug industry is normally embroiled in law cases, often suing each other for various reasons, all of course to do with money, big money. Johnson & Johnson won $1.67 billion, the largest payment verdict in U.S. history, from Abbot Laboratories. This was over a formula used to produce an arthritic drug. It appears that Johnson's were owed $1.17 billion in lost profits and $504 million for royalties.

The facts and figures mentioned in this book, *Selling Sickness!*, **about the pharmaceutical drug making multinationals and their role in the Sickness Industry, give very much food for thought.** In 2008 the drug giants Pfizers won a case in the High Court which meant keeping a much cheaper statin out of Ireland for the following three or more years. Pfizers chemical statin which sells under the brand name Lipitor, the worlds biggest selling drug, would have been competing with a generic drug. The prescribing of the latter mentioned would have saved millions for the Irish users and taxpayers, also the H.S.E. To read about one of the greatest cons of all time, which is being perpetrated on the unwitting users, see **Cholesterol** also **Statins** captions.

As more and further sickness is being promoted, sold and in some instances invented worldwide within the Sickness Industry, the mighty chemical drug manufacturers are setting up directly and otherwise in foreign countries. This is partly because no drugs of any consequence, no blockbusters, are coming through the system in the western world, as it now operates. Allied to their problems is the fact that the sales of the cheaper generic drugs are eating into their profits.

We learn that Novartis, the Swiss drug giant, is to invest $500 million in Russia, as they try to establish a stable base in what is regarded as a growing market. An interesting question is, "How did the inhabitants of Russia manage previously?" Are they too to become a sick nation as we are now, all because of the unnatural, or let's add, unparalleled promotion and prescribing of chemical drugs and more drugs, this only happening here in recent years? Nycomed, Novo Nordisk and Glaxo Smith Kline are also in the process of making their entry too. Can they do as heretofore, where with hype, propaganda and prescribing in Europe, it has been akin to hitting the jackpot for the chemical drug conglomerates. Similar efforts are being made to enter the Chinese market, here again a huge emerging market. Will they too become another sick nation or huge cog in the wheel of the carousel, which goes to make up the Sickness Industry, as we see it now?

The amazing part of the workings of the pharmaceutical chemical drug producing companies, in their quest for profits, is that so much of what is prescribed is useless. Many have little if any scientific basis. The drug companies themselves fund the studies and then tell us what suits them. When tested for approval it is what they did, not do (i.e. harm somebody), that helps them become licensed. What they can or will do is seemingly irrelevant to the licenser, the licensing body. It is absolutely wrong that a proliferation of chemical drug compounds, readily available as pills, capsules or vaccines, can be obtained or prescribed when there is no evidence whatsoever of the long term consequences. Indeed in many instances there is no confirmation of short term outcome or aftermath.

Some time ago an almost year long E.U. investigation concluded that drug-manufacturing companies intentionally interfered with the importation of cheaper drugs. Anti trust laws were supposedly planned against several companies. At the time of writing, some years later, we learn of drug manufacturers offices being raided, as the E.U. seeks further evidence regarding the matter. The carry on allegedly involved various 'criminal' and wicked ways of interfering with the introduction of generic drugs, which are much cheaper and equally as good as the patented products which the huge chemical concerns are trying to protect from competition.

The E.U. has also conducted raids where widespread abuses were found in relation to drug firms *'Trying to keep prices high'*. One of the manoeuvres is to buy up companies that compete and sell their drugs for less. We learn of a drug company taking out over 1,250 patents for one drug. This makes it virtually impossible for a rival company to produce the drug when the official patent expires.

In almost all cases of conniving in cases bordering on, if not criminal, we are informed that action will be taken against offenders. What happens in this kind of case? As with much in the Sickness Industry **'LITTLE OR NOTHING'**.

Over the years I have followed with interest a case where Pfizers, after much procrastination and time wasting, eventually agreed a settlement of $75 million with a Nigerian State. This followed a legal battle, of many years standing, over allegations that children were harmed by an experimental drug, Trovan. There was of course no admission of liability by Pfizer. One cannot see Pfizer or any business parting with $75 million if innocent. When Pfzier was sued back in 2004 for illegal promotion of Neurontin, the case was settled for $430 million. The last case I was informed of, in which Pfizer transgressed, this time criminally, it cost them $2.3 billion, plus. **The outcome of the criminal prosecution was that as part of the settlement Pfizers would pay almost $1.2 billion, the largest criminal fine ever imposed in the U.S.A.** They also agreed to pay $1 billion in civil damages and penalties to compensate for false claims submitted.

I am very much against informers. We have had all too many of them in Ireland in the past, with terrible consequences for our people. In the case of Pfizers or indeed any drug combine I only wish we had more whistle-blowers like those who informed on the criminal actions of this multinational. **The six whistle-blowers in this instance shared $51.5 million, also from the coffers of Pfizer.** They are to be congratulated for the exposure of this criminal outfit.

The mentality of those who run this now criminalised business is startling. A Pfizer vice president said afterwards *"We regret certain actions taken in the past but are proud of the action to strengthen our internal controls and pioneer new procedures".* It is my opinion that those in control at Pfizers have nothing to feel proud about. They should be ashamed of themselves. The fines and payments mentioned mean nothing to the enormous drug manufacturers, whose sales to the Sickness Industry are astronomical. Extreme law-breaking chances are taken, as they promote, sell, market, all too often making false claims about their drugs. Off label marketing of unapproved drugs also misrepresentation, plus other illegal and criminal acts seem to mean little to the giants of the chemical, medical drug producers.

Recent laws, now signed in by President Obama in the U.S., mean that informers on non-law abiding conglomerates will be entitled to awards of 10% to 30% of what is paid in fines or other settlements. This to be in relation to financial or other fraud cases such as the drug manufacturers have been involved in. Hopefully they will expose certain of the drug-manufacturing companies, let's call them manipulators, for what they are.

In 2010, we learn about Johnson and Johnson being caught and dealt with in the courts. Yes, Johnson & Johnson again, which led to what to them is a paltry fine, with meagre change to their bank balance.

Two subsidiaries or units of Johnson & Johnson had to pay more than $81 million. This is because they were found to have promoted for psychiatric uses a drug, which was unapproved.

If it had not been for more 'whistle blowers' the company would have continued to carry on in a criminal manner.

Not long ago, shortly after the turn of the century, Elan, Ireland's largest pharmaceutical company, was almost at the top of the list on the Irish Stock Exchange, being a high flier. Ten years later the shareholders could only look on as the shares languished.   Elan were found guilty of illegally paying doctors to prescribe their epilepsy drug Zonergan to children, but for different and wrong purposes. These included obesity, weight loss, migraine, headaches, eating disorders, also as mood stabilisers for manic and bipolar disorders. As a result of their wrong-doing Elan had to pay $203 million, plus huge costs, the biggest part being criminal fines.

Like other drug-manufacturing consortiums mentioned, this was not Elan's first illegal performance, having been prosecuted before on whistleblower evidence. Fines, which to the unscrupulous giant drug producers are trivial, will not deter them from committing criminal offences. They are at no loss except for the very small dent in their bank balances. **The jailing of certain of the leading directors, those at the top, who all too often automatically pass the buck to lower or sometimes middle management, as do all too many business leaders, might lead to much more serious thought being given to running their chemical drug industries honestly.**

The *Irish Independent*, commenting on the Elan fiasco, put it concisely in a hard-hitting editorial, part of which reads, *'There are many losers in this sorry tale; the adults and children who used Zonegran without proper oversight, the American doctors who allowed themselves to be persuaded to prescribe the drug with trips to Bermuda and Florida, the Irish regulators who took no action despite Elan's base here, the pension funds who invested in the company despite the strong smell that has emanated from Elan for years and of course, the executives inside Elan who were responsible'.*

To read of the payments to those who run the drug-manufacturing empires is an eye opener. We find that the Chief Executive of one chemical processing company has seen his annual salary rise by 13% to nearly $3 million. Will somebody tell me what overseer is worth this kind of obscene payment? I can mention various other outlandish bonuses and salaries, all of which proves that the drug-manufacturing companies profits are immoral. These are the giant operators who are legalised drug pushers. Some of them invent sickness. Cholesterol is a clear illustration. They sell drugs, often harmful, mostly with side effects, none of which guarantee a cure. Patent power is defended strenuously as they go in search of more profits.

Disease mongering for humans, as used in the Sickness Industry, is now being hugely promoted for animals by the drug conglomerates referred to. We have tranquillizers, weight-loss and many other drugs being highlighted and publicised for cats and dogs. **The Food and Drugs Administration in America has approved Prozac for use on dogs. It does not cure humans, then why promote or sell it for treatment of or**

administering to a pet?

The chemical drug processing industry will continue to conjure up ideas at the expense of the health of man and beast to build up their bank balances, to please their shareholders. Selling more and more sickness is the huge brief of the almighty drug fat cats.

In May 2007 we learned of how China's former top drug regulator had been sentenced to death. This was for taking bribes to approve untested medicines. If that happened here in all probability it would be hushed up. As a drug regulator he might even be 'promoted'! Nothing surprises me anymore. Like much within the Sickness Industry nothing would be done. In November 2007 we learned that this man had been executed.

Recently there was a highlighted heading on the front page of a 32 page pharmaceutical industry tabloid type publication. It read, *'WHY MEDICINES MATTER'*. Another headed, *'A HEALTHY PHARMA FUTURE'*, tells us *'For employers and students the pharmaceutical sector represents a highly attractive career option as the industry here moves into a new phase of its evolution'*. By using the word evolution, which means growth, expansion, enlargement, this can only lead to much more of the same of which we already have far too much. I stress again we are already a sick nation, does this evolution mean that we will become sicker? I further stress *"WHAT IS THE POINT OF PRODUCING MORE PILLS, MEDICINES AND OTHER CHEMICAL DRUGS IF NOTHING, YES, IF NOTHING WE HAVE SEEN USED IS A CURE? IT IS EVIDENT THAT WE ARE TO REMAIN WITH CROWDED SURGERIES AND OUR HOSPITAL RESOURCES STRETCHED TO THE LIMIT"*. All concerned with the running of the ever expanding industry must be fools if they can't see or don't realise that the Sickness Industry in its present format cannot be maintained or allowed to expand as it has done in recent years.

Yes, no chemical or synthetic drug is a cure. Perhaps somebody can prove beyond all doubt that I am wrong. I have yet to see one for cancer, heart disease, diabetes, kidney disease, Alzheimer's, depression, vascular disease, including varicose ulcers or indeed any of the hundreds of ailments with which we are now plagued. I have seen many natural remedies and aids to better health, obtainable from the Health Food Store, which work and cure.

Health problems, which in past years were looked upon as mild, are now being treated as extremely serious, with drugs being prescribed where none were ever used. It is obvious that many are under the influence of the Sickness Industry, in the guise of all too many drug companies. With vested interests, such as theirs, it is in their remit to keep people unwell.

Visit a Health Food Store where you will hear or see a homoeopathic doctor, a naturopath or one of the other alternative practitioners. In most cases appointments have to be made. Here you will find excellent remedies and cures. Yes, CURES. This is more than can be said of the vast majority of the medical profession, who of course have allied to the drug companies, as they promote their products and sell more sickness.

Now that doctors are being allowed to advertise, in order to promote and **sell sickness,** we are certainly moving into a new phase of evolution, which is a pointer to the future enlargement of the Sickness Industry. My thoughts on the Sickness Industry we now have can be evaluated in a few words *'It is one of, if not, the biggest cons or swindles known.'* The chemical drug-manufacturing industry, which is a huge part of the Sickness Industry, has grown at a phenomenal rate in both Ireland and Britain, all in a very short time. Is it a fluke, coincidence or correlation that in that time we have witnessed an enormous upsurge in the incidence of sickness, ailments and disease? Does all of this not confirm my insinuations regarding the **selling of sickness**, as now being witnessed regularly?

When all consider the terrible implications of the use and over use of chemical and drug intake into the human body surely it is apparent that we go down the wrong road. Who gives thought to the use of Paracetamol, Neurofen Plus, Aspirin, Panadeine, Solpadeine or hundreds of other off the shelf, non-prescription, so called medicines, being used? 'Harmful' legalised drugs are easily purchased in the supermarket or at the filling station, with some being regarded as if they are sweets, all too often being consumed carelessly. They are taken for the slightest thing wrong, often given to children indiscriminately. Taken by adults who drink alcohol they are an extremely dangerous health hazard. There are often side effects, some serious, which go with taking almost all chemically processed drugs.

Consider just one of these branded chemicals such as Solpadeine. The millions spent on purchasing this analgesic and temporary reliever of pain is astronomical, unbelievable. How many taking the drug realise that it must not be taken with paracetamol or anything containing this chemical. Here is a prime example of a drug, which does not cure. It is like so many others on the market. It is just a stopper of pain as well as being a huge money-spinner for the drug barons who produce it. Here again people give no consideration as to what chemicals enter the human body, which I repeat is super natural, a marvel, a wonder unparalleled.

If one has pain there is a reason. Find the cause, then the pain in many instances will not be there if the origin is treated. There is a wholly excellent painkiller available from the Health Food Store. It is

pure and natural with no side or after effects, no long term consequences. It is called White Willow Bark. This is not promoted as a cure being just another pain aid. The advice is to find the cause of the pain and treat with a natural remedy.

When will those who appear to worship the doctor, who believe there are pills, capsules or medicines for all ills, finally learn that there is a natural remedy available at the Health Food Store, which will match any chemical so called remedy. I reiterate that many natural treatments, all of which are produced under stringent rules, being registered as medicines, food supplements, alternative or homeopathic remedies, are far superior to the chemical drugs. There will certainly be no side effects when taken as prescribed.

All who are interested in the natural health way of living are acutely aware of the E.U. and American Government campaign to restrict Vitamins and minerals levels to idiotic or far too-low dose levels. Driven no doubt by their love for the huge money-spinner which is the chemical pharma drug making industry, one cannot help but feel that it is the intention of the E.U., aided by the American Congress, to destroy the health food business as we now know it. A big majority of the bureaucrats are allied to the almighty drug lobbies which work in conjunction with the giant pharmaceutical drug-manufacturing industry. As already mentioned, the question will soon be answered in America "Are we being ruled by the Government or the chemical drug processing conglomerates?" See *Natural Remedies & The Efforts Being Made to Ban Them* caption

The nameless faceless bureaucrats who make E.U. directives have apparently been granted more power than ever. Ireland's Yes vote gave them full autonomy to rule as they wish. The voters were foolish enough to change their minds. What benefits have they derived from doing so?

There would be little need for any remedies, either chemical drugs or the natural, if all those who take these pills and medicines just took a little time to learn of natures non or little cost elixir or panacea. It means just using one's common sense, putting into practice the nine words I harp on consistently – '**WE ARE AS WE EAT, DRINK, SLEEP AND EXERCISE**'. Thousands of times I have advised people with various kinds of sickness and ailments to live simply by simple change of lifestyle. Prescriptions and other drugs have been left aside, now to be forgotten about, as the many helped have returned to good or better health.

A change of lifestyle can work wonders. I know I keep repeating this, but the message must be driven home, therefore repetition is often necessary.

Our Government, the physicians, and those within the Sickness Industry will tell us nothing about natural remedies and change of lifestyle. It will not generate money for the economy, the drug companies and the others who make up the Sickness Industry.

When one looks at the expansion of the drug industry, the big entry of private hospitals and nursing homes through the Sickness Industry, even the huge expansion of the hospital car parks, it is obvious that we are to become a sicker nation.

Recently a gentleman telephoned me and his first words were *"Ronnie, you were right"*. This family man has suffered from manic-depressive psychosis (Bipolar Disorder), commonly known as manic depression. For over two years I had talked with, cajoled and oft times argued with the person. In the beginning I thought he was a lost cause. He was on seven different forms of chemical drugs. He could see no way out of his depressive mania and head thumping state. Neither could I, because he appeared to be really badly effected. I had helped other similar cases before curing them, dare I use the word, because the medical bods will have a fit. None were as badly affected as the person who telephoned me. Over the months I had driven him to see my way of thinking. To change his lifestyle, diet, drinking, eating and sleeping habits, took much patience and discipline, as one by one he came off the drugs. Yes, he is on five or six varying items of pure natural, no side effect remedies, now. He can be referred to as a valued customer by his local health food store. What a difference in the medication and what a difference in the man. The Hay Diet was his liberator as well as the natural remedies obtained from the health store.

At no time when dealing with people who come to me with their health problems do I suggest, advise or recommend coming off whatever medication they are on. I just tell people what others have done, what I have done and what I would do, it is entirely up to them what form of treatment they take. Speaking on the telephone, the man I am writing about partly explained why I was right. He told of how pure natural food, including some meat and plenty of fresh white fish, had helped. He cut out alcohol and coffee. He did everything I had said worked when treating various forms of manic depression. He followed the three words assiduously, *'CHANGE YOUR LIFESTYLE'*. His words to me before leaving down the telephone were *"I can't thank you enough"*. Very often I hear these words as people get off the many slow 'killing' chemical drugs, then regaining much better health by using natural remedies.

How did we manage in the past, say up to 20 years ago, before the Sickness Industry imploded on our lives? The minds of all too

many healthy people have been manipulated. The drug companies and the medical profession are responsible for turning many who were well into permanently sick people, those who take the legalised chemical drugs. Only last week I had a letter from a lady who had experienced terrible trauma over the previous 12 months, where I had been able to help two families, both herself and a sister. Neither mother could control their two sons because of what they were told was Attention Deficit Hyperactivity Disorder (A.D.H.D.). They attended two different doctors who prescribed amphetamine-related drugs including Ritalin and two others. All in my opinion are dangerous and should not be given to children or indeed anybody. We hear of some idiotic Bioethics expert – note the word expert – saying that the terrible drug Ritalin should be taken by healthy people. This is utter nonsense. Another case of *selling sickness*, another example of making healthy people ill.

Let's return to my two lady friends, although I only know them for little more than a year. Only one of the mothers visited me, and that on four different occasions. We were regularly on the telephone to discuss the situation. She acted as the information carrier. Having had much success in similar cases over the years, with quite a number of hyperactive young people, even teenagers, being helped, I had the answers. I had warned the mothers of the danger of psychotropic drugs such as Ritalin. They had not allowed them to be used. The advice was to change their lifestyle, but more so than when dealing with an adult. This was difficult but was made easier because the boys and the mothers were at home. It was the beginning of the summer holidays. Inferior diets and drinks were at the top of the list for changing.

Sugar, fizzy and energy drinks, sugary products, crisps, fries, all processed foods, sweets, chocolate, coffee and anything unnatural being taken were totally banned. Both played hurling and football. Their coach/trainer was roped in to help. He was given a list of 'do haves' and 'do not haves'. A water filter from Simply Water in Dublin was installed in the pipelines of both homes. This was fitted to eliminate the chlorine and fluoride, which are detrimental to better health. These chemicals are enemies of A.D.H.D.

The two boys became enthusiastic about the changes to their lifestyle as time went on. Their coach was probably listened to, more so than the parents. Much discipline was required. The result was an eye-opener. The boys calmed down, became more friendly, and sat and listened when asked to. The letter told me some of the story, but I needed filling in on exactly what had happened, so I visited the mother. She related much about the huge success of the natural treatment, which I had suggested some 12 to 18 months previously. She spoke about the goodness of pure unadulterated, unsweetened, additive free foods and drinks and of the various changes to their lifestyles. She was ecstatic, being delighted that the problems appear to have been solved. She related to me her delight in having both families all on natural foods and drinks, of the vast improvement in the health and outlook of all. She said and I quote her words *"I had to rule with an iron will, especially at the outset, but it worked"*. She thanked me at length. Like many I have helped to better health she wanted me to accept money. I told her, as I tell others who offer payment for advice, to give it to my favourite charity, Saint Vincent de Paul.

What is set out elsewhere in this book, ***Selling Sickness!***, I repeat at 80 odd years of age, on no medication, and with thousands like me who have been weaned off prescription and other drugs, **"Anybody who takes them should stop and think seriously before doing so"**. That is if they wish to enjoy better health. There may be some who cannot do this. The vast majority can refuse them. It is their prerogative what they do.

What hope is there of converting people to a healthy way of thinking that '**WE ARE AS WE EAT, DRINK, SLEEP AND EXERCISE'**, if the Government and the majority of the politicians, the E.U., the drug companies and their cohorts, the medical profession and the Sickness Industry in general, don't wish to know about living simply or how to enjoy better health naturally. Money appears to be their *god*, as more and more chemical drugs and medicines are promoted. Nowhere does this circulate more freely than in the Sickness Industry, to which so many are dedicated.

The 'pills for all ills' mentality is too strong for many reasons, certainly the monetary way. Yes money rules. **YES, yes, MONEY RULES.** The health of the people is of little importance, being shown lip service by all too many concerned. Prevention of sickness is unheard of.

I repeat, and I make no apologies for doing so **"OUR HEALTH IS OUR OWN RESPONSIBILITY"**. There is a much, much better way of enjoying good or better health than by using chemical drugs or medicines. Without doubt we are moving in the wrong direction when we decide to use legalised chemical drugs. There are times when certain medicines have to be used. **In the majority of cases of sickness or illness a natural remedy will cure, which is more than can be said about chemical pharma DRUGS.**

FIZZY DRINKS. ARE THEY UNHEALTHY?

The long term 'harm' of fizzy, sports, isotonic or so-called energy drinks is incalculable and will remain untold. These sugary, artificially and otherwise sweetened drinks can create major health problems in later life. I respectfully suggest that the drinker reads the ingredients labels. If they are not understood and one wishes to have good or better health, then learn about them. They are additive-filled, a 'danger' to health, if not now, then certainly in the future. Many of the ingredients can lead to clogging up the veins, arteries and capillaries. They can affect kidneys, liver, teeth and many other parts of the body.

Granted there are many who wish for more energy. Drinking these kinds of liquids is certainly a 'dangerous' and unhealthy way of obtaining energy or of trying to be more vigorous or active. They are certainly not a thirst quencher. Because of the ingredients many are just another form of harmful drug. Very soon after drinking one of the additive and sweetened drinks, some with the dreaded caffeine or aspartame included, there is the urge for another. It is repetitive. The 'harm' of Bisphenol-A, which is in the make-up of the plastic bottle, is another reason to forget about these 'unhealthy' concoctions. See **Bisphenol-A** caption. I squirm when I see the sports bodies, also the leading sports men, promote the sugar or sweetened-filled drinks, many being paid for the endorsement.

Handed to me recently was a bottle which contained **a so called sports drink.** In very small print on the label **"Products quality assured for athletes. For adults participating in active sport and exercise".** The ingredients label does not bear out anything which suggests that this additive laden mixture is health improving. It reads as follows: *Water, Glucose Syrup, Citric Acid, Acidity Regulators (Sodium Citrate, Calcium Carbonate). Flavouring, Preservatives (Potassium Sorbate). Sweeteners (Aspartame, Acesulfame K.). Stabiliser (Acacia gum). Vitamins (Niacin, Pantothenic Acid, B6, B12).* It contains a source of *Phenylalanine,* which on its own can be dangerous to health. There is no comparison between this stuff and pure water. The over sweetened, additive, 'quality assured' liquid was poured into the septic tank.

These sort of drinks, as mentioned elsewhere, can only be a forerunner of ill health especially in later life. To me they are evil, to be avoided. Drinks like this can lead to diabetes and other illness. Good food and pure drinks, such as water, are the energy givers.

FOOD

There is a big difference between pure food and food products.
Pure is food, processed is a product

THE MEDICAL CONSULTANT'S MONEY WRANGLE SAGA

Many like myself have watched, over a period of five or six years, the saga of the medical consultant's contracts, before they were finally agreed. The Government, The Health Service Executive, (H.S.E.), The Irish Hospital Consultant's Association (I.H.C.A.), and the Irish Medical Organisation (I.M.O.) were all involved. The I.M.O. and I.H.C.A. are amongst the most powerful, autocratic and dictatorial unions in the country. The I.M.O., the real protagonists, procrastinated and talked down to their employers as they demanded, pronounced and laid down what they would accept, will do or will not do. Imagine any businessperson or employer accepting this when the terms of future employment are discussed. It has been like the heated exchanges of a soap opera.

Having one union such as the I.M.O., which can almost hold our country to ransom, is serious. Having two unions, as in this instance, is extreme.

Their members, of what is a closed shop, know that our Government and the Health Service Executive can draw on no other source of qualified personnel. When I say they can almost hold all to ransom it is no wild statement. At one time, during the years of parleying, the I.H.C.A. decided to ballot for a campaign of industrial unrest. If this is what living in a democratic state is like, where the medical welfare of all is at stake, then you are welcome to it.

What are we to expect from this lot when the former leader of the Health Service, a doctor and medical professor, told us, including those who work for him, that even though paid €360,000 plus per annum, with an €83,000 bonus tagged on, he would be better off working as a doctor. This is certainly far from proper diplomacy for one in his position and a sad reflection of current money grabbing ideas.

Near the end of what appeared to be a never-ending saga the I.M.O. walked out of the negotiations with the agenda only half discussed. This tactic backfired on them badly as the I.H.C.A. stayed and negotiated a deal, deserving credit for this. To save face the I.M.O. had the audacity to state that **"Their organisation or union, by withdrawing, resulted in a sense of realism and movement from the health employers"**.

This was an idiotic, but excellent and well thought out excuse, for what can only be seen as child-like behaviour and impetuosity. It reminds one of the tantrums of youngsters who cannot have their way. A member of the I.M.O. has since told me that because of the walk-out most were hoping that the talks would collapse again.

Later we learn that the I.M.O. indicated that the salary scales as set up and agreed, are unfair and insufficient. The mind boggles as one wonders if there is any limit to the doctor's union and organisation's demands. This domineering and all-powerful body contends that the *'poor'* consultants will have to work a longer week also being rostered for duty early in the morning or late in the evening. The unlucky *creatúrs* will have to work certain weekends, receiving overtime for this. One can be certain it will not be just single time rates, or a pittance. This all shows that because the I.M.O. was now left out in the cold, they could only pick holes in the agreement made between the Government and the I.H.C.A.

The mind-set of many responsible for the health of the population leaves much, very much, to be desired. I have not yet mentioned the salaries being offered because I just could not comprehend that the telephonic numbers, denoting euro, being flashed on our T.V. services and written about in the media, were true. The consultants in this country are on remuneration, which in many instances is almost 50% higher than U.K. medics with similar qualifications. Just imagine being paid up to six to eight times the average industrial wage, as they bickered for more, acting as I have said, like school kids.

The I.H.C.A. are on record as referring to the high and obscene pay as 'Mickey Mouse'. Yes, this was the term they used. Their greed for money is appalling. These professional members and their unions have, over the years, put every possible obstacle in the way to hinder the restructuring of the contracts. There were issues brought up at every debate or meeting, all to delay or even halt the proceedings. Things like doctor/patient relationship, clinical indemnity, their rights to advocate on behalf of patients, and much else trivial and often silly interpolation. When this bickering was going on between the I.H.C.A., the I.M.O., the H.S.E. and the Government, we were listening to and reading about proposed drastic monetary cuts to be made throughout the country.

Almost daily we heard of costs being pared, of workers being laid off in industry, the realisation being that we are no longer competitive. Much has been put across about benchmarking, the cost of living and the old chestnut, the inflation figures. All this is accepted by the general public without a word of public outcry or protest.

Then the consultant's are offered salaries, which can be well over €5,000 per week. We also find that some of these consultants, who have almost pleaded poverty, are grossly overpaid as they double job. To many of them the contracts must be just a piece of paper of no legality. These are the ones who show contempt for the contracts, also those who employ them, as they treat too many private patients. The contracts set out the firm, stringent rules on the number of private patients they are allowed to treat, when working in public hospitals. This is being blatantly ignored. One of the results is that the taxpayer is unwittingly paying hundreds of thousands of euro in respect of private patients in the public hospital system. The public patients are also losing out.

Here is another illustration of **why the Sickness Industry thrives**, as many professionals stack up the huge, immorally gained lucre. It used to be that if an employee did something 'dishonest', as many of these public servants are doing, there would be disciplinary action taken. This is not so any more as industrial relations governance becomes more idiotic daily, especially where professional or white collar workers are concerned. The ordinary person in life would not be allowed to get away with this kind of 'dishonesty'. With these professionals, contempt for the rules is the norm all too often. **Within the Sickness Industry, despite the Government pleading poverty, there is this element of thinking that when there is much, take all you can, and when there is little, take the lot.**

The taxpayers once common sense or public outrage has certainly dissipated, as all remain silent. There seems to be no limit to the ingenious and indeed the disingenuous mindset of consultants who can earn thousands of euros in extras and payments, which increase the salary figures. With overtime, allowances for work on Saturdays and Sundays, provision of out-of-hours emergency services, standby payments, being called if rostered to visit patients in emergency cases, additional charges in some instances can be from €100 to €200 per hour. All this, with perhaps more I have not learned about, on top of the upped thousands of euro plus salaries, as already mentioned. Oh, to be younger than my 80 odd years and to be a consultant!

Some can say, *"What business is this of yours"?* The answer is **"I don't like usurpers".** In my lifetime, when I was never out of work, like many of my breed and character, the idea was to obtain an honest day's pay for an honest day's work. As far as the Sickness Industry is concerned and this includes the medical consultants, all too many are driven by the seemingly unappeasable greed for money. There is a huge element of 'Mé Féinism' in what I refer to.

One of my mottos is *"DON'T FIND FAULT, FIND A REMEDY".* On my own I can't find the remedy to curb the Sickness

Industry we have now, but I can try. Voices are not being heard in this respect. My still lone cry may be heard if I can shout loud enough and long enough. **Perhaps you too might join in?**

It has been disclosed that almost one in five consultants treated patients in private hospitals when they had originally been on the public waiting list. We are told that in some cases consultants are being paid twice – in both the public and private system – for treating the same patient. Who raises a voice to decry this 'roguery'? Who disciplines a professional bod who transgresses? Until somebody proves differently to me, the answer is '**NOBODY**'. The same '**Ms Nobody** who has so much to do with the Health Service Executive, which is the Sickness Industry.

Speaking with friends who have had reason to visit medical consultants, also from my own experience, their ways of making money can only be admired. My visits entailed dealing with vascular, hearing and lung specialists. Very often, one is spoken with by the consultant's aide, his assistant. On all visits there was quick turn around, with further appointments being made. Very often there is no need for further consultancy because they can do nothing by way of remedy. Here again one could liken their further reappointment procedure to a well-organised conveyer system. This is highly obvious where the patient or client has private health insurance.

The consultant's saga, which took years to settle – if it is fully settled, shows what can be done by tenacity and doggedness. They now line their pockets monetary wise. Instead of fighting for more and more money, I would prefer to fight for and have good and better health. All can do this on their very own.

We were informed that 'The Health Service Executive had told over 200 consultants in the Sickness Industry that they are continuing to practice privately in public hospitals, grossly ignoring their contracts'. **Plans to name and shame the biggest offenders have been thwarted**. People like this make their own rules, many being in dispute as to how the ratios of conniving or 'stealth' are being calculated. In days past, except of course for those chosen, where dishonesty was found, those implicated were fired. Fired or sacked are not politically correct words anymore, or so it appears.

At the expense of the Government, the Health Service Executive which is the Sickness Industry, the tax payers and the patients, the consultant's now laugh all the way to the bank simply because the majority don't give a damn about their health or lifestyle.

THE CARES OF LIFE

It is not the work but the worry
that makes a person grow old
That shortens the years of many
before half their life is told

It is not the work but the worry
that places on life a ban
The cares and fears that crowd the years
which break the heart of man

It is not the work but the worry
that causes the stress and strain
If only all would remember
with worry there is nothing to gain

It is not the work but the worry
that leads to an early grave
So change the way you are living
You'll be surprised at your strength to be brave

GOVERNMENT SILLINESS IN WITHHOLDING THE LONG AWAITED NATIONAL POLICY ON NUTRITION

Early in this century, in 2005 to be exact, somebody in our Government thought that proper nutritional directions for all should be studied, offered and used. This was at the time the now almost forgotten about and certainly not acted upon, **'National Task Force on Obesity Report'** was issued. This was placed before the limp willed Government of the day. This is another report where the over 90 recommendations are gathering dust. Then an Oireachtas Sub-Committee was instructed by the Government of the day to produce a **National Policy on Nutrition**. It appears that no time was lost by the people who drew up the important **National Policy on Nutrition** because it was presented to the Government in 2005, the year it was decreed that it should be prepared.

The vast majority are unaware of this extremely important Policy on Nutrition and the huge improvements its findings could have on the health of our people.

Not only that but the savings to the nation, because of the resultant improvement in the well-being of so many, could run into billions of euro.

Most of our people are unaware of the fact that our rulers and those who often appear as dictatorial bureaucrats will not release the findings and recommendations. The words nutrition as well as prevention appear to be despicable to the Government, also to the Health Service/Sickness Industry. I repeat drugs and more chemical medicines are all they wish to know about. **There is no money in nutrition, prevention or the advice in the National Policy on Nutrition which they are concealing**. It would hinder the quest for more money, their apparent sole interest, because the sale of chemical drugs would fall away.

The *Health Plus Weekly Supplement*, which is with '*The Irish Times*' each Tuesday, tells in a fair and impartial article of the scandalous carry on. This was in January 2010 some five years after the promised report was presented to the Government. Here is **Paul Cullen's '*Irish Times*'** exposé. Note the official heading and the excuse that it is delayed because of cutbacks. **This is untrue.** It has not been made public for the simple reason that it would seriously affect the workings of the Sickness Industry, including the Pharmaceutical Drug Industry also the Medical Profession. It would only headline my slogan *"WE ARE AS WE EAT DRINK, SLEEP AND EXERCISE"*. I repeat what **Hippocrates**, the father of modern medicine said: *"Let food be your medicine, let medicine be your food"*. You the reader can form your own conclusions when this caption has been read. In my humble opinion those who govern are a national disgrace, in this as well as many other instances. The country and that includes our Health Service Executive, which is the Sickness Industry, is rudderless, in need of guidance. Here '*The Irish Times*' wording is given verbatim.

Long-awaited Nutrition Policy delayed by cutbacks.
Initial draft on plan to tackle obesity did not find favour with Department of Health officials.

The development of a promised National Policy on Nutrition has been put on the back burner because of a lack of resources and differences within the Department of Health overall drafts. The Department says: "A National Nutrition Policy remains an ultimate objective but there are no immediate plans for its publication. This is in spite of repeated promises by Ministers and the Department in recent years that publication of the policy was imminent".

A National Policy on Nutrition was first proposed after the National Taskforce on Obesity report was completed in 2005 and is seen by experts as an important plank in efforts to promote healthy eating and to counteract the rise in obesity.

*The Department last month refused a Freedom of Information request by '**The Irish Times**' for documents relating to the policy, saying* *the public interest would be better served by the non-release of the information at this time. When the schedule of documents not being disclosed was sought, this newspaper was told there were none.*

In refusing the Freedom of Information request, the Department said the document was being reviewed "Against a background of competing priorities for the Department and the availability of the necessary resources". Since the completion of the obesity taskforce reports, the focus had begun to shift towards delivering practical nutritional guidelines for specific sectors of the population.

It is understood that the initial draft of the policy did not find favour with Civil Servants. "It was too long on back ground and short on concrete measures, so it was (sent) back to the drawing board", an official with the department's health promotion policy unit told 'The Irish Times'. The official said no committee of experts had been set up to oversee the preparations of the document, as is normal, and admitted that it was "strange" that there were no documents on file apart from drafts of the policy.

In November 2005, Seán Power, the Junior Minister in the Department, promised the policy would be published early 2006 and would provide strategic direction on nutrition for the next decade.

In February 2008, Taoiseach Brian Cowen said it would be published "in the coming months". Two months later, junior minister Pat the Cope Gallagher said it was "in the final stages" of development, and his successor in the department, Mary Wallace, said in May that year it would be published "later this year".

In June 2009, the department said the policy would be published by September. However, according to the official, there was "No reality" behind any of these dates. More than 60% of Irish people are overweight or obese and consumption of alcohol in Ireland is among the highest in OECD states.

We certainly have been fobbed off for years, but at what cost to the health of all? Releasing this Policy and its recommendations immediately would help to ensure that there would be much less need for cut backs. Why? Because if put on natural diet of good food and drink the health of millions would improve dramatically. Billions of Euro could be saved. This is what tantalises the Sickness Industry. The medics who run it are afraid that the carousel, the merry-go-round, the money-spinner, would stop.

I have in front of me several reports issued over the years, all pertaining to health, all making suggestions as to how to improve the well-being of the nation. None get any further than the archives. I mean the

Governments archives. This procrastination is usual, where after a time the lot is put to sleep, filed away, never to be looked at again. This is not to be wondered at because many of the recommendations or suggestions are long-winded, loaded with the usual bureaucratic jargon, much of it drivel. I say this because there is little, if any sense, in putting much of this kind of information before the ordinary person. The all too over elaborated grammar and language is not easily understood by most. The Sickness Industry is notorious for this kind of lark, with most reports gathering dust. Millions of euro has been spent on their preparation. Most of them have been shelved.

A former Minister for Health, Mícheál Martin T.D., who helped create the ogre which is the Health Service Executive, which quickly mushroomed into a Sickness Industry, had a huge capacity for setting up groups, committees, sub-committees and delegacies. These groups, some small, others quite large, where all individual members had to be paid, turned out reams of paperwork. They were responsible for having large volumes of reports and other ideas printed, with the big majority of them cast aside, unclassified, being unwanted paperwork. The cost of this has been ridiculous, but when it is a part of the H.S.E. it is no wonder, being just another example of how the minds of many of our bureaucrats work. Martin, despite much opposition from many strong lobbies and others, did one valiant deed during his term in office when almost single-handed he banned smoking.

Mothers, parents, guardians and the majority responsible for the future health of the young cannot read into or absorb the kind of information given in the reports referred to which are available

They are not written in simple language, which can be absorbed easily. It appears to be almost secretive, as is so often the case with the Sickness Industry Service information. What is in some of these reports can be viewed on the internet, but very often cannot be printed off. Perhaps this is another of their secret ways of operating.

In May 2005 the Government was presented with their demanded report showing 93 recommendations to tackle obesity and being overweight. On reading this long winded report which sets out so much which will never be put into practice or retained, it seems obvious that the people who issued this are lacking in common sense.

Re-reading the report now, I feel like tearing the hairs out of my head. It is evident that almost all just pay lip service to the our health, just sitting on their backsides, doing '**NOTHING**'. I quote just three of the recommendations. Remember these are just three which accompanied the other 90 suggestions.

• The Department of Environment, Heritage and Local Government should develop coherent planning policies for urban/rural housing, transport, amenity spaces and work place settings to encourage spontaneous increases in physical activity in adults and children.

• The Irish Financial Services Regulating Authority should examine the high costs of public liability and their impact on physical activity. It should foster initiatives to address these costs.

• The Health Services, in their strategic planning and delivery, should advocate and lead a change in emphasis from the primacy of individual responsibility to environments that support healthy food choices and regular physical activity.

Remember this is in connection with obesity or being overweight. Do we need these affective and over the top words and sentences to tell us what could be put into much simpler and understood briefing or advice? They should be short and to the point. The third suggestion has firm advice, if drafted in simple words, so that the ordinary person might understand the guidance.

Until such time as we, the general public, regain our sense of outrage, demanding action regarding the Sickness Industry/Health Service Executive, all will canter on leisurely, as the money pours into the medics accounts, the drug-manufacturing companies, the pharmacies and all who draw from the seemingly inexhaustible funds provided by the tax-payer.

Where better to let our voices be heard than to demand that our silly Government make public the long promised National Policy on Nutrition. Furthermore and of extremely vital importance is that they and the general public act on it.

GET UP AND GO

Those who do not have the inclination, or cannot make time for exercise, will make time for illness in the future.

OBESITY
BEING OVERWEIGHT, STOUT, OR IF WITH SURPLUS FAT

To some these words may appear harsh as they go far to describe how many of our citizens appear. Much is said, written and shows up, on or in the media, about obesity.

Working on the need for exercise, the required and extremely necessary sleep and sleep pattern, the use of natural additive, colour, preservative and sugar free foods and drinks, with elimination of fast and take away foods, using only pure water, will lead to a sudden and highly effective health change.

Where possible I like to eat in vegetarian or whole food restaurants. Often I remark on never seeing an obese or overweight person in any of them. This gives much food for thought, being a pointer to where many might be going down the road to eventual ill-health.

In 2005 the **National Taskforce on Obesity** handed the head of Government a report which politicians had propositioned the previous year. The 27-member committee, the majority of them connected to the Sickness Industry/Health Service Executive, made ninety-three recommendations to tackle the problem of obesity or being overweight.

These proposals, some of them long-winded, many of them unworkable, could easily have been summed up by using my slogans *"WE ARE AS WE EAT, DRINK, SLEEP AND EXERCISE"* or *"A CHANGE OF LIFESTYLE WORKS WONDERS"*, with recommendations to work out from there. The suggestions given are in language and words which to the ordinary layperson are mostly just lingo. They are typical of the political jargon we are all too familiar with. In some ways the report itself could be described as 'obese'. There is much intelligent and sensible advice set out in their recommendations, if only it had been made simple reading. As already mentioned, many of them are unworkable. This is because so many with vested interests in food, drinks, marketing, advertising, education, medicine, including the Health Service Executive/Sickness Industry and much else related, would find ways of opting out of or disagreeing with all too much of the advice.

The more often one reads the proposals or suggestions the more obvious this becomes. It is also highly evident that all, and all in this instance means everybody in the country, would have to co-operate and work fully together to ensure the successful outcome of the 93 proposals put forward. There is not the slightest chance of all working as a team to eliminate obesity or being overweight.

The report tells us about submissions from Tesco (Ireland), Burger King, Coca Cola, Irish Sugar, McDonalds, Tayto, amongst other fast food or food additive purveyors and manufactures. **We are not told what is in their submissions. Probably the usual evasive drivel, as they try to defend themselves from their major exploitation of the serious overweight problems we have.**

Here again I am being repetitive when I say, *"What is needed on a National basis is education about prevention of illness, this to include advice on proper nutrition, with huge emphasis on eating, drinking, exercising and sleeping habits. This would encompass the enormous and unhealthy problem of unwholesome diets, the use and over use of sugar and sugar products, including fizzy and additive-filled drinks and processed 'foods', lack of exercise, too little sleep and other minor problems which lead to ill-health and obesity or being overweight".*

When the Report of **The National Taskforce on Obesity** was presented after being compiled, some sensible person or persons advised, that to enable the recommendations, or at least as many as possible of them, to be put into practice, it would be a good plan to have a **National Nutrition Policy.** The suggestion or idea was accepted by the powers that be. An Oireachtas Sub-Committee was set up to prepare the policy. Its members drew up the code or scheme within less than nine months. This Policy was also handed to our government. **It was a brilliant idea, if and when used in conjunction with the Obesity Taskforce recommendations.**

BUT, and here the almighty big **BUT** is headlined. Our Government refused to allow the **National Nutrition Policy** to be presented, read, or made public. For information on this scandalous withholding of the Policy see *'National Policy of Nutrition and Government Silliness ' caption.*

Our Government through the Health Service Executive should countrywide be highlighting, promoting and advertising the need for proper nutrition through use of natural pure food and drinks. They could tell us, as I do to all, *"Sugar is evil as are many unnatural processed food and drinks".* Without natural food, drink, exercise and regular sleep we are and will continue to be a sick nation.

What hope have we of either the Health Service Executive or the gutless Government implementing any plan when the latter will not even release the long awaited and regularly promised **National Nutrition Policy Document** of 2005, first decided upon because of the obesity problems we have. They have not done anything to highlight, to publicise **The National Task Force on Obesity Report's** 93 recommendations issued in 2005, or the **World Cancer Research Expert Report**, available and in the archives since 2007. I repeat all are suppressed because the subject matter of the findings are as focused on in this book, *Selling*

Sickness! It is apparent that constituents are treated as uncaring fools.

I don't believe all the hype written or promoted by the Sickness Industry that we are as obese a nation as they make out. Nevertheless this is all the more reason why the Government, including the Health Service Executive, circulate this **Nutrition Report,** at the same time kick-starting a system of education regarding the need for proper nutritional food and drink, also the necessity for exercise and proper sleep. Once again the *'experts'* make entrance, telling us that children spend an average of five and a half hours daily in front of the T.V. In this respect it would take more than the Government to move the couch potatoes.

Many who had cooking skills have lost them. Look at the T.V. to realise this. As a cook, a lover of good food, I become annoyed when I see the chefs, cooks and their assistants and tasters, as they endeavour to show the viewers how to cook. So too the many hacks who give recipes for various dishes. This is seen on the box or in many magazines, particularly those that come at weekends. My annoyance is because most of what is written about and shown is too complicated, taking too much time for preparation and cooking. Note how much of the food has been almost fully prepared before these culinary 'experts' labour through the further preparation and necessary cooking.

People want simple education or instructions about plain, no-frills cooking, of health-giving and nutritious food. The food can be simple, natural, and nutrition-filled, quickly and easily prepared and above all it can be cheap. Micro-waved *'food'* is an insult to better health. I would dearly love to visit every school in the land and explain about pure food and drinks, with all being natural, all simple to prepare, eat, drink and enjoy. See *Eat Well On A Limited Budget* caption.

Best of all with regard to natural food, everybody, no matter how susceptible to putting on weight, can fill or over fill their plates with what I advocate. There is no danger of weight increase where pure food and drinks are taken. Yes, diet is number one, with exercise on a par. We hear from *'experts'* that the main reason for obesity is over eating. They are ignorant of the full facts. They are like so many who do not understand what a balanced diet is. They are probably like those referred to elsewhere in this book who have an additive-filled food imagination, where a balanced diet could be a nutrigrain or mars bar in one hand and a bottle of lucozade, some kind of coke or other fizzy drink in the other hand. I know this is mentioned elsewhere and while it may seem outlandish, what I speak about is visible daily. **These so called *'experts'* should have continued by telling us that one of the chief reasons for being overweight is over-eating or indeed eating or drinking unnatural foods and liquids. Food and drink which is processed, additive and sugar**

containing, leads to obesity and is a slow killer. It is as dead food. It cannot be and is not nourishing.

How many with overweight problems or unable to control their weight know about Bisphenol-A and its relation to weight problems? It is used in plastic bottles to maintain flexibility. It has now been discovered that it is leaching into the bottled water, fizzy drinks, microwaved foods and other plastic packaged food and drink products. It may be toxic, with many world reports telling us that it probably is a cause of obesity. See *Bisphenol-A* also *Healthy Body Weight* captions.

It is noticeable that margarine, which is the epitome of processed foods, being additive laden, is in plastic containers. Nowhere amongst all the wording on all these boxes are we told that the plastic is Bisphenol-A free. Flahavans now promote a breakfast size amount of porridge in a thin plastic container, which we are told is microwave suitable. **These tubs are free from Bisphenol-A in their makeup.** Flahavans are the only food providers I know of to date who arranged for this. The highly questionable additive is not allowed in the container's make-up. We do know it is not allowed in plastic baby bottles, but as yet only by some manufacturers.

It is when liquid becomes warm that the real danger of Bisphenol-A leaching into food or drinks occurs. Cling-film over foods, microwaved foods, especially those in plastic containers made up with Bisphenol-A, are some of the causes of obesity if we are to rely on the reports of their dangers. In my talks and in my books I decry the use of the microwave. My advice is to use one of my slogans, *'IF IN DOUBT, LEAVE OUT, DO WITHOUT'*. My family, like many we know, will not allow microwave use. The vast majority know little or nothing about the stuff they purchase and eat or drink as food or liquid. I repeat much of it is 'foodless', perhaps harmful, especially if microwave heated.

A capital or first class example of idiotic promotion, with money the all important factor for both, is the recent tie-up between McDonalds, who can be looked on as one of the fastest fast foods outlets in the world and Weight Watchers, who promote weight loss although they call the outfit 'weight watchers'.

Like most of the so-called weight losing promotions, the flab returns again unless the customer is terrible disciplined. *'The Guardian'* reports: *'As part of the deal, which is the first of its kind in the world, McDonalds will use the Weight Watchers logo on its menu boards and Weight Watchers will promote McDonalds to dieters'*. It is blatantly obvious that all of this is in the pursuit of money. As the well known natural health promoter, **Mike Adams**, known as the **'Health Ranger'**, sets out in his daily writings and advice, *"The bizarre and inexplicable decision has made Weight Watchers the laughing stock of the health* *world, where nutrition and weight loss experts normally don't use 'McDonalds fast food' and 'weight loss' in the same sentence".*

Looking at weight watchers branded and franchised *'foods'* on the shelves of some food stores or supermarkets, the ingredients labels show us that much is additive-containing. Many of the processed products they allow their weight watchers name to be added to are far from natural.

In the past and as an over eighty years young bod, I remember that some were ill and grew up sick because of lack of food. Now too much so-called food is the cause of much illness. As I have pointed out much of it is not wholesome or health giving. I repeat, *"All too much of what is put into the body today can sometimes be likened to garbage".*

Recently I read an article put together by a nutritionist. It was about super foods. The lengthy article, much of it nonsense, could have been issued in less than twenty words, as follows: *"ALL FOODS WHICH ARE NATURAL, ADDITIVE, COLOUR, PRESERVATIVE AND SUGAR FREE, NON PROCESSED, ARE SUPER FOODS".* This to include vegetables, fruit and pure water. The writer mentioned power foods, calories, low fat, glycaemic index, high soluble fibre content, very much of which the ordinary person does not understand. I asked myself *"How did I get this far in life and remain young even if old".* I ate simply and lived simply as do my family and many friends also the many whom I have helped to enjoy better health. Amongst other things I drank plenty of pure water.

The nutritionist referred to, mentioned yoghurts and probiotics. Try finding any that are pure and natural, non processed. Of the hundreds on the supermarket shelves only three or perhaps four brands are natural, without sugar or additives. Even then the ingredients labels have to be scanned. Of the many yoghurts and probiotics lined up on the shelves in the supermarkets, I cannot help touching again on the excellent Glenilen probiotic yoghurt. It is made by Glenilen Farm in West Cork. The description on the carton **reads 'HAND MADE NATURAL PROBIOTIC YOUGHURT – UNSWEETENED. ABSOLUTELY NO ADDITIVES'.** There are three purely natural ingredients in the make-up – and nothing else. I do like their three words on the product container, **'AND NOTHING ELSE.'** See **Probiotics** caption.

Try reading the labels on the containers, mostly plastic, of the many additive-filled so called yoghurts or probiotics, to find the print ridiculously small, often unreadable even when wearing glasses. Many of our nutritionists and health hacks who write for profit should dwell on these facts.

One thing about the obesity problem, which has helped turn it into a money-spinner, is that the Sickness Industry prescribes obesity drugs.

We find that the number of children in the U.K. who take prescribed weight loss drugs increased by 1,500% between 1999 and 2006. Drugs like this show up the ignorance of those who allow them to be used. Very often the parents or guardians should realise that simple corrective dietary measures are all that is needed. Hence the call for education and prevention for all health problems, including obesity or being overweight. On enquiry, figures for 2006 onward were not available. They are probably more frightening!

We hear of dieting, slimming, weight watching and the other fads, all money-spinners, where those fat, obese and overweight are targeted. Read the caption in this book which is wonderful advice, *'Healthy Body Weight, How to be the Right Weight and Brimful of Energy'*. I don't stand to make anything out of the guidance given, I just pass on the advice. Like everything else I write about, it works extremely well. Through the advice given in the caption, thousands have told me that using the suggestions made has proved for them a marvellous way of living and it costs little. If disciplined to put the advice into practice, read it. If without restraint or unwilling to learn how to be your correct weight, then it is best forgotten about, because as with any method of dieting a stop start attitude is wrong.

At the present time our Government, because of their silliness, pig-headedness and obstinacy, are responsible for **The Report of The National Taskforce on Obesity** also **The National Nutrition Policy** gathering dust because the latter **Policy** is withheld. The latter is not even available on **Freedom of Information** request. Their lame dog excuse is that *"The public interest would be better served by the non release of the information at this time"*. If pressurised they would probably issue a watered down version which in all probability would be of little use in the fight to eliminate obesity or its causes.

Of the 93 recommendations issued by the Obesity Taskforce, the very first one, yes number one, tells us that *"The Taoiseach's Office should take the lead, responsibility and provide an integrated and consistent pro-active approach to addressing Overweight And Obesity and to the implementation, monitoring and evaluation of The National Strategy On Obesity in conjunction with the Government departments, relevant bodies and Agencies, Industry and Consumer Groups"*. If ever there was balderdash issued then this is typical. This lot will do nothing to address anything, except to spend most of the time trying to extricate themselves from giving us the economy we have, or to politically out-manoeuvre the opposition parties. It is obvious that the health of all is far from their thoughts.

What a charade. What a useless bunch of bureaucrats we have to govern us. Lip service is freely pouted. To put it bluntly **"It is all words and little if any action in too many instances, including the fight to reduce obesity and being overweight"**.

I repeat; those who have a weight problem must realise, that like their health, it is their own responsibility to set the matter right where possible. There is no better way to do this, easily and naturally helping to achieve better health and lose weight, both at the same time, than by following the advice set out in this book under *Healthy Body Weight* caption.

ILL HEALTH

Ill health means wealth for the Sickness Industry,
which includes the Doctors, Consultants and the
chemical drug-manufacturing multinationals

AMALGATION WITHIN THE SICKNESS INDUSTRY

Not so long ago it was suggested and discussed amongst our bureaucrats that the Food Safety Authority of Ireland (F.S.A.I.) and the Irish Medicines Board (I.M.B.) should merge. Luckily some common sense prevailed resulting in the daft thought being rejected. This was a hair-brained idea and points to the ill-thinking of those in authority. This idiotic idea of a merger between the two bodies referred to could be likened to putting two alcoholics together to run a bar.

KINDNESS

Kind words can be short and easy to speak,
but their effects are truly endless

CHILD AND INFANT HEALTH

Doctors, parents, and those responsible for a child's or infant's health should give very serious thought before prescribing or administering any medicine or remedy, be it chemical or natural. Children's immune systems and other inborn disease or ailment fighting methods can be damaged or perhaps even destroyed. The result is that in later years there is little if any resistance to illness. This is a major reason as to why there is now little base or support to fight off disease or ailment in many children, teenagers and adults.

Few, if any, appear to give sufficient thought to what is put into the human body, the most intricate and complex system in the universe. It is a marvel, but all too often treated despicably, something very many should be ashamed of. **Giving children of any age medicines or pills is to be regarded with horror except in extreme cases of illness**. Speaking with grandmothers, elderly mothers and pooling our experiences, we cannot accept or understand the present day mentality of pills for all ills. Yes, a good natural tonic, given to children, also teenagers, from October to March is a must. See *Tonics* caption.

Being without exercise, on inferior diet, such as the processed, sweetened or sugary so-called foods or drinks being provided now, also without sufficient or proper sleep and especially a good sleep pattern, leads to much of the illness children appear to have all too frequently. Imagine feeding a baby with something like the off the shelf, proprietary branded liquids or often foodless foods, where the carton or container shows anything up to a 12 month hence sell-by date. Reading the ingredients labels should be enough to put any mother off using most of these processed additive-filled and unnatural baby 'foods'. Imagine anybody allowing a young person to be prescribed chemical cosh drugs such as Ritalan. It is evil.

Many youngsters are starting out as obese, then with much ailments which are preventable. Some children's health problems are as a result of passive smoking in the home.

As mentioned elsewhere, it appears that children are now to be exploited, as the makers of Lipitor, a statin drug, are supposedly about to promote a chewable form. This is entirely wrong because with statins being used to lower cholesterol, it is idiotic to promote this kind of thing amongst children. As mentioned more than once cholesterol and the lowering of it by statins is one of the biggest cons being promoted by the Sickness Industry. See *Cholesterol* also *Statins* captions.

Many children are sent to school or college without the all-important **BREAKFAST.** Very often they are given money to buy food, which is regularly spent on snacks, some supposedly healthy, which can contain up to 65% sugar. Health experts are demanding that the food industry adopt a different stance regarding fast foods. One can endlessly complain about the 'rubbish' food being provided. Asking the fast food-snack food industry to change falls on deaf ears. In almost all instances of providing healthy food and drinks for school-goers, the onus must rest with the parents or guardians. Sadly the advice to provide nutritious, healthy, whole and pure foods is all too often not listened to, being ignored. Many, like myself, brought the sandwiches, a bun or scone if we were lucky, and a bottle of milk, untreated and natural, straight from the cow, in our schoolbags. I have school-day companions, all in their 70's and 80's, still alive. I'll not comment further!

Staff at Alder Hey Children's Hospital in Liverpool said recently that the number of avoidable complaints could lead to a generation dying before their parents. Dr Steve Ryan, the medical director of the hospital, said **"Children should not be suffering from these problems."** It is obvious that the health problems have only arisen in very recent years. Here is a pointer to the dramatic increase in and consuming of fast and additive-filled 'foods' and 'drinks', also lack of exercise and proper sleep requirements. The all too easily obtained prescribed and over the counter chemical drugs have harmed many, especially children. The old way of doing things was right.

There are few restaurants one can walk into today and order a nutritious meal, especially for children. The restaurants are not always to blame. Very much of the problem is that parents have allowed themselves to become dictated to, as youngsters demand what they want, not what is nutritious or good for them. The foods, mostly fast, have been concocted, made up, to appeal to the taste buds of the youth. Television adverts promote all too much which is of no food value, being without nutrition. Children and teenagers are brain washed, believing the many advertising plugs. Many parents allow themselves to be dictated to as the youngsters demand fast, processed, additive-filled or pretentious, so called foods or drinks. Boiled oil saturated chips, chips and more chips are the usual fancy or fad, all wholly and totally unhealthy.

When the mothers, grandmothers and myself, as referred to, were given home-cooked, nutritious food and delicacies we did not complain. If we did we were bluntly told "eat it or you'll get nothing". The result is that today, and always, we have been partial to pure, nourishing and wholesome food. I well remember as a youngster having food put on my plate and refusing to eat it. My mother told me "You can eat it or leave it on the table." I sat for a period, and then said "I think I like it now" and proceeded to eat. To this day, I never refuse good food.

Visiting homes at mealtimes, I have witnessed the processed, sweetened and one can safely say dead, nutrient-empty, so-called foods being served. Very often children demand what they like, not what the parent or guardian deems good. In a family of five there can be three different menus used as the spoiled and demanding siblings dictate to the cook, usually the mothers, who all too easily give in to their whims.

It takes just discipline and a simple change of lifestyle to lead to a happy, healthy and wonderful outlook on life. The lives of all, especially our children, our future generation, would be changed dramatically. Fast and quickly prepared, processed, additive-containing food is unnatural. It may be cheap. It can work out to be terribly expensive.

CHILDREN'S MEDICINES

WARNING

Parents should carefully check the instructions or seek advice from health food store staff before administering to or allowing children to use complementary medicines or natural remedies. There are many health giving children's natural remedies available from the health food store. These writings are not intended as a substitute for professional advice. Anyone who has a medical condition or is concerned about their health is advised to consult with a qualified practitioner, homeopathic doctor, herbalist, complementary therapist or health food store personnel.

MILK

Speaking with some local dairy farmers, they outlined the scandalous way they are being treated regarding both wholesaling and retailing of milk. The farmer's return is miniscule compared to those who get it to the users. These seven day workers, and sometimes many nights also, told of how it is deplorable to see water costing more than milk. The milk being purchased off the shelf is processed, having been pasteurised, homogenised, bleached, with much of its goodness gone. Those same farmers are not allowed to retail their milk from the site it is produced on because of the rigmarole of red tape the Department of Agriculture has introduced and implemented over recent years. There are severe penalties for such practice, as fresh milk is deemed to be dangerous for one's health!

Some States in America, because of legal action having been taken, are now allowing fresh untreated milk to be sold at the farm. People there are refusing to purchase what to them is additive-containing milk. It is a fact that the pasteurisation destroys more that is good than bad in milk, also eliminating many elements which are vital for the health of the immune system.

WHEN ONE CONSIDERS THAT TESCO OFFER UP TO 38 KINDS OF BRANDED MILK, SOME WITH ADDITIVES, MUCH OF IT IMPORTED, OFTEN WITH MANY HUNDREDS OF FOOD MILES LOGGED UP, AS THE LIQUIDS ARE TRASPORTED ENORMOUS DISTANCES, the question must be asked **"WHEN DID MILK CEASE TO BE MILK?"** When I was a young person there was cow's and goat's milk. There was little need for the doctor! I don't ever remember visiting one

Many times I have mentioned that we have lost our sense of outrage. Here is a typical example. The gullible public accept the hype from the relevant bureaucrats about the good of pasteurisation, homogenisation, colour altering, when all of the time they are using another additive-containing product. When milk was delivered to the doorstep, as in the glass bottle era, we were a very much healthier nation. Milk was milk then and not interfered with as at present before being purchased in a chemical made-up plastic container or carton. To learn of the 'harm' of *Bisphenol-A* turn to that caption. It is in the make-up of all semi-rigid plastic containers, including those which hold milk.

There is only one pure milk, whether it is obtained from cow, goat, ewe, or that provided by a mother. There's also the fact that a container of milk can have the words '**FRESH**' or '**FRESHEST**' on a printed label, at the same time showing a ten days hence sell by date, When I was a boy fresh milk would last no longer than two days in the winter and less in the summer. It did not last very long in most cases because we were always consuming it, as a refreshing drink, just as we did with buttermilk, also water which was fresh from the well. **Pure milk, unadulterated and untreated, is a complete food for young and old and is used for rehabilitation by many when recovering from illness.**

WORRY

Worry does not empty tomorrow of its sorrow, it empties today of its strength. It is the interest we pay on trouble before it comes. Worry does not rid any day of its sorrows. It robs today of its joys.

UNCLUTTERING THE HOME AND THE MIND

The things we possess do not and will not define us, nor bring us peace or happiness. Some may still believe abundant possessions bring happiness or that they are a sign of GOD'S favour, but most of us know that when we are least reliant on material things, we are happiest. A friend of mine who is materially very well-off made major changes in her home recently. By keeping what she only needed on a daily, weekly and monthly basis and giving away everything else, she has discovered the secret of living simply. This woman's attitude is a very simple one: 'People are more important than things'. She has discovered that 'I have' is the greatest threat to 'I am'. My friend has also discovered that it is so much easier to keep the home tidy. A big uncluttering was the remedy. From '*Gardening the Soul*' by Sr. Stanislaus Kennedy. See **Bibliography** section

DON'T FIND FAULT - FIND A REMEDY

Some people on reading this book must think that my thoughts are like those of a complainer, a moaner. I am not complaining, merely setting down facts, all pertaining to the health problems many have to face up to daily. If I am judged to be finding fault or kicking up a fuss then I will be delighted. *'Don't find fault, find a remedy'* is a slogan which appears in my writings on numerous occasions. I hope that I can be judged to be finding remedies too. Again I persist, when I state that if I shout loud enough and long enough somebody will take notice and that others might consider doing likewise. In offices where I worked, attached or pertaining to civil engineering projects, I always had this slogan prominently displayed for all to see. It was first used by Henry Ford. Now, when friends or acquaintances who worked with me telephone, they tell how they never forgot the wording of the slogan.

If those who go down the road of negative thinking, wrong eating and drinking habits, living without exercise, insufficient or proper sleep, wish to continue this way, so be it. It will not cost me a thought, even though I think they are extremely foolish. It is their prerogative. Without scare mongering I can do no more than set down facts, of which there are many, hoping that the much which I see wrong in the sickness, chemical drug, 'drink' and 'food' industries will be corrected. **Michael Davitt's** words or advice to **"Leave politics and economics out of the world."** could only lead to a much healthier or better society. Reading this book, *Selling Sickness!,* tells of how our Government gives little thought and direction to the health of all. Politics, back-biting, complaining and the economy take up the little time they give to governing us. *'Don't find fault, find a remedy'* is the least of their thoughts. If all who are in a position to do so adopted this slogan, putting it into practice when possible, the results would enable many to live stress free lives, being with less worry.

BUTTER.

In my book *'Health is Wealth'* I had a caption headed Butter. I promised not to duplicate. I am not duplicating, just giving more facts. The alleged collusion or conniving between a giant margarine factor's public relations agency, despite their denials, and a heart surgeon named Kolvekar is typical of how big businesses will stop at nothing to promote their processed 'foods'. For those who do not know, this multinational produces many additive-containing 'foods'. Their margarines and pretentious spreads are touted as 'healthy' alternatives to butter. Margarine is not food. It contains additives, is processed, being unnatural. See *Margarine* caption

Shyam Kolvekar, perhaps 'aided' by the manufacturer's promotional agency, got worldwide headlines, telling the population that we should *"Ban butter"*. Like many who have lived life the natural way, including eating butter, we can all ask Kolvekar to prove what he says. Failing this he should seek the same publicity to undo the harm he has done to the dairy industry. He also indirectly told the brain washed public to eat processed, unnatural margarine, all of which contain additives. It would be interesting to know if Doctor Kolvekar received remuneration for his 'sales patter', despite his denying this.

If approached, the relevant public relations agency might not be so co-operative, because a stunt which gave free publicity, coverage and advertising, in the highly untruthful rant against the natural food which is butter, was a huge success from their point of view.

I rest my case for promoting butter, something which I have eaten all my life, by stating, *'Statistics show the rate of heart disease has increased enormously as butter consumption has decreased'.*

MOUTHWASHES – ARE THEY 'DANGEROUS?'

THE SAME QUESTIONS CAN BE ASKED ABOUT TOOTHPASTES.

Before proceeding further, querying what is in the make up of the chemical and additive-containing liquids which are mouthwashes, I ask a question, **"How did we manage in the past without these so called antiseptic mouth washes?"** It is not coincidence that we had little sickness or ailment such as we see now and that includes cancer. Our teeth and mouths were as good, or perhaps much healthier, when we had less chemical concoctions. There is huge doubt about the contents or make up of mouthwashes or of their effectiveness.

Professor Michael McCullough from Melbourne University tells us *"Mouthwashes can cause oral cancer and should be removed from the shelves"*. He says, amongst other worrying factors, that *"We see people with oral cancer who have no other risk factors than the use of alcohol-containing mouthwash, so we have reviewed all the evidence that is out there"*.

Who gives thought to the use of these washes, many of them chemical laden, perhaps doing more harm than good, apart from the cancer scare? Most people have much good bacteria in the body, including the mouth. Millions of euro or pounds are spent annually on mouthwashes. The chemical and alcohol containing liquids supposedly fight bad breath and prevent gum problems by reducing plaque or allegedly cutting tooth decay. We are informed that these 'harmful' solutions are now being promoted for children.

Like antibiotics and other chemical drugs, which kill much of the good bacteria or micro-organisms, so it is with mouthwashes. The makers of the chemical filled mouthwashes will not entertain these conclusions. The spokesperson for Johnson & Johnson, which makes Listerine, dismissed the findings. He would, wouldn't he? Does he think that all are fools and should not listen to Professor McCullough? Cancer, of whatever kind, is not something to be treated in this off-handed, know-all manner. Here is another bod who should keep his mouth shut, as he too, makes a fool of himself.

Mouthwashes and many toothpastes are others to add to the list of undesirables, to follow one of my mottos, *WHEN IN DOUBT, LEAVE OUT, DO WITHOUT.* Until proved otherwise, many mouthwashes and toothpastes can be 'dangerous'. Indeed many of the hyped up toothpastes as seen stacked on the supermarket shelves are best avoided. **Try reading the ingredients labels, very often in small or perhaps illegible print. The list of chemicals and other additives is frightening to those who understand about them. This includes the terrible chemical which is fluoride, known as fluorosilicic acid.**

In the Health Stores there are purely natural toothpastes and mouthwashes with no danger regarding their use. *'Optima'* is an excellent brand. **Optima Aloe Dent** mouthwashes contain Vitamin K, Tea Tree also grapefruit extract, with other herbs and purely natural ingredients. Their toothpastes and mouthwashes are just two of a large range of natural health helping products they formulate. They are no more expensive than the chemical and alcohol containing stuff, which is highly advertised and promoted. Everything sold in the Health Food Store is natural, pure and safe. See *Teeth Care* caption

LIFESTYLE.

Who gives this word or their own lifestyle much thought? Many who are ill with any type of ailment or disease, no matter what it is, can benefit enormously from a **change of lifestyle.** It is a slogan I use frequently and am well qualified and informed to speak about.

At the stroke of a pen, three words, yes, just three words, could put into practice in Ireland and the U.K. a plan to save billions for the Health Service Executive, the National Health Service and the taxpayer. The Sickness Industry could be liquidated. The three words are, *CHANGE YOUR LIFESTYLE.* Used in conjunction with my motto – *WE ARE AS WE EAT, DRINK, SLEEP AND EXERCISE* – the changes overall would be dramatic. So many who took my advice about improving or changing their way of living, 'modus operandi' or lifestyle have told me of their experiences. A full book could be written about return to good or better health, how difficult it was at the beginning, but later so easy when more healthy, to give up cigarettes, hay fever gone, with concentration and memory improved, also much, much more. Almost all tell of how energy levels have improved. The result of following my advice about weight loss, and keeping it so, by eating pure and natural food, as set out under *Healthy Body-Weight* caption, is often repeated to me.

People who were told they had diabetes and many of those who had the disease are now free from it. Blood pressure, depression, headaches, circulation, insomnia, lethargy and hundreds of health problems, little and large have vanished. By changing to and following rigidly, using natural food and food supplements, the Hay Diet has improved and **cured** Psoriasis and Myalgic Encephalomyelitis (M.E.). This diet, as promoted by Dr. Hay, is a marvellous remedy for many serious health problems, especially as a wonderful aid for serious depression, which includes the treatment of bipolar disorders   Certain food supplements must be used in conjunction with the Hay Diet. There are several books which explain much about this wonder diet. See *Bibliography* section

To attain healthy lifestyle need not be hard work. Just a little thought, diligence and some discipline is all that is needed to allow one feel better.

Those interested in better health are pestered and almost besieged daily as they are told to eat this, drink that, try the other, as the do-gooders and so-called '**experts**', all too many of them with monetary and vested interests, try to get their messages across. The vast majority of them have little, if any, understanding or knowledge about natural foods or drinks. I doubt if they would know how to describe or set out a pure, nutritious food balanced diet. My simple message is to be selective. If the food or drink is processed, with colour, additive and preservative, with Es or other constituents with unpronounceable names, just leave all on the shelf. Use only that which is natural food or drink.

The question of drinks, exercise and sleeping habits must be given much food for thought. This will lead to simple action having to be taken to put one on the right course.

If I had listened to my doctor some years ago, I would be on a walking stick, as I was then, taking no exercise, because I was unable to walk properly. I went down the road of treating myself. It has worked for me and thousands like me. *I changed my lifestyle completely.* Many whom I have advised about change of lifestyle were on chemical medicines and drugs. The majority have been able to come off them. They now live much more healthy and better lives.

Depression is an example, where change of lifestyle works wonders. Try explaining this to the doctor, as I have on numerous occasions. I have listened to people who told the doctor what they have done by way of treating themselves naturally. They related to me the results of trying to tell of their good fortune. Like myself they just got an answer or a remark which could be attributed to a political bureaucrat. Call it a brush off. The well-oiled wheels of the Sickness Industry will not be stopped or interfered with. The doctor and his beloved prescription pad, his cash till, will not part company. **I have been told harrowing stories about side effects of anti-depressants or other drugs which people have taken.** In some instances it took months, even years, to overcome the withdrawal symptoms. One can only guess the long-term harm that has been done. See *Depression* caption.

Sometime ago I had a telephone call from a grateful lady in the U.K. She followed the advice to help lose weight and to use a cliché *'She was over the moon'.* Having weighed over 15 stone, changing the diet to natural food and drinks, as advised, walking for an hour each day, sleeping regular hours, and following the advice given about *Healthy Body Weight* as set out under that caption, she has lost 42 pounds, (almost 20 kilos.), in 19 months. This nice person followed the advice diligently and persistently. She told of how it was rather expensive having to buy correct fitting clothes regularly, as she shed the pounds, both in weight loss and purchase of fashion wear!

Like others, who have followed the recommendations, the lady told of how she never felt so well, having lots of energy. This can be attributed to her losing weight slowly and not having to cut down on the natural foods which I advise. Also mentioned was a change to better skin, hair and nails, saying how her hair used to be dull, also with breaking and white spotted nails, all now looking healthy.

The lady conversed on the telephone for over 45 minutes as she went into details. She finished by saying that having tried several diets and weight loss plans, none of which worked, there was big doubt about my plan at first. What makes it a winner, and many have told me as this person did, **"I can eat all I wish to and not put on weight, with the other diets there was always a feeling of being hungry and listless"**. *A CHANGE OF LIFESTYLE CAN WORK WONDERS FOR ALL.*

THE CHEMIST AND PHARMACY LUCRATIVE BUSINESS.

Chemists, pharmacists and the drug stores or shops they run are an integral part of the Sickness Industry. They are the middlemen. To be politically correct, as we are expected to be in this era, I will also add, the middle-women. Regularly, as the chemists stringently fight for what they alone deem to be their rights, we see and hear of their demands, confrontations and arguments with the Government, the Health Service Executive or the National Health Service.

The pharmacies seek expanded roles in patient services. They whimper and moan about the proposed cuts in their profits. **Their union or licensed closed shop which had been set up, was calling for, note the word 'calling for', more medicines to be available without prescription. Their calls have now been answered, allowing them to do just that.** They say the deregulation of certain medicines or drugs would enhance patient care and save time and money for patients. To put it bluntly, *"They're all the time looking for another slice of the rich cake which sickness brings for them"*. In other areas there are the serious issues of wrong prescribing, often with calamatious results or consequences, almost all of which go unreported. We learn of the many deaths caused by misuse of medication, some of it wrongly prescribed. **Is this not sufficient and serious warning that pharmacy demands, especially in this area of medicine, should have been and must be treated as nonsense?**

Put in simple terms, the pharmacies seek to add further to their very huge range of over the counter drugs. There is a big and worrying aspect of further addiction, with many already hooked on prescribed drugs and unable to break their habits. We do not hear about this. The idea of keeping quiet within the chemical drug-manufacturing and allied Sickness

Industry works well, for those concerned.

The chemist or pharmacy set up should settle for what they have in the highly lucrative and often rip-off business they run. At the height of what most regarded as a boom in 2007, more than 50 new pharmacies were opened in Ireland. Some years later the pharmacy regulator told us *"We have the highest figure ever for this professional sector"*.

The profits are obscene at 50%, often very much more. One can hear loud spurious denials of this, the favourite one is that 50% is quickly turned into 33%. If an article is purchased at a certain price, with 50% added by the retailer, this is a mark up of 50%. The chemist will tell us it is 33% because that is the profit on the drugs or medicines sold. No matter how one argues this, there is a mark up of at least 50% of the cost, often very much more.

The charging set up is nefarious. For instance here in Ireland if one purchases Nexium, to give an example, the State pays approximately €50 if supplied to a medical cardholder. If registered under the drug payment scheme the State pays approximately €59. If one, as a private individual, purchases the same item the charge can be over €70. The ratio of charges is all according to the strength. Nefarious is too nice a word to describe this rip-off.

Why is Ireland the most expensive place in Europe to buy prescription drugs? I know from travelling through Europe that certain drugs are over fifty per cent dearer in Ireland than the U.K. Many drugs purchased in Spain are very much cheaper. Considering that Ireland is the chemical drugs-manufacturing capital of Europe there is certainly big, very big food for thought, in this revelation?

The wholesale mark up is far too high as is the pharmacy mark up. The distribution costs are another factor. They are also far too costly.

Drugs, which have come off patent and are therefore much cheaper, are called generic drugs. These are conveniently forgotten about in the pharmacies, with sales not pushed to the forefront, because the profit margin gives less incentive to do so.

The story of the scandalous methods of charging for prescription drugs, as against generics, is described in the fact-finding and chemical drugs sales shenanigans and exposures in the writings of *'Jeffrey Robinson'*. His book *'Prescription Games',* as listed in **Bibliography** section, tells about how the chemical drugs processing industry has those within the Sickness Industry, also the Government, conned into the belief that they are all supreme. This is why the almighty synthetic drug-manufacturing barons are treated with extreme courtesy. If they upped sticks and took the pharma-drug processing industry from the country, we would be up the creek as far as the economy is concerned. I read this book twice, saying to myself, *"These so and sos are not interested in cures, seeking nothing other than money"*. I repeat, "Money is *god* like to those at the helm of the chemical drug selling industry".

Over the years we have been told of deregulation, of restrictions on chemists revoked, of a shake-up in the pharmacy sector, of how this would lead to cheaper drugs. This was just false thinking. Over the past 20 years many drug prices have increased by over 400%. In 2009 the headlines were that there would be a 40% reduction in certain branded medications. Note the word certain. Little has changed since then.

Why the spiralling costs of drugs, medicines and pills? Read the Irish Pharmaceutical Union's pathetic explanation, as they tell us *"That the increases in the past 10 years aren't surprising".* They give us this jargon:
• Population has increased.
• People living longer.
• Fantastic developments in medicines – new cancer treatments, etc.
• Focus on preventative therapies, like statins, to control cholesterol.
• All patients over 70 years of age getting a medical card.

What has population increase or people living longer got to do with the cost of drugs? Our population is now decreasing, as many emigrate from our shores. The union gives the excuse of *fantastic developments in medicine – new cancer treatments, etc.* Drugs don't cure. Neither do these worthless excuses bear a whit of significance.

What has the focus on **Preventative** therapies to do with the spiralling costs? **Only 0.07 per cent of the total budget of nearly €14 billion spent in the Sickness Industry is allocated to prevention and education about sickness. This outlay on prevention and health education is a mere triviality. The World Health Organisation states that 10%, yes 10%, of our total health budget should be spent on education about and prevention of ill-health**. It is laughable to say the least. Note how statins are referred to as **Preventative** therapy. All too many of the gullible or trusting public lap this up as they accept statins, which are harmful as well as being useless. See **Statins**, also **Cholesterol** captions.

The number of prescriptions issued in 2009 was nearly 16.25 million; the figure for 2010 is nearly 18.5 million.

The idea that all patients over 70 have a medical card is a fallacy. Many of these have been withdrawn because of means testing. How unions have the gall to issue statements like this I cannot understand. Is there any honesty or integrity left in our world? It is mind-boggling that here in Ireland, the bill for drugs dispensed at time of writing is between two and two and a quarter billion euro annually and rising rapidly. This comes from released H.S.E. figures.

Veterinary medicine is another huge money-spinner for vets, pharmacies and drug companies, but again this is a story for another day.

Our chemists and pharmacies run a lucrative and gainful business as part of the Sickness Industry. They are well organised to stand up for what they believe to be their rights. They are pleased with and well looked after by the Irish Pharmaceutical Society, their autocratic union.

Many complain, but few stand up and do anything about much which is wrong in the Sickness Industry. I repeat and I repeat again and again *"We have lost our sense of outrage"*, just as the majority have lost their sense of nationalism. Here lies much food for thought as we fork out for over prescribed drugs, which in many cases are just a money **RIP-OFF.**

DEMENTIA

Where a change of lifestyle has been accepted and used, I have seen many cases of dementia and depression reversed, as effected people returned to normal or much better health. I have cried at times when people have thanked me, especially the relatives.

Good nutritious natural food meals, with natural water, plus some exercise, such as walking, and a proper sleep pattern, are the answers to many of today's health problems including dementia and depression.

A small drink of good port, with honey on three or four Choice Grain crackers is an excellent tonic, taken an hour before bedtime. Sometimes it can be three or four fingers of wholemeal bread. It helps one sleep and is an aid to dementia.

If eating nutritious food, a good **natural** Multivitamin also a Vitamin D3 and a Rhodiola supplement, obtainable from the health food store, are an added bonus to help the body and brain. What has been terribly obvious in my observations of many, is that elderly and indeed some younger, who should have some common sense, are all too often under the misapprehension that they can live on little food. Some say how they are dieting. This is very often an excuse for not eating. By living under this cloud they neglect their bodies. This can only lead to illness. As we used to say and indeed still do, **"Three square meals of good, pure and natural food daily, is nature's greatest medicine"**.

Some of those who do eat, whether more or very little, buy cheap, additive-filled, processed so-called foods. Many look at the price labels instead of looking at the ingredient labels. Because it is fast 'food', much of which can be stuck into a microwave, it is easily heated. Very often, no preparation is required. They should read the ingredients labels to see that much of it can be regarded as 'rubbish'. I repeat again and again, cheap 'food' can be expensive in the long term. Turn to *Eat Well on a Limited Budget* caption.

As with much other illness and ailments, the response to natural treatment by those with dementia has to be seen to be believed. For much helpful advice which can aid dementia, see *Depression* caption.

TELEVISION

"What has this to do with the Sickness Industry"? It has nothing to do with anything natural, only having an enormous amount to do with ill-health of mind, body and soul. It is open to debate by many, but it has been one of the most evil things to come into viewers lives.

The goggle box is another cog in the wheel of the huge Sickness Industry, as we now know it. It is one of the reasons for much of the ill-health of mind and body we have now.

TELEVISION is responsible for glazed eyes, bored expressions, false imaginations, diminished reasoning, obesity, very often a need for speech therapy, social isolation, fragmentation of life particularly to couch potato children and young people, with all too much apparent laziness of mind and body.

Many, whom we would not consider inviting into our homes, supposedly entertain us. It is an enemy of good health, as many lay about or snooze in front of the goggle box, with young children especially at risk.

Exercise, which the vast majority took in the past, is now turned into inactivity of both body and mind. Except for news, weather, sport and the odd topical item or documentary we are best without television. The off button is one of its best features. The teletext, which my family use, is the answer to all of this. We read the news, weather and sport in that order. Just scroll down to what is of interest, read it and switch off. Don't clutter up the brain or mind with very much which is irrelevant to daily life. Life is too short to waste on much of the idiocy which television bombards us with. It is no coincidence that the upsurge in thuggery, rape, murder, robbery and much of the evil we see today, has only occurred since the advent of commercial television.

We expect that a child's character is formed between the ages of two and eight. This may begin even earlier in life. They are then most vulnerable, when they learn the difference between right and wrong, good and bad. Sadly to-day many children's lives are dominated by television. In some homes babies are regularly to be seen viewing the screen.

The foundation for the individual's traits, mannerisms and outlook on life was, and should now be properly laid down by the parents. As stated, the characters of our young people are all too often formed in front of the box, where shooting, killing, maiming, and very much more, all alien to a child, is colourfully transmitted. The adverts are sometimes more deranged than the other, very often being nasty programmes, which children look upon as being the real thing.

Children in their formative years need nurturing, training, speaking with, instructing, disciplining and providing for – all to be combined with a big amount of loving.

Most parents seem unaware of the harm that T.V. is to infants, children and young people. It is a cause of belligerent and aggressive attitude, bad behaviour and much hostility. Good manners and courtesy to others has almost disappeared since the arrival of television. All of this can lead to depression, stress, juvenile delinquency, and in later life perhaps criminal tendencies.

Irregular and bad eating habits are often a result. Loss of vital sleep, also irregular sleep pattern, can lead to illness and malfunctioning of the brain. Television leads to much distraction and can certainly be regarded as time wasting. Many parents are addicted to the television, resulting in the family being neglected.

With figures given for viewing hours of averages of five to seven hours daily, this makes sad news. It points to the fact that young people are being neglected intellectually. There is little or no conversation, debate, reading or communication between members of the household. All too much of what is viewed is inappropriate and of no educational value. Noel Coward said many years ago *"Time has convinced me of one thing, Television is for appearing on, not looking at"*. See *Books* caption.

Do you remember when children could roam safely or went to school by themselves? All could walk our streets fearlessly. House doors could be left open. You saw policemen walking or cycling in the neighbourhood. There were no rowdies. Football matches were carefree and good games, with sport being sport, not business, as it is now. Senior citizens, teachers and others in authority were respected. **Honesty and integrity was the hallmark of the majority then, even amongst doctors, politicians and bankers.** We took regular exercise, ate proper nutritious, additive free food and made our own enjoyment. People were certainly much healthier than they are now. There was little need for the doctor or medicine. **THERE WAS NO TELEVISION.** Taken from *'Health* is **Wealth Encyclopaedia'**

BALANCED DIET

Here are two words which make me angry when I see them, usually used if or when those with monetary interests are promoting unnatural, processed, additive-containing, often what can be regarded as 'rubbish' foods. Frequently we hear or read of what has turned into a cliché, **'As part of a balanced diet'.** This is often used in media food advertisements, health articles or on containers, such as the plastic boxes which hold additive and processed margarines or substitute butter spreads, also so-called probiotics. Often, in very small print, where many people have to use glasses, sometimes magnifying glasses, to read the often illegible wording, well set out from the advertising or promotional blurb, one sees the words *'If, or when taken with, or in conjunction with a balanced diet'* or a sentence to that effect. Newspaper articles tell us of the need for a balanced diet. Frequently we see the balderdash from the medical profession or health journalists who set out that there is no need for food supplements, including vitamins or minerals, if we have a balanced diet. The big problem with this is that all too often many don't have a clue as to what a proper balanced diet is.

Officially we are informed that over 75% of the food sold in the supermarkets, can be classed as junk food. I don't think that it is as bad as that. There is much natural and good on their shelves. It just needs looking for and reading the ingredients labels, leaving anything that is processed, fast, or containing additives, on the shelf. Within a very short time, one recognises what is good, what is bad, for reasonable or better health.

I repeat, the vast majority don't understand or know what makes up a balanced diet. The doctors or Sickness Industry personnel will not sit one down to explain what is the biggest requirement of good health, our greatest medicine, good food. They too are probably amongst the majority who do not understand the requirements for nutritious natural food meals.

All that is required to provide a balanced diet of three nutritious meals daily is pure natural, additive free, non-processed food. It must be prepared and cooked properly. Meat used in moderation, fish, vegetables, including potatoes and greens, grains including brown rice, fruit and pure water, also the excellent health giving rolled grains of oats, which is porridge, provide the base for a balanced diet.

Visit the supermarkets and see the trolleys laden with junk foods and drinks. See the additive, salt and sugar filled things purchased as *'food'* for the purchaser or their families. *Do any of these people understand what a balanced diet is?*

There is no need to ask, *"WHY ARE WE A SICK NATION"?* Sadly the chief reasons are that the vast majority do not understand, especially the younger generation, about the two words, **'BALANCED DIET.**

To eat, drink and therefore have a sense of well-being, turn to *Eat Well on a Limited Budget* caption, then realising that one can enjoy simple nutritious meals with little outlay if a target is set and the priorities are right.

COPYRIGHT

BIBLIOGRAPHY

Many of the following books, magazines, periodicals and papers contain much which can help one to attain, regain or maintain reasonable health, through the use of homoeopathic, herbal or natural remedies. Natural remedies can be complementary or alternative to man-made drugs. I have derived enormous pleasure, also learning much from the writings in the literature listed hereunder.

These writings are not intended as a substitute for professional advice. Anyone who has a medical condition or is concerned about their health is advised to consult with a qualified practitioner, homeopathic doctor, herbalist, complementary therapist or health food store personnel, and then to proceed down the road they choose.

ARTHRITIS AND COMMON SENSE, by Dan Dale Alexander, Worlds Work Ltd, Kingswood, Tadworth, Surrey, England. ISBN 457-00500-3.

AWAKE magazine, available from Jehovah's Witnesses, Newcastle, Greystones, Co. Wicklow or The Ridgeway, London, NW7 1RN, or their voluntary distributors in your area.

BEAT DIABETES NATURALLY, by Michael Murray, N.D. and Michael Lyon. M.D.. Pub. by Rodale. ISBN 101-59486-315-6.

BETTER EYESIGHT WITHOUT GLASSES, by W.H. Bates. (M.D)., Pub. by Thorsons. IBSN 10-0-00-710900-8.

BIBLE DIARY, Chlarentian Publications, U.P. P.O. Box 4, Diliman, 1101 Quezon City, Philippines. ISBN 971-501-332-5.

29 $ BILLION REASONS TO LIE ABOUT CHOLESTEROL, by Justin Smith. Pub. by Matador, 9 De Montfort Mews, Leicester, England LE1 7FW U.K   ISBN 978-1848760-714.

BIOCHEMIC HANDBOOK ON TISSUE SALTS, Pub. by Thorsons, Harper Collins. ISBN 0-7225-0613-9.

CHINA STUDY, THE by T. Colin Campbell. PhD & Thomas Campbell 11. Pub by Benbella Books, Dallas, Texas, ISBN 1-932100-66-0.

CHOOSING THE RIGHT FATS, by Dr.Udo Erasmus,   Pub. by Alive Books. ISBN 1-53312-035-3. Also by the same author, **FATS THAT HEAL, FATS THAT KILL.** ISBN 0-920470-38-6.

CLARE COURIER, THE Unit 4 Ballycasey, Shannon, Co. Clare.

CLOSE YOUR MOUTH (ASTHMA CARE) BUTEYKO CLINIC HANDBOOK, by Patrick McKeown. ISBN 0-9545996-1-6.

COMPLETE CIDER VINEGAR, THE   Pub by Thorsons. ISBN 0-7225-1876-5.

COMPLETE HERBAL, THE   by David Hoffman. Pub. by Mustard, an imprint of Parragon, 4 Queen Street, Bath, England BA1 HE. ISBN 1-84164-167-7.

COSMETICS UNMASKED, by Dr Stephen and Gina Antczak. ISBN 978-000-733-571.

CURATE'S DIARY, THE Rev. Fr. Thady Doyle, Shillelagh, Arklow, Co. Wicklow.

DAILY TELEGRAPH, 1 Canada Square, London, England E14 5DT UK.

DEVIL'S CLAW, by Hildesgard Pickles.   Reforma AG, Postfach, Switzerland 6300 ZUG.

E FOR ADDITIVES, by Maurice Hanson with Jill Marsden.   Pub by Thorsons, an imprint of Harper Collins, 77-85 Fulham Palace Road, Hammersmith, London   W6 8JB ISBN 0-7225-1562-6.

EAT WITH JOY – ON A WHEAT FREE, GLUTEN FREE DIET, by Ann O' Dowd Fogarty, Pub. by A and A Farmer, Beech House, 78 Ranelagh Village, Dublin 6. ISBN 1-899047-73-5.

EAT YOUR HEART OUT, by Felicity Lawrence. Pub. by Penguin Books. ISBN 978-0-141-02601-5.

ENCYCLOPEDIA OF HERBAL MEDICINE, by Thomas Bartram, FWIMH. Pub. by Grace Publishers, Mulberry Court, Stour Road, Christchurch, Dorset, England BH23 1PS U.K.   ISBN 0-9515984-1-4.

FAMILY GUIDE TO HOMOEOPATHY, THE   by Dr. Andrew Lockie. Pub. by Penguin Books, ISBN 0-241-13572-9.

FEARFULLY AND WONDERFULLY MADE, by Dr. Paul Brand and Philip Yancey. Pub. by Zondervan, Grand Rapids, Michigan, 49530, U.S.A. ISBN 978-0-310-35451-2.

FLOURIDE – DRINKING OURSELVES TO DEATH, by Barry Groves. Pub. by Newleaf, an imprint of Gill & McMillan Ltd, Hume Avenue, Parkwest, Dublin 12, Ireland. ISBN 0-7171-3274-9.

FLUORIDE DECEPTION, by Christopher Bryan, Pub. by Seven Stories Press. ISBN 1-58322-526-9.

FOOD COMBINING (THE ORIGINAL HAY DIET), by Kathryn Marsden. Pub. by Thorson, Harpur Collins, 77-85 Fulham Palace Road, London, England W6 8JB.

FROM DUN SION TO CROKE PARK, by Mícheál Ó Muircheartaigh ISBN 978- 1844-880-454

GARDENING THE SOUL, by Sr. Stanislaus Kennedy. Pub. by Townhouse & Country House Ltd, Trinity House, Charleston Road, Ranelagh, Dublin 6, Ireland. ISBN 1-903650-05-4.

GOVERNOR, THE by John Lonergan. Pub.By Penguin Books. ISBN 978-1-844-88240-3.

GRACE MAGAZINE, Quarterly, by subscription, from Grace Publishers, Mulberry Court, Stour Road, Christchurch, Dorset, England BH 23 IPS UK.

GREAT CHOLESTEROL CON, THE by Dr. Malcolm Kendrick, Pub. by John Blake Publishing Ltd. 3 Bramber Court, 2 Bramber Road, London W14 9PB U.K. ISBN 978-1-84454-360-1.

GUARDIAN, THE 119 Farringdon Road, London, EC1R 3ER.

GUIDE TO VITAMINS, MINERALS AND SUPPLEMENTS, Readers Digest. ISBN 0-276-42448-4.

HAY DIET MADE EASY, THE by Jackie Habgood, Pub. by Souvenir Press. Also **GET WELL WITH THE HAY DIET**, ISBN 0-285-63535-2.

HEALTH IS WEALTH, by Ronnie Plant. An A to Z Encyclopaedia of Over the Counter Natural Remedies and Good Food. Pub. by St. John Publishing, 10 St. John's Court, Wellingtonbridge, Co. Wexford, Ireland. ISBN 0-9551051-0-2.

IRELAND'S OWN, Channing House, Rowe Street, Wexford, Ireland.

IRISH EXAMINER, Academy Street, Cork, Ireland.

IRISH FARMERS JOURNAL, The Farm Centre Bluebell, Dublin 12, Ireland.

IRISH INDEPENDENT, Middle Abbey Street, Dublin 2, Ireland.

IRISH TIMES, 24-28 Tara Street, Dublin 2, Ireland.

LET THEM EAT PROZAC, by David Healy, Pub. by New York University Press. ISBN 0-8147-3697-1.

LIVING DANGEROUSLY by Pat Thomas. Pub. by Newleaf, an imprint of Gill and McMillan Limited, Hume Avenue, Park West, Dublin 2. ISBN 0-7171-3600-0

NATURAL FOOD REMEDIES, by Lelord Kordel. Pub. by W.H. Allen, London, England. ISBN 0-491-01742-1.

NATURE DOCTOR, THE by Dr. Alfred Vogel. Pub. By Mainstream Publishing Co., 7 Albany Street, Edinburgh, Scotland. EH1 3UG. ISBN 1-85158-274-6.

PRESCRIPTION GAMES, by Jeffrey Robinson, Pub. by Simon & Schuster U.K. Ltd. Africa House, 64-78 Kingsway, London WC2B 6AH. ISBN 0-684-85837-1.

ST. MARTIN'S MAGAZINE, 42 Parnell Square, Dublin 1, Ireland.

TIMES, THE 1 Virginia Street, London, E98 1XY.

TRICK & TREAT, By Barry Groves. Pub. by Hammersmith Press Limited. 496 Fulham Palace Road, London, England, SW6 6JD U.K. ISBN 978-1-905140-22-0.

VITAMIN D CURE, THE by E. Dowd M.D. and Diane Stafford. Pub. by John Wiley & Sons Inc. Hoboken, New Jersey. ISBN 978-0-470-13155-8.

WHEN THE GAME IS OVER IT ALL GOES BACK IN THE BOX, by John Ortberg. Pub. by Zondervan, Grand Rapids, Michegan, 49530, U.S.A. ISBN 978-0-310-23519-8.

WHILE THE KETTLE BOILS, by Thomas Bartram, F.W.I.M.H., Pub. by Grace Publishers, Mulberry Court, Stour Road, Christchurch, Dorset, England BH23 1PS U.K.   ISBN 1-903604-00-1.

WORD FOR TODAY – YOUR QUIET TIME COMPANION, P.O. Box 255, Stoke-on-Trent, Staffordshire, England ST4 8YY UK. or P.O. Box 784 Dun Laoghaire, Co. Dublin, Ireland.

YOUR BODY'S MANY CRIES FOR WATER, by J. Butmanghelid. Pub. by Tagman Press. ISBN 1-903571-49-9.

YOUR LIFE IN YOUR HANDS, by Prof. Jane Plant. Pub. by Virgin Books. ISBN 0-7535-0850-8.